NEUROLOGICAL EPONYMS

NEUROLOGICAL EPONYMS

Edited by

PETER J. KOEHLER
GEORGE W. BRUYN
JOHN M. S. PEARCE

OXFORD
UNIVERSITY PRESS
2000

OXFORD
UNIVERSITY PRESS
Oxford New York
Athens Auckland Bangkok Bogotá Buenos Aires Calcutta
Cape Town Chennai Dar es Salaam Delhi Florence Hong Kong Istanbul
Karachi Kuala Lumpur Madrid Melbourne Mexico City Mumbai
Nairobi Paris São Paulo Singapore Taipei Tokyo Toronto Warsaw

and associated companies in
Berlin Ibadan

Published by Oxford University Press, Inc.,
198 Madison Avenue, New York, New York, 10016
http://www.oup-usa.org
1-800-334-4249

Library of Congress Cataloging-in-Publication Data
Neurological eponyms / edited by Peter J. Koehler, George W. Bruyn, John M. S. Pearce.
p. cm.
Includes bibliographical references and index.
ISBN 978-0-19-513366-0
1. Neurology—Terminology. 2. Eponyms. I. Koehler, Peter J. II. Bruyn, G. W. III.
Pearce, John, 1936-
[DNLM: 1. Neurologic Examination—Terminology—English. 2.
Eponyms—Terminology—English. 3. Nervous System Diseases—Terminology—English.
4. Neuroanatomy—Terminology—English. WL 15 N494 2000]
RC343 . N434 2000
616.8'01'4—dc21 99-088374

Printed in the United States of America
on acid-free paper

PREFACE

> Be not the first by whom the new is tried, nor be the last to throw the old aside.
>
> Thomas Carlyle, "Sartor resartus est"

Medical eponyms are again in vogue, after a period of 50 to 60 years, lasting through the 1980s, when would-be-scientific doctors disdainfully rejected eponyms as obsolete. This seems to have been a feeble attempt to emulate the "real" sciences such as mathematics and physics. The medical world has now made a *volte face* that is curious, if one sits back and reflects on the underlying forces.

We boldly suggest that it is precisely because medicine has recently acquired a scientific status that it can afford again the luxury of eponyms. We can put it quite simply: the silent revolution of molecular biology in identifying mutations, deletions, frame shifts, and the like—as the explanation of certain phenotypes—has raised the rational power of medicine to a scientific level. Of course, we can add to this other factors such as statistical sophisticaton, stricter methodologies, computerized imaging techniques, and advances in electronic and chemical technology.

Liberated from its inferiority complex vis-à-vis the hard-core sciences, medicine became aware of two situations which reinforced the newly acquired attitude:

1. It now transpires that physics, chemistry, mathematics, astronomy, geography, paleontology, botany, and the like, command a plethora of many hundreds of eponyms.

2. Many terms chosen in place of eponyms are unwieldy and awkward, both in argument and conversation, at conferences and at the bedside. Consider the scientific diagnosis "the clinical phenotype produced by the point mutation at Val127/Leu128 position in codon 192 of exon 6 in chromosome 39q27-ter, coding for the omega-subunit of the potassium-ionophore protein"; substitution of a simple eponym like "Koehler–Bruyn–Pearce syndrome" is in most circumstances apt and concise. Even if the descriptive term is correct, it sounds ludicrously pedantic.

This book is derived from *Eponyms in Neurological Examination,* a text composed for the centenary of the Netherlands Society of Neurology in 1995. Since the book was well received in the Netherlands, a revision and expansion to other aspects of clinical neurology for a broader international audience seemed worthwhile. Whereas the Dutch edition was confined to eponyms in neurological examination, with this book we had to face the problem of making a considered choice from the many existing neurological eponyms.

Several criteria were applied to the choice of eponyms to be included. We considered frequency of occurrence, familiarity of the clinical neurologist with the notion or concept, and the importance for neurology of the person behind the eponym. Furthermore, we attempted to include eponyms from several fields that are relevant for the neurological clinic. Starting at the base (neuroanatomy) and working up to well-defined diseases we arrived at five classes of neurological eponyms: anatomy and pathology, symptoms and signs, reflexes and tests, clinical syndromes, and finally diseases and defects. Of course there will be readers who wonder why certain eponyms were included and others not. Selection is always arbitrary. But this anthology covers the history of clinical neurology in sufficient depth to show the problems confronting our predecessors.

The authors were asked to follow the same format for their respective chapters, in order to achieve uniformity. They were invited to write a short biography and to discuss the original or key publication as well as the subsequent evolution and significance of the eponym.

This book aims at both education and entertainment. They are best intermingled so that where the first ends, the second starts. Enjoyment of the unknown and unexpected, we hope, will enhance the teaching of neurology's heritage in this age of CD-ROM and Internet. We still need an appreciation of the human, cultural factor in today's chilly technocracy. If this book succeeds in such purposes, its making was not in vain.

We would like to acknowledge the contributors, who were prepared to offer a good deal of their time to write one or more chapters and to suffer the editing process. We are grateful to Mirjam Wetzels, librarian, for searching and ordering numerous articles; to Frans Goutier, photographer, who helped in the preparation of many figures; and to the secretaries Chantal Broers, Chantalle Dinther, Marion Spaans-Metz, and Gaby Wijsman, who provided administrative assistance.

September 1999

P. J. K.
G. W. B.
J. M. S. P.

CONTENTS

PART III REFLEXES AND OTHER TESTS

PART IV SYNDROMES

CONTRIBUTORS

H. AUGUST M. VAN ALPHEN, MD, PHD
EMERITUS PROFESSOR OF NEUROSURGERY
OUDERKERK AAN DE AMSTEL
THE NETHERLANDS

MICHAEL J. AMINOFF, MD, FRCP
PROFESSOR OF NEUROLOGY
UNIVERSITY OF CALIFORNIA
SAN FRANCISCO, CALIFORNIA
UNITED STATES

PIERO G. ANTUONO, MD
PROFESSOR
DEPARTMENTS OF NEUROLOGY, PHARMACOLGY, AND TOXICOLOGY
MEDICAL COLLEGE OF WISCONSIN
MILWAUKEE, WISCONSIN
UNITED STATES

NICOLAAS J. M. ARTS, MD
NEUROLOGIST
NIJMEGEN
THE NETHERLANDS

PAUL E. BARKHAUS, MD
ASSOCIATE PROFESSOR
DEPARTMENT OF NEUROLOGY
MEDICAL COLLEGE OF WISCONSIN
MILWAUKEE, WISCONSIN
UNITED STATES

HENRY J. M. BARNETT, MD
THE JOHN P. ROBARTS RESEARCH INSTITUTE
LONDON, ONTARIO
CANADA

HARM BEUKERS, MD, PHD
PROFESSOR OF HISTORY OF MEDICINE
UNIVERSITY OF LEIDEN
LEIDEN
THE NETHERLANDS

BEN A. BLANSJAAR, MD, PHD
DIRECTOR OF TRAINING AND RESEARCH
ST. JORIS GASTHUIS PSYCHIATRIC HOSPITAL
DELFT
THE NETHERLANDS

GEORGE W. BRUYN, MD, PHD
EMERITUS PROFESSOR OF NEUROLOGY
UNIVERSITY OF LEIDEN
LEIDEN
THE NETHERLANDS

RICHARD P. M. BRUYN, MD, PHD
DEPARTMENT OF NEUROLOGY
DIAKONESSEN HOSPITAL
UTRECHT
THE NETHERLANDS

DAVID CORTES, MA
DOCTORAL CANDIDATE IN THE HISTORY OF MEDICINE
UNIVERSITY OF WISCONSIN
MADISON, WINCONSIN
UNITED STATES

ANNELIES J. E. DALMAN, MD
DEPARTMENT OF NEUROLOGY
WILLEM ALEXANDER HOSPITAL
'S HERTOGENBOSCH
THE NETHERLANDS

Ernst M. H. van den Doel, MD, PhD
Department of Neurology
Medisch Centrum Molendael
Baarn
The Netherlands

Paul Eling, PhD
Department of Comparative and Physiological Psychology
University of Nijmegen
Nijmegen
The Netherlands

Jos A. M. Frederiks, MD, PhD
Neurologist
Eindhoven
The Netherlands

Jan van Gijn, MD, FRCP, FRCP(Edin)
Professor and Chairman
University Department of Neurology
Utrecht
The Netherlands

Christopher G. Goetz, MD
Professor of Neurological Sciences and Pharmacology
Rush University/Rush Presbyterian St. Luke's Medical Center
Chicago, Illinois
United States

William Gooddy, MD, FRCP
Neurologist
Godalming, Surrey
United Kingdom

Samuel H. Greenblatt, MD, FACS
Professor of Neurosurgery at Brown University
Chief of Neurosurgery at Memorial Hospital
Pawtucket, Rhode Island
United States

Peter Hudgson, FRCP, FRACP
Emeritus Consultant
Regional Neurosciences Centre
Newcastle General Hospital
Senior Lecturer in Neurology
University of Newcastle upon Tyne
Newcastle upon Tyne
United Kingdom

Hansruedi E. Isler, MD
Department of Neurology
University Hospital
Zurich
Switzerland

Ernest H. Jellinek, MD
Emeritus Consultant of Neurology
Edinburgh
United Kingdom

Axel Karenberg, MD
Privat-Dozent
Institute for Medical History and Ethics
Universtiy of Köln
Germany

Jan M. Keppel-Hesselink, MD, PhD
University of Witten/Herdecke
Faculty of Natural Sciences
Department of Pharmacology
Witten
Germany

Antoine Keyser, MD, PhD
Department of Neurology
Academic Hospital
Nijmegen
The Netherlands

Peter J. Koehler, MD, PhD
Department of Neurology
Atrium Medical Center
Heerlen
The Netherlands

Ernst H. Koppejan, MD
Department of Neurology
St. Laurentius Hospital
Roermond
The Netherlands

Hendrikus G. J. Krouwer, MD
Associate Professor
Departments of Neurology and Neurosurgery
Medical College of Wisconsin
Milwaukee, Wisconsin
United States

Howard I. Kushner, PhD
Professor of the History of Medicine
San Diego State University
Visiting Scholar
University of California
San Diego, California
United States

Boleslav Lichterman, MD
Chair of Pediatric Neurosurgery
Russian Postgraduate Medical Academy
Moscow
Russia

John B. Lyons, MD, FRCPI
Professor of History of Medicine
Royal College of Surgeons of Ireland
Dublin
Ireland

Heather Meldrum, BA
The John P. Robarts Research Institute
London, Ontario
Canada

David Moffie, MD, PhD
Amsterdam
The Netherlands

Hans J. G. H. Oosterhuis, MD, PhD
Emeritus Professor of Neurology
Groningen
The Netherlands

John M. S. Pearce, FRCP
Emeritus Consultant of Neurology
Hull
United Kingdom

Charles M. Poser, MD, FRCP
Visiting Professor of Neurology
Department of Neurology
Beth Israel Deaconess Medical Center
Boston Massachusetts
United States

Victor M. Riccardi, MD
The Neurofibromatosis Institute
La Crescenta, California
United States

Allan H. Ropper, MD
Professor of Neurology, Chair of Neurology
Tufts University School of Medicine
Chief of Neurology
St. Elisabeth's Hospital
Boston, Massachusetts
United States

Frank Clifford Rose, MD
Director
London Neurological Centre
London
United Kingdom

Francis Schiller, MD
Department of History of Health Sciences
University of California
San Francisco, California
United States

Franz Seitelberger, MD
Emeritus Professor of Neurology
Klinisches Institut für Neurologie
Universität Wien
Vienna
Austria

Chris U. M. Smith, PhD
Vision Sciences
Aston University
Birmingham
United Kingdom

Frank Spaans, MD, PhD
Professor of Clinical Neurophysiology
Academic Hospital
Maastricht
The Netherlands

Jan Stam, MD, PhD
Professor of Neurology
Academic Medical Center
Amsterdam
The Netherlands

Alan H. Sykes, MD
Chapel Stile, Ambleside
Cumbria
United Kingdom

Anton Valkenburg, MD
Department of Neurology
Atrium Medical Center
Heerlen
The Netherlands

Jan Voogd, MD, PhD
Emeritus Professor of Anatomy
Erasmus University Rotterdam
Rotterdam
The Netherlands

Conor Ward, MD, FRCP, FRCP(Glasg), FRCPI, FRCPCH (Hon)
Emeritus Professor of Pediatrics
Teddington, Middlesex
United Kingdom

Rianne J. Wennekes, MD
Department of Neurology
Atrium Medical Center
Heerlen
The Netherlands

Eelco F. M. Wijdicks, MD
Professor of Neurology
Mayo Medical School
Medical Director
Neurology–Neurosurgery Intensive Care Unit
Consultant
Department of Neurology
Mayo Clinic and Mayo Foundation
Rochester, Minnesota
United States

George K. York, MD
Clinical Professor of Neurology
University of California at Davis
Chief of Neurology
Kaiser Permanente Stockton
Senior Fellow
The SÅa Institute
California
United States

I

Structures and Processes

1

ADAMKIEWICZ'S ARTERY

Boleslav Lichterman

Albert Adamkiewicz was born to a Jewish family, the son of district physician Adolf Adamkiewicz and Zuzanna Jacobson, on 11 August 1850 in Zerkow in the Poznan region of Prussia (presently situated in Poland).[1–3] He received a German education at secondary schools in Bydgosh and Rastenburg and was never able to speak or write good Polish.[2,4] He studied medicine in Königsberg (the present Kaliningrad, Russia), and subsequently in Breslau (present-day Wroclaw, Poland), where he worked in Rudolf Peter Heinrich Heidenhain's physiology laboratory. His study was interrupted by the Franco-German war in 1870–1871, as he had to serve in the German army.

After the war, Adamkiewicz continued his studies in Würzburg, visiting the clinics of Heinrich von Bamberger, Wenzel von Linhart, and Friedrich Wilhelm Scanzoni and worked at Friedrich D. von Recklinghausen's laboratory. He was awarded the first prize of Würzburg University and the doctorate degree for his work *Die mechanischen Bluttstillungsmittel* [The mechanical bloodstemming agents]. He returned to Breslau in 1873, where he was graduated at the medical faculty. From 1873 to 1876, Adamkiewicz worked as an assistant in the physiological laboratory of Königsberg University, and later in the clinic as a *Dozent* (associate professor), teaching medical diagnostics and pathology. He moved to Berlin in 1876, where he was appointed senior physician in the clinic of nervous diseases of Carl Westphal (1833–1890) at the Charité and lecturer in diagnostics and neuropathology. In 1880, he was invited to Jagellonian University in Krakow, Poland, where a new chair of general and experimental pathology was established. Despite his poor Polish, he soon became famous as an outstanding teacher and researcher. Influenced by his wife Kazimiera Reichmann, who was from a banker's family in Warsaw, he converted to Roman Catholicism in 1889.[2]

Adamkiewicz published about 100 papers (mostly in German) covering different branches of medicine and became internationally known. However, he ruined his scientific reputation by his overconfidence. In his 1885 publication "New Nervous

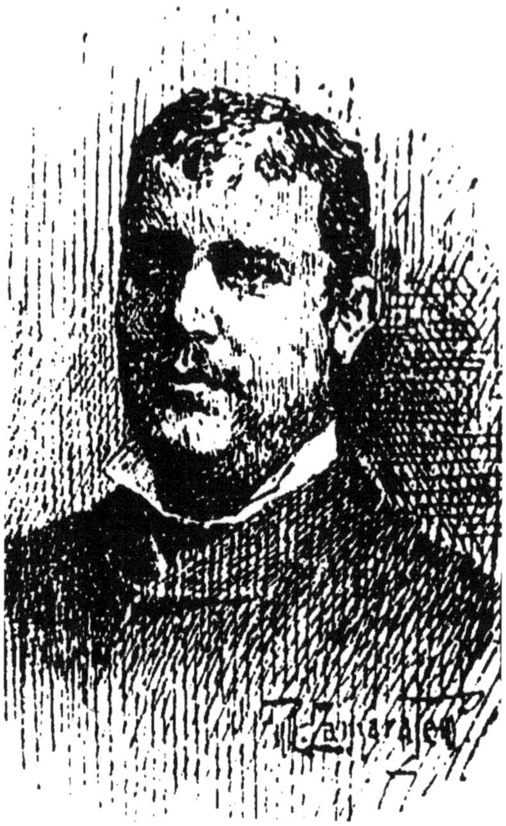

Figure 1–1. Albert Adamkiewicz (1850–1921). From Wielka Encyklopedya Powszechna. *Warszawa: Naklad i Druk S. Sikorskiego, 1890, vol. 1, p. 137.*

Cells: Previously Unknown Morphological Components of Peripheral Nerves,"[5,6] for instance, he described crescent-shaped cells beneath the neurilemma of myelinated nerve fibers (the so-called demilune of Adamkiewicz), which most of his contemporaries considered to be artifacts or ordinary Schwann cells.

In 1891, he claimed that cancer is poisonous and caused by a parasite named "coccidium sarcolytus." Its toxin is directed to nervous cells and causes death due to brain damage, but it might be inactivated by disinfection using carbolic acid or by boiling. He also claimed the discovery of a new anticancer serum, which would eliminate metastases: "We created our own method of treatment which is available and safe for everybody. . . ."[4] The "discovery" was sharply criticized by his colleagues at the medical faculty, who accused him of self-advertising. The Ministry of Education allowed Adamkiewicz a sabbatical year and in 1892, he started to study the anticancer serum in Prof. Eduard Albert's surgical clinic in Vienna. Adamkiewicz published ten monographs on the anticancer serum during his life.[2] These publications made his return to Jagellonian University impossible. In 1893, he applied for early retirement because of health problems. He worked as an ordinary physician at the Rothschild Jewish hospital in Vienna until his death on 31 October 1921.[2,3] His death went unnoticed by the international medical community. He was survived by two sons—Jerzy and Wlodziemerz. Both of them became lawyers and made diplomatic careers in the new independent state of Poland, emerging after World War I in the backyard of two disintegrated empires, the Russian and Austro-Hungarian.

In Kelly's *Encyclopedia of Medical Sources,* Adamkiewicz's name is eponymously mentioned with respect to the above-mentioned demilune and anticancer serum ("a suppressed alexin, obtained from cancer tissue and used hypodermically for the treatment of cancer"), a safranin stain for myelin, and a test for proteins.[7] The artery of Adamkiewicz is not listed.

Until the end of the nineteenth century, the blood supply of the spinal cord was thought to be provided by anterior and posterior spinal arteries originating from intracranial segments of the vertebral arteries. It was erroneously argued that each spinal cord segment has an additional blood supply via radicular arteries (Willis, 1664; Vieussens, 1685).[8–10] The spinal cord was thought to be supplied by three longitudinal arterial trunks—one anterior and two posterior spinal arteries, which accompany the spinal cord over the whole length and carry blood in caudal direction. Radicular arteries were thought to branch symmetrically to each spinal cord segment and to play a secondary role.[10]

Haller's 1754 anatomical pictures show that the anterior parts of thoracic and lumbosacral regions of spinal cord are supplied by three radicular arteries (Fig. 1–2).[10,11] This observation was largely neglected until Adamkiewicz published "Die Blutgefässe des menschlichen Rückenmarkes" [The bloodvessels of the human spinal cord], in two parts (1881–1882).[12] Spinal cord vascularization is shown on a series of colored anatomical plates reproduced here in black and white (Fig. 1–3). Adamkiewicz demonstrated the reduction of radicular arteries by injection of colored solutions into the vessels. He named them aa. spinales and gave a detailed description of anterior and posterior radicular arteries. The number of aa. spinales anteriores varied from 3 to 13. Among them, he always noted one large vessel in the lower part of spinal cord, which he called "arteria magna spinalis." It is this artery that was later named for Adamkiewicz in the French literature. It passes most often at level T9–T12, reaches the anterior spinal fissure, and afterwards divides into ascending and descending branches. These branches had been called "aa. spinales anterior" since their description by Willis (1664). Adamkiewicz renamed them the "anterior anastomotic chain." Circumferential vessels with small transverse branches were named "vasocorona spinalis" (the spinal vascular crown) by Adamkiewicz. Similarly, the so-called aa. spinales posterior were renamed "posterior anastomotic chain". The two chains communicate with each other via transverse anastomoses ("rami cruciantes"), the largest of which is located at medullary conus and is called the "crux vasculosa" (the vascular cross).

Adamkiewicz utilized the injection technique of Professor Ludwig Teichmann, who was director of the Anatomical Institute in Krakow. Teichmann's assistant Henryk Kadyi (1851–1912) had been working in the same field. His monograph on spinal cord vascularization was published in 1889.[13] Kadyi explained this delay in publication by the fact that he had to leave Krakow for Lemberg (now Lvov, Ukraine) in 1881, which made his work more difficult. In the introduction to his monograph, Kadyi wrote:

> I have been given the initiative to the work below by my revered teacher, Professor Teichmann, as a result of Professor Adamkiewicz's statement expressed in one of

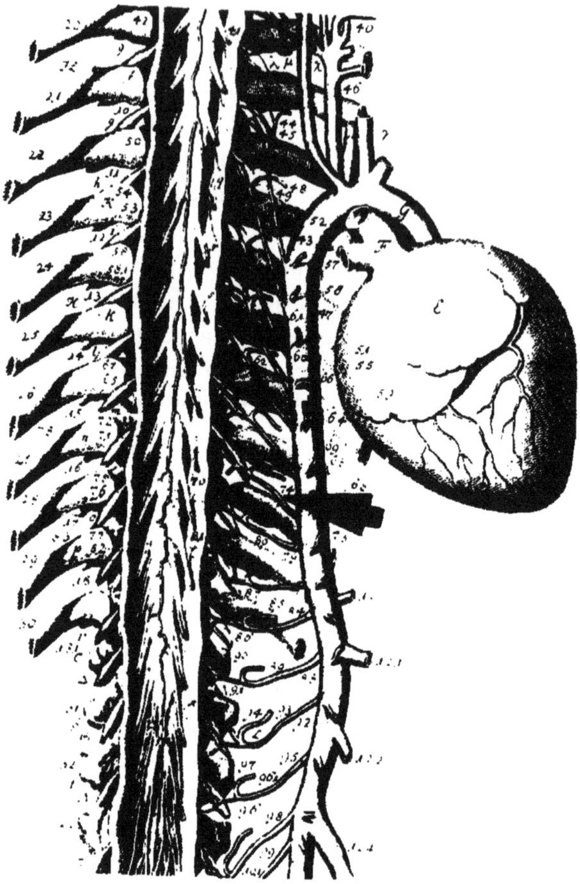

Figure 1–2. Illustration from Haller (1754), detail. Several principal arteries running along the spinal roots are visible, including the arteria radicularis magna (indicated by arrow) accompanying the left ninth thoracic root.

> his dissertations, that certain degenerative changes of the spinal medulla spread with the arterial blood flow. As it was the clear wish of Professor Teichmann, whose assistant I was at that time, I was at first to study blood vessels of the spinal medulla together with Professor Adamkiewicz. Because of reasons beyond my control, however, neither our work together, nor publications, nor even Professor Adamkiewicz's later suggestions for Professor Teichmann to develop this subject with him, without my participation, were accepted. Professor Teichmann requested us to conduct studies on the spinal medulla separately, with a motive that if two researchers undertook independent studies on such an important subject, it would certainly be beneficial for science. (Cited in Ref. 14)

Adamkiewicz accused "ein gewisser Herr Kady" [a certain Mister Kady] of plagiarism. This unfounded accusation has brought shame on Adamkiewicz, because Kadyi was known for his scientific honesty and anatomical skills.[4] The original name "arteria magna spinalis" was not accepted by Kadyi. He argued that the adjective "spinalis" means "vertebralis" and does not relate to the spinal cord but to the spinal vertebrae. The vessel was renamed "arteria radicalis magna." "Crux vasculosa" was transformed by Kadyi into "rami anastomotici arcuati."

Figure 1–3. Illustration from Adamkiewicz (1882). The arteria radicularis medullaris magna is running to the anterior spinal artery along the left eighth thoracic root.

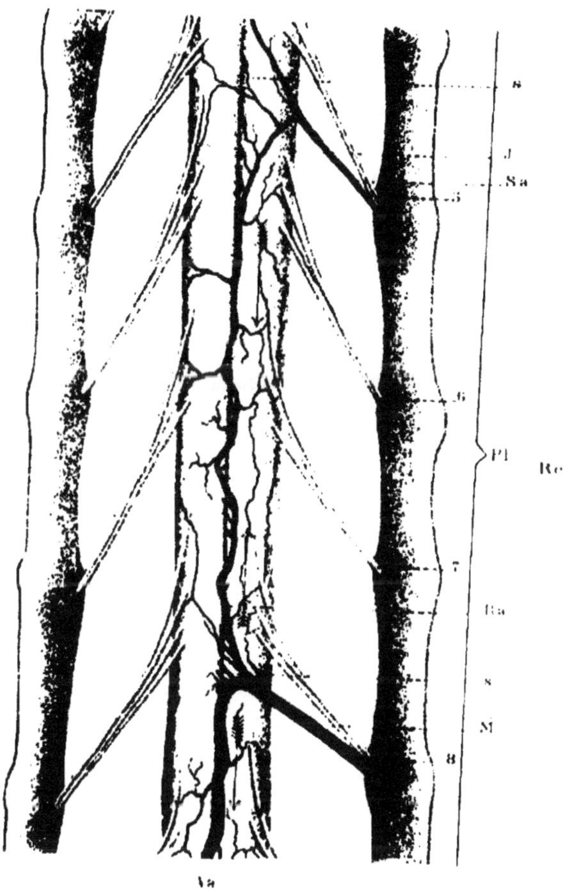

Kadyi's terminology helped to get rid of chaos in naming segmental and longitudinal spinal cord vessels. It is used in the modern literature for naming Adamkiewicz's artery in a slightly changed transcription: "a. radicularis magna" or "a. radicularis anterior magna." Lazorthes et al.[15,16] called this vessel "a. intumescentia lumbalis," arguing that such a name well defines the region of blood supply. Bogorodinsky and Skorometz suggested the name "a. radiculomedullaris magna anterior."[8] Nowadays, the "artery of Adamkiewicz" and "a. radicularis medullaris magna (ARMM)" are the most widely used terms, although neither one corresponds to international anatomical nomenclature.[9,17]

Adamkiewicz's artery is the main feeding vessel of the lower or thoracolumbar-sacral region of the spinal cord. In 75%–80% of cases it starts at the left side of the T8–T12 vertebrae.[16,18–20] That is why this level is sometimes recommended for performing angiography in paraplegic patients with suspected spinal arteriovenous malformations (AVMs).[21,22] An occlusion of ARMM is usually caused by aortic pathology, sometimes caused by surgery. It may result in ischemic spinal cord infarcts, the onset of which is either sudden or progressive with clinical signs of lower motor deficit and spinal pain of short duration.[8,23] Unlike cerebral vascular events, emboli of cardiac origin are rarely involved.

References

1. *Biographisches Lexicon der hervorragenden Ärzte aller Zeiten und Volker.* 2nd ed. Berlin: Urban & Schwarzenberg; 1929;1:24–25.
2. Mieses M. *Polacy: chrescijane pochodzenia zydowskiego.* Pt. 1. Warszawa: Wydawnictwo M. Fruchtmana; 1938:1–2.
3. *Polski Slownik Biograficzny.* Pt. 1. Krakow: Polska Academja Umiejetnosci; 1935:25–26.
4. Herman E. Albert Wojciech Adamkiewicz (11.8.1850–31.10.1921). *Neuropat Pol.* 1968;6:1–10.
5. Adamkiewicz A. *Die Nervenkörperchen: Ein neuerer bisher unbekannter morphologischer Bestandtheil der perischen Nerven.* Wien: Gerold's Sohn; 1885.
6. Adamkiewicz A. Cialka nerwowe nowe, dotychczas nieznane skladniki morfologiczne nerwow obwodowych. *Przegl Lek.* 1885;24:12–16.
7. Kelly EC. *Encyclopedia of Medical Sources.* Baltimore: Williams & Wilkins; 1948:3–4.
8. Bogorodinsky DK, Skorometz AA. *Infarkty spinnogo mozga.* Leningrad: Meditsyna; 1973.
9. German DG, Skorometz AA. *Narushenija spinnomozgovogo krovoobrashenija.* Kishinev: Shtiintza; 1981.
10. Luyendijk W. The arteries of the spinal cord: the history of a paradigmal shift. *Acta Neurochir (Wien).* 1982;61:25–41.
11. von Haller A. *Iconum Anatomicarum. Quibus Aliquae Partes Corporis Humani Delineatae Traduntur.* Göttingen: Apud viduam Abrami Vandenhoeckii; 1754.
12. Adamkiewicz A. Die Blutgefässe des menschlichen Rückenmarkes, I: Die Gefässe der Rückenmarksubstanz. *Sitzb Akad Wiss.* 1881;84:469–598; II: Die Gefässe der Rückenmarksoberfläche. *Sitzb Akad Wiss.* 1882;85:101–130.
13. Kadyi H. *Über die Blutgefässe des menschlichen Rückenmarkes.* Lemberg: Gubrynowicz & Schmidt, 1889.
14. Sokolowska-Pituchowa J. Two monographs on the spinal cord vascularization. *Folia Morphol (Warsz).* 1980;39:1–8.
15. Lazorthes G, Gouaze A, Zadeh JO, et al. Arterial vascularization of the spinal cord: recent studies of the anastomotic substitution pathways. *J Neurosurg.* 1971;35:253–262.
16. Lazorthes G, Gouaze A, Djindjian R. *Vascularisation et circulation de la moelle épinière.* Paris: Masson; 1973.
17. Skorometz AA, Tissen TP, Panyushkin AI, Skorometz TA. *Sosudistye zabolevanija spinnogo mozga.* Sankt-Peterburg: Sotis; 1998.
18. Alleyne CH, Cawley MC, Shengelaia GG, Barrow DL. Microsurgical anatomy of the artery of Adamkiewicz and its segmental artery. *J Neurosurg.* 1998;89:791–795.
19. Illuminati G, Koskas F, Bertagni A, et al. Variazioni di origine dell'arteria di Adamkiewicz. *Riv Eur Sci Med Farmacol.* 1996;18:61–66.
20. Rodriguez-Baeza A, Muset-Lara A, Rodriguez-Pazos M, et al. The arterial supply of the human spinal cord: a new approach to the arteria radicularis magna of Adamkiewicz. *Acta Neurochir (Wien).* 1991;109:57–62.
21. Tissen TP. *Selectivnaya spinal'naya angiographija.* Moskva: 1975. Thesis.
22. Djindjian R, Hurth M, Houdart R. En hommage a Albert Wojciech Adamkiewicz (1850–1921): étude arteriographique normale et pathologique de l'arteria radicularis anterior magna. *Rev Neurol (Paris).* 1971;125:211–218.
23. Masson C. Les accidents ischémiques médullaires. *Presse Méd.* 1994;23:1723–1728.

2

BRODMANN'S CORTICAL AREAS

Chris U. M. Smith

Korbinian Brodmann was born at Liggersdorf, Hohenzollern, on 17 November 1868. He was educated at Gymnasia in Sigmaringen and Konstanz and studied medicine at, successively, Munich, Würzburg, Berlin, and Freiburg-im-Breisgau. He passed his final medical examinations at Freiburg on 21 February 1895. It seems that his ambition after passing his medical examinations was to work as a doctor in the Black Forest region. To this end he enrolled at the Munich Pediatric Clinic and Polyclinic, but he was prevented from taking up the time-consuming duties of general practitioner when he contracted diphtheria. Instead, in May 1896, he assumed the less demanding position of assistant in the Neurological Clinic at Alexanderbad-im-Fichtelberg (northern Bavaria), whose director at that time was Oskar Vogt. This was a crucial moment in Brodmann's career.

Oskar Vogt was at that time working to establish an Institute of Brain Research and the young Brodmann quickly caught the enthusiasm. Vogt was impressed by his assistant's broad scientific interests and careful, methodical work habits. Vogt's efforts to establish a brain research laboratory finally bore fruit in 1898 with the formation of the Neurobiologisches Universitäts-Laboratorium in Berlin. Brodmann briefly followed Vogt to Berlin and then went to Leipzig to study pathology. Here he completed his medical training with a doctorate awarded in 1898 for a thesis entitled *A Contribution to the Understanding of Chronic Ependymal Sclerosis.* Brodmann's next appointment was at the University Psychiatric Clinic in Jena, directed by Otto Binswanger; he then transferred to yet another position and, in this case, a post that would confirm him in his choice of specialty. This position at the Städtische Irrenanstalt at Frankfurt-am-Main lasted for 18 months, from 1900 to 1901.

In the last decades of the nineteenth century Frankfurt was full of excitement for a budding neuroanatomist.[1] Brodmann came under the influence of a galaxy of like-minded scientists. Carl Weigert, expert in staining cells and inventor of many

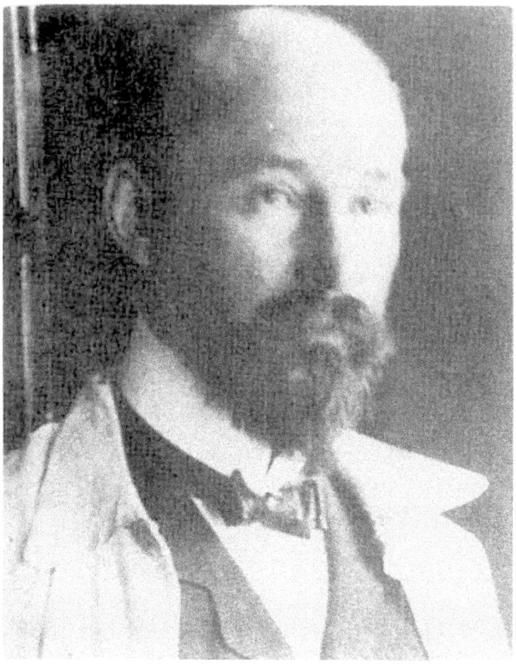

Figure 2–1. Korbinian Brodmann (1868–1918). From Ref. 9.

histological techniques, including the perfection of celloidin embedding, had worked in Frankfurt since 1885. Franz Nissl, who had worked closely with Weigert in developing neuroglial stains, had left for Heidelberg only a few years before the young Brodmann arrived. Ludwig Edinger had settled in Frankfurt in 1882 and, making use of Weigert's technique for staining myelin sheaths of the central nervous systems of lower vertebrates, had become one of the founders of comparative neuroanatomy. But the neurologist who influenced Brodmann more than any other was Alois Alzheimer. Alzheimer had arrived in Frankfurt in 1882 and remained until 1902. He had collaborated closely with Nissl in analyzing the histopathology of the cerebral cortex. Alzheimer possessed an outstanding gift for explaining clearly and vividly his microscopical observations.

In the autumn of 1901 Brodmann rejoined Oskar Vogt in the newly established Berlin Neurobiologisches Universitäts-Laboratorium. Here he met and collaborated with Max Bielschowsky and Richard Henneberg. Bielschowsky had developed the technique of silver impregnation of nerve fibers, a technique which now bears his name. The two neurohistologists published a joint paper on the histology and histopathology of the cortex in 1905.[2] The years in Vogt's laboratory, from 1901 to 1910, were by far Brodmann's most productive. Between 1903 and 1908 he published seven papers in the *Journal für Psychologie und Neurologie* (of which he was editor) describing the fine structure of the cerebral cortex in a number of mammals, especially primates. These papers formed the basis of his great 1909 publication *Vergleichende Lokalisationslehre der*

Grosshirnrinde [Localization in the cerebral hemispheres: a comparative study] Although he was far from the only investigator interested in cytoarchitectonics,[3,4] his maps and, in particular, the numbers he attached to the various cytoarchitectonic regions have entered the neuroanatomical literature and are frequently quoted.

The first edition of *Vergleichende Lokalisationslehre der Grosshirnrinde,* published in 1909,[5] is now very rare. A second edition was published in 1925, seven years after its author's death, and Barth Verlag, the original publisher, reissued the 1909 edition in 1985. An English translation by Laurence J. Garey was published by Smith-Gordon in 1994,[6] and it is this translation that I use in the following quotations. In the Foreword Brodmann describes the origins of his investigation:

> When I began my work in the Neurobiological Laboratory of the University of Berlin eight years ago the task befell me to undertake a topographic analysis of the human cerebral cortex based on its cellular structure, in the context of the research program of this institute.

He distinguishes his work from that of his co-workers in the Berlin laboratory. Fiber architecture (fibrilloarchitectonics) was undertaken by Bielschowksy and myeloarchitectonics (based on the onset of myelination in different brain regions) was of particular interest to Oskar Vogt.[7] Brodmann took cytoarchitectonics as his responsibility. He defined this as the localization of the individual histological elements, their layering, and their arrangement in the adult brain.

The practical aim of cytoarchitectonics, he writes, is to provide a minute description of the cortex, which would be of value to neuropathologists and clinicians. But he soon saw that it was necessary to take a much wider perspective. Here his experience of working alongside the comparative neuroanatomists at Frankfurt must have been valuable. For, he says, it quickly became obvious that in order to understand the "extremely complicated and unfathomable human brain" it was essential to first examine the cortex in simpler forms. His research was thus broadened to include the histological examination of brains from representative examples of the whole mammalian class, from prototherians *(Echidna acuelatus)* and metatherians (marsupials; *Macropus rufus:* red kangeroo; *Macropus dorsalis:* black-striped wallaby) to numerous eutherians: hedgehogs, rabbits, mice, rats, cats, dogs, lions, tigers, seals, bats, and a wide variety of primates. Altogether 64 different species of mammal are included in Brodmann's investigation. He acknowledges the great help and encouragement that he received from the Berlin Zoological Gardens in providing, as he says, "valuable specimens" for use in his research.

Brodmann's investigations were by no means all qualitative. Although statistical analysis is lacking, he gives much quantitative information relating to brain-body ratios, cortical thicknesses in different areas compared across different mammals; ratios of cortical thicknesses to body mass in different animals; and so on. He concludes that it is by no means clear that any of these quantitative measures can be related straightforwardly to a mammal's taxonomic position. But his major contribution is undoubtedly in the arrangement of the cortex according to the mix of morphological types of histological element present.

The value of Brodmann's approach depends on two assumptions: (1) cells of similar morphology can indeed be recognized in different parts of the cortex and (2) similarity in morphology implies similarity in function. But, as he admits, this is easy to specify but difficult to confirm. "First and foremost," he writes, "we still lack clear criteria for the recognition of anatomically equivalent cellular elements." Brodmann is also quite clear about the dangers of identifying individual neurons with specific psychological or behavioral functions. "There has been occasional talk of 'sensory cells' located in particular regions, or of sensorial '*special cells.*' People have invented acoustic or optical special cells and even a 'memory' cell, and have not shied away from the fantastic 'psychic cell'" (emphasis in original). Brodmann will have nothing to do with this. He "refutes it energetically" and insists that even the most primitive psychic phenomena are to be correlated not with "individual *cell type* but *cell groupings.*"

At the end of his treatise Brodmann sums up his work. A knowledge of the cytoarchitectonics of the normal brain is, he writes, essential if we are to understand the neuropathology of the diseased brain. He looks forward to a broad, collaborative investigation, for he recognizes that he has given only a "sketchy outline." He is optimistic that brain scientists are "at the threshold of a new field of research." He is dismissive of those who wish to study the functions of the brain by methods involving extirpation. "Functional localisation," he concludes, "without the lead of anatomy is utterly impossible." He ends by quoting Bernhard Gudden, whom he designates as an earlier master of brain research: "first anatomy and then physiology; but if first physiology, then not without anatomy."

As mentioned above Brodmann was not the only neuroanatomist interested in cytoarchitectonics at the end of the nineteenth and beginning of the twentieth century. His analysis, detailed but not too detailed, has stood the test of time and his enumeration of cortical areas (e.g., Fig. 2–2) is still used by neuroscientists.

Brodmann completed the introduction to *Vergleichende Lokalisationslehre der Grosshirnrinde* with the usual acknowledgments, singling out Oskar Vogt and his colleagues at the Berlin Neurobiological Laboratory and the trustees of the Berlin Municipal Benefaction (Stiftungsdeputation der Stadt Berlin). He notes, with some bitterness, that his thanks to these individuals and organizations is all the greater as he had repeatedly failed to obtain funds from the Science Research Fund of Berlin University because of the opposition of the Medical Faculty. It seems that this animosity between Brodmann and the Berlin Medical Faculty (which had rejected his thesis for *Habilitation* [a qualification for teaching there]) lies behind his departure for Tübingen in 1910 to work with Robert Gaupp. He began to make his work more widely known by presentations in Stuttgart (1911), Munich (1912), and Vienna (1913). His presentations showed that he was no narrow specialist.[9] Indeed, perusal of his 1909 treatise shows that this was always a misrepresentation. His interests ranged widely over neurology, psychiatry, neuroanatomy, anthropology, zoology, evolution, and physiology. His presentation in Vienna 1984, for instance, described his research into cortical anatomy with respect to problems in anthropology.[10] Finally, on 1 May 1916, the 48-year-old Brodmann obtained his first secure and permanent appointment. This was the position of pro-

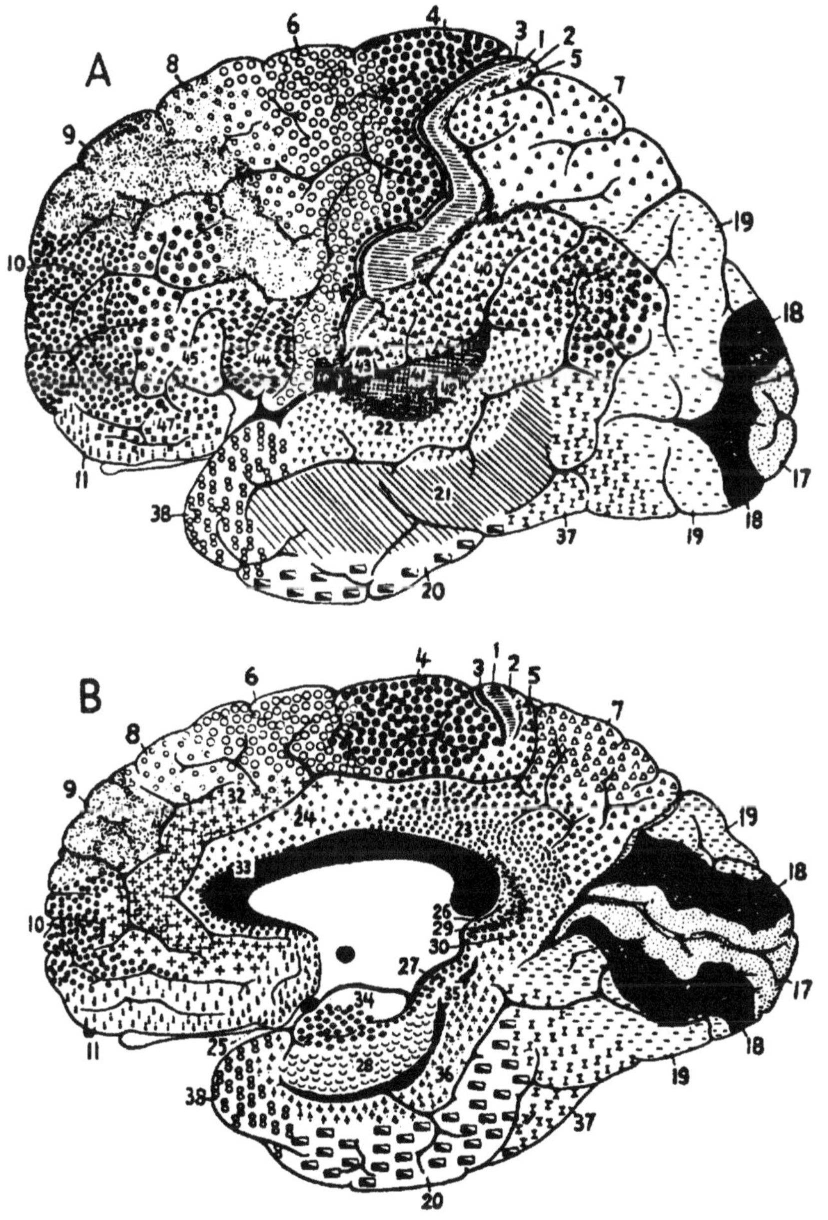

Figure 2–2. Cortical areas of the (A) *lateral and* (B) *medial surfaces of the human brain.*[5,8]

sector at the Nietleben Mental Asylum in Halle, under the directorship of Berthold Pfeiffer.

Brodmann was now at last in a position to develop his career and his scientific ideas. Furthermore, he had met and on 3 April 1917 married Margerete Francke. A daughter, Ilse, was born in 1918. In 1918 also, as the war was drawing to its end, Brodmann was offered and accepted a highly prestigious appointment. This was to the Deutsche Forschungsanstalt für Psychiatrie, which Emil Kraepelin, in collaboration with Franz Nissl and Walther Spielmeyer, was organizing in Munich. The opportunity to work with Nissl and Spielmeyer, the author of *Technik der mikroskopischen Untersuchung des Nervensystems* (1911) and, later (1922), *Histopathologie des Nervensystems,* was auspicious. Brodmann accepted the chair of architectonics and topographic anatomy. In spite of the bleakness and chaos of the war's end, the scientific future must have seemed bright and full of possibilities. But it was not to be:

> At this moment when he had begun to live a happy family life, when, after years of distraction due to war work, he was at last able to take up his research activities again in independent and distinguished circumstances, just when his friends were looking forward to a new period of successful research from him, a treacherous infection took him from us after a short illness on 22 August 1918.[11]

According to Spielmeyer[12] Brodmann was "an intense and earnest man, reserved to the point of timidity, but who could flare, on occasion, into a temper." His long period of untenured and insecure employment possibly explains some of this introversion. Whether it also accounts for the standoff with the Berlin Medical Faculty is impossible at this distance in time to ascertain. It is tragic that he died just as the clouds were lifting on his life. He is survived, however, by his *Localization in the Cerebral Cortex,* which has provided illustrations for countless subsequent texts and papers in neuroanatomy. Its 1985 reissue and 1994 English translation may bring it to the notice of a new generation of readers who will savor it not only as a historical document but also for its wide intellectual survey of a still fascinating topic.

References

1. Haymaker W, Schiller F, eds. *The Founders of Neurology.* 2nd ed. Springfield, Ill: Charles C Thomas; 1970.
2. Bielchowsky M, Brodmann K. Zur feineren Histologie und Histopathologie der Grosshirnrinde mit besonderer Berücksichtigung der Dementia paralytica, Dementia senilis und Idiotie. *J Psychol Neurol.* 1905;5:173–199
3. Kemper T, Le Brun T, Galaburda AM. Principles of Cytoarchitectonics. In: Peters A, Jones EG, eds. *Cerebral Cortex.* New York: Plenum; 1984;35–57.
4. Smith CUM. A century of cortical architectonics. *J Hist Neurosci.* 1992;1:201–218.
5. Brodmann, K. *Vergleichende Localisationslehre der Grosshirnrinde in ihren Principien dargestellt auf Grund des Zellenbaues.* Leipzig: Barth; 1909.
6. Garey LJ, ed-trans. *Brodmann's Localisation in the Cerebral Cortex.* London: Smith-Gordon; 1994.
7. Vogt O. Der Wert der myelogenetischen Felder der Grosshirnrinde (Cortex pallii). *Anat Anz.* 1906;29:237–287.
8. Brodmann K. Bermerken über die Fibrillogenie und ihre Beziehungen zur Myelogenie mit besonderer Berücksichtigung des Cortex cerebri. *Neurol Centralbl.* 1907;26:338–349.
9. Bogaert L. van. L'Institut Korbinian Brodmann a Tübingen (Allemagne). *World Neurol.* 1961;2:846–848.
10. Brodmann K. Neue Forschungsergebnisse der Grosshirnrindeanatomie mit besonderer Berücksichtigung anthropolischer Fragen. *Verhandlung der anatomischen Gesellschaft;* 1913.
11. Vogt O. Korbinian Brodmann. *J Psychol Neurol.* 1918;24:i–x.
12. Rose JE. Korbinian Brodmann. In: Haymaker W, Schiller F, eds. *The Founders of Neurology.* 2nd ed. Springfield, Ill: Charles C Thomas; 1970.

3

HEAD'S AREAS

Ernst M. H. van den Doel

> It is the great merit of the English neurologist Henry Head to have drawn our attention to the fact that diseases of the inner organs frequently produce painful sensations (referred pains) or even hyperesthesias of the skin in those radicular areas that correspond to the spinal segment from which the said internal organ draws its *rami communicantes.*

Thus the Swiss neurologist Robert Bing summarized in his *Textbook of Nervous Diseases* (1952)[1] the work to which Henry Head (1861–1940) had devoted the greater part of his life. For the modern neurologist, especially at a time when complaints not directly understood can be analyzed with the help of innumerable diagnostic devices, the concept that a pain need not originate at the place of the body where it is felt may seem superfluous. Yet the common medical knowledge that pain between the shoulder blades may originate in the thoracic aorta is largely due to Henry Head. "The dwarf sees farther than the giant, when he has the giant's shoulder to mount on" (Samuel Taylor Coleridge, 1772–1834). We present-day dwarfs sometimes seem to have lost sight of our giants altogether.

Henry Head was born on 4 August 1861, at 6 Park Road, Stoke Newington, London, now a borough of Greater London.[2–6] He was educated at Charterhouse School.

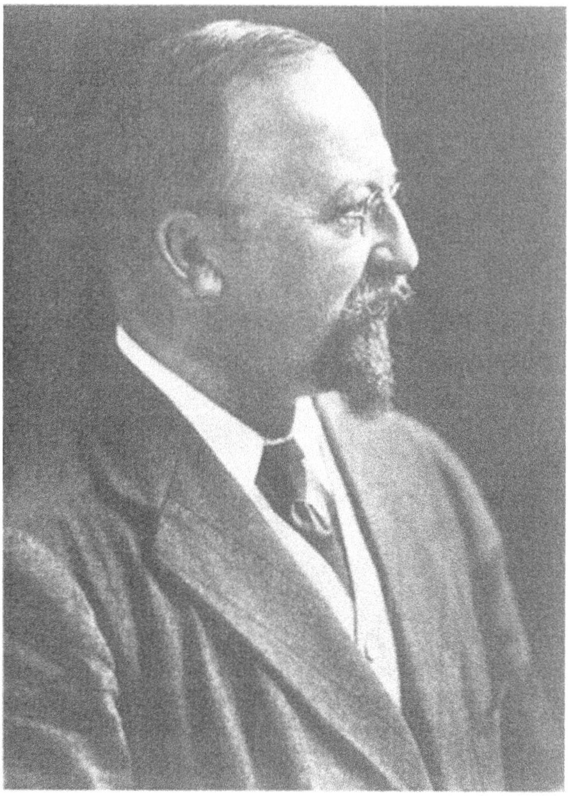

Figure 3–1. Henry Head 1861–1940. From Ref. 5 with permission from Thieme Verlag, Stuttgart, Germany.

Head's parents were affluent Quakers, which enabled him to spend two months at the Martin Luther Universität of Halle-Wittenberg in Germany before starting his studies at Cambridge. He was elected to a scholarship at Trinity College, of which he later became an honorary fellow. Michael Foster (1836–1907), Walter Gaskell (1847–1914), and John Newport Langley (1852–1925) were among his teachers. Lord Lister, founder of surgical antisepsis, was Head's cousin.

After obtaining his B.A., Head spent some time at the German University in Prague, where, under the supervision of Ewald Hering (1834–1918), the discoverer of the Hering-Breuer reflex, he studied the physiology of the regulation of breathing in newborns. As a result of frequent visits to the continent Head became proficient in German as well as French, an asset for a neurologist at the turn of the century.

Once back in Cambridge, Head took his M.A. and M.D. in 1892. His M.D. thesis was founded on his work at University College Hospital in London, where the neurologists Henry-Charlton Bastian (1837–1915) and William Gowers (1845–1915) and the surgeon Victor Horsley (1857–1916) were practicing. This thesis, on disturbances of sensation with special reference to the pain of visceral disease, was extended later and published in three parts in *Brain* in 1893, 1894, and 1896.[7] It established the term "Head's zones" or, more commonly (and in Head's own terminology), "Head's areas."

In 1886 Head started practicing in the London Hospital. He also worked for a time in the Rainhill County Asylum. Until the end of his career he continued to study the physiology of human sensation. In 1900 he published his findings in 450 cases of herpes zoster, in 21 of which an autopsy was performed. Head demonstrated that the skin lesion corresponded with the cutaneous distribution of a dorsal nerve root.[8]

Head's way of working was very time-consuming and in some patients his examinations led to exhaustion. In 1905, frustrated by his patients' lack of ability to describe their sensations, he had the superficial branch of his left radial nerve transsected and sutured, to study the effects of nerve healing during the six months that followed. He was assisted by the psychologist William Halse Rivers (1864–1922). As a result of his experiences he distinguished two kinds of sensitivity, *protopathic* (gross pain and temperature discrimination) and *epicritic* (fine pain, temperature and tactile discrimination), next to deep sensibility (gross actile sensation and proprioception). This classification has not, as we know, withstood the test of time. Head's work with Gordon Holmes (see Chapter 27) resulted in publications regarding disturbances of sensation in various afflictions of the brain, among which we find an early description of the thalamic syndrome that was later to be named named for Jules Dejerine (1849–1917) and Gustave Roussy (1874–1948). From 1918, Head became increasingly interested in aphasia, especially of traumatic origin. The Great War, alas, gave ample opportunities for this kind of research.[9,10]

Head was the editor of *Brain* from 1910 to 1925. Unfortunately, he suffered from Parkinson's disease in the last 20 years of his life. He withdrew to his home in Reading in 1925, where his wife Ruth cared for him. He dedicated his collection of poems, *Destroyers and Other Verses,* to her. His obituary by Robert Nichols in the *Times* of 1940 describes him as a conversationalist who could talk with knowledge in the course of an evening on Goethe and Mozart, symphonic music, looping the loop, coordination in a golfer, Ninon de Lenclos, Joseph Conrad, religious ecstasy, and social customs in Melanesia. Nichols further wrote: "Sir Henry Head possessed the fullest as well as the wisest mind I have ever known . . . He had Leonardo's lofty human compassion, humility and patience, and profound serenity of spirit." Henry Head died in 1940, 17 months after his wife.

Some years before his thesis of 1892, Head had noticed that the usual descriptions of the pains of stomach disorders were far from complete. This brought him to explore pain and sensation in disorders of all the internal organs, and so to his famous three articles in *Brain.*[7] The first article concerned the abdomen, the second the head and neck, the third the heart and lungs. He had noticed that diseases of different organs produced pain and tenderness to pressure in other specific parts of the body, without directly influencing the nervous sytem. These sensitive areas often were found quite remote from the diseased organ. He also found that these areas corresponded with the dermal representation of specific peripheral nerves or nerve roots. Head extensively describes his observations in individual patients and his conclusions from these cases. In a great number of specific disorders—stomach ulcer, sinusitis, lung abcess, diseases of the valves of the heart, aortic dissection and

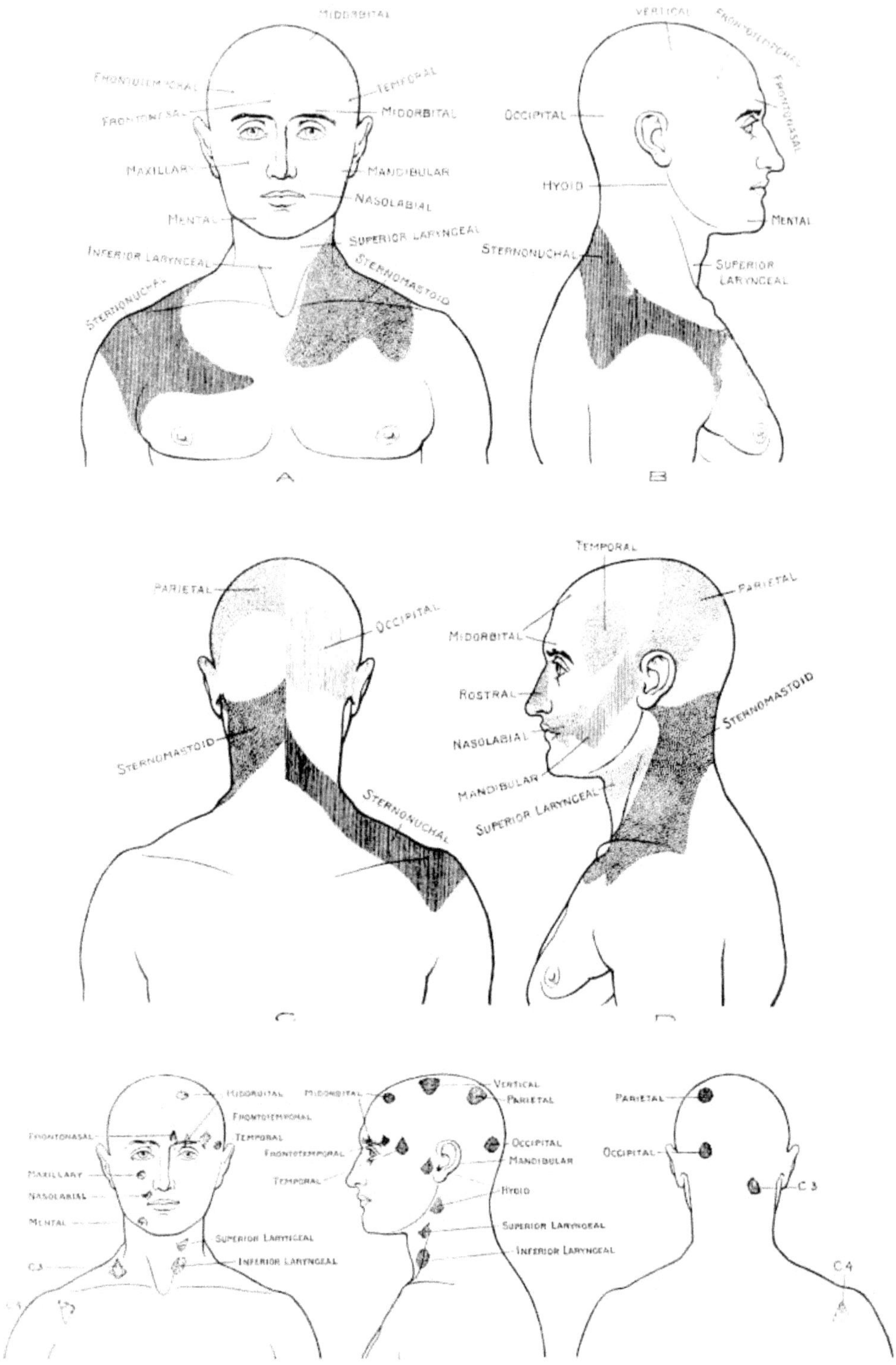

Figure 3–2. Head's areas for the head and neck. The third plate gives the points of maximum intensity. From Ref. 7.

aneurysms, liver diseases, and so on—the sites in the body are described where pain is felt and where tenderness or hypersensitivity to touch exists. The present-day physician is aware of the fact that an aneurysm of the descending aorta can cause pain between the shoulder blades, but Head has drawn attention to the fact that in those cases a quite circumscribed area, extending to the left arm, is painful to pressure, and he describes this vividly:

> The commonest situation for the pain is down the inner side of the arm. Sometimes it only extends to the inner condyle of the humerus, but occasionally and not infrequently it extends over the ulnar side of the forearm to the little finger. . . . The pain is usually of a dull aching character, relieved by pressure or rubbing. Thus patients who suffer from this pain frequently make the following characteristic movements: The left arm is somewhat adducted so that the elbow lies over the cardiac area of the chest. The right palm is placed over the left arm, so that the fingers reach over to that aspect of the left arm which is now outwards. (Owing to the rotation of the left arm which accompanies the adduction this portion which now lies outermost is in reality the inner aspect of the arm.) The right hand is then rubbed up and down over the outer part of the left arm.[7(pt2,p169)]

Head observed how gallbladder disease can result in pain dorsally in the left shoulder; pharyngeal disorders can produce occipital headaches. He conceived the idea that these *referred pains* had their origin in the sympathic nervous system and that the pain originated in the dermatome from which the rami communicantes toward the afflicted organ came. Thus the area for the heart was found in the first thoracic dermatome and the area for the bronchi in the second to fourth thoracic dermatomes. Based on this theory, however, the area for the bladder should consist of the dermatomes L5 to S3, a very large area indeed.

One of the reasons for the obscurity of Head's areas is that there are so many of them. Reading Head's extensive caserecords, one is not always convinced that the diagnosis of the diseases upon which his conclusions are based stand up to modern standards. Our diagnostic tools have rendered Head's areas largely redundant. And yet, at a time when pain blockading techniques are becoming increasingly popular, the general idea that pain need not originate at the place where it is felt merits close attention. One is surprised, therefore, to see that Head's areas and the concept of referred pain have largely disappeared from neurological textbooks as well as those on general anesthesia and pain management. When the name "Head's areas" is mentioned it is as the concept of referred pain, and a specific area is not described.

Head's present obscurity is belied by his appearance in Pat Barker's *Regeneration Trilogy*, the third part of which (*The Ghost Road*) received the Booker Prize (a British award for fiction) in 1995. Here he is introduced as the teacher of one of the main characters, the psychologist Rivers (e.g., in Ref. 11, part 2, *The Eye in the Door*, p. 145–149). Dr. David Barker, the author's husband, informed me that both he and his wife have been familiar with the lives and works of Head and Rivers for many years, he from his thesis on the recovery of proprioceptor function and she from interest in Rivers's work at Craiglockhart War Hospital. They visited Rivers's room at St. John's College, Cambridge, where the tests on Henry Head regarding nerve regeneration were carried out. So we see that truly great figures are never far away: may this serve as a reminder in evaluating pain in neurological practice, as well as a stimulant for reading and traveling.

References

1. Bing R. *Lehrbuch der Nervenkrankheiten.* Basel: Benno Schwabe & Co Verlag; 1952:620.
2. Denny-Brown D. Henry Head (1861–1940). In: Haymaker W, Schiller F, eds. *The Founders of Neurology.* Springfield, Ill: Charles C Thomas; 1970:449–452.
3. Sir Henry Head. *Brain.* 1940;63:205–208. Obituary.
4. Sir Henry Head. *Arch Neurol Psych (Chicago).* 1941;45:698–702. Obituary.
5. Critchley M. Henry Head. In: Kolle K, ed. *Grosse Nervenaerzte.* Stuttgart: Thieme; 1970;2:173–179.
6. Brain WR. Henry Head. In: *Doctors Past and Present.* London: Pitman; 1964:100–108.
7. Head H. On Disturbance of Sensation with especial Reference to the Pain of Visceral Disease. Part 1: *Brain.* 1893;16:1–133. Part 2: *Brain.* 1894;17:339–480. Part 3: *Brain.* 1896; 19:153–276.
8. Head H. The Pathology of Herpes Zoster and Its Bearing on Sensory Location. *Brain.* 1900;23:353–389.
9. Head H. *Studies in Neurology.* 2 vols. London: Oxford University Press; 1920.
10. Head H. *Aphasia and Kindred Disorders of Speech.* 2 vols. Cambridge: Cambridge University Press; 1926.
11. Barker P. *The Regeneration Trilogy.* London: Penguin Books; 1992–1996.

4

THE FORAMEN OF MONRO

Ernest H. Jellinek

Alexander Monro "Secundus" (1733–1817) was, according to Guthrie, born to greatness. His grandfather John Monro (1670–1740), who had studied medicine at Leyden under his fellow Scot Archibald Pitcairne (1652–1713), became one of the protagonists of the foundation of a medical school at Edinburgh. John Monro trained his son Alexander Monro "Primus" (1697–1767) to become the first professor of anatomy at Edinburgh at the age of 22 in 1719, after periods with Hermann Boerhaave (1668–1753) in Leyden and with William Cheselden (1688–1752) in London. Monro Primus was joined in the chair by his son Alexander Secundus in 1768. Secundus later also occupied chairs in medicine and surgery, passing on his chair in anatomy in 1798 to his son Alexander Monro "Tertius" (1773–1859), who occupied the chair until 1846, keeping it a "family chair" for 126 years.[1–4]

Alexander Monro Secundus began his medical studies at Edinburgh in 1752; in London he became a pupil of William Hunter (1718–1783), who, in his turn, had been taught by Monro Primus. Secundus began to give evening lectures in anatomy for his father in his second year as a medical student (1753). He took his degree of M.D. in 1755 and was made assistant professor of anatomy and surgery in the same year. He studied with Johann Friedrich Meckel (1714–1774) in Berlin, and when his father became ill in 1758, he took over the Edinburgh anatomy chair at age 25. In addition to teaching students anatomy, medicine, and surgery over a 50 year stretch, increasing from about 60 to over 400 students per annum by 1800—some 14,000 in all[2]—Monro Secundus became one of the leading Edinburgh practicing physicians. He was elected president of the Royal College of Physicians of Edinburgh, retaining that honor from 1779 to 1782.[5,6]

Although professor of surgery as well as anatomy and medicine, Monro Secundus practiced little surgery. His failure to teach surgery and surgical anatomy adequately led the Edinburgh surgeons to petition the government in 1777 to found a separate

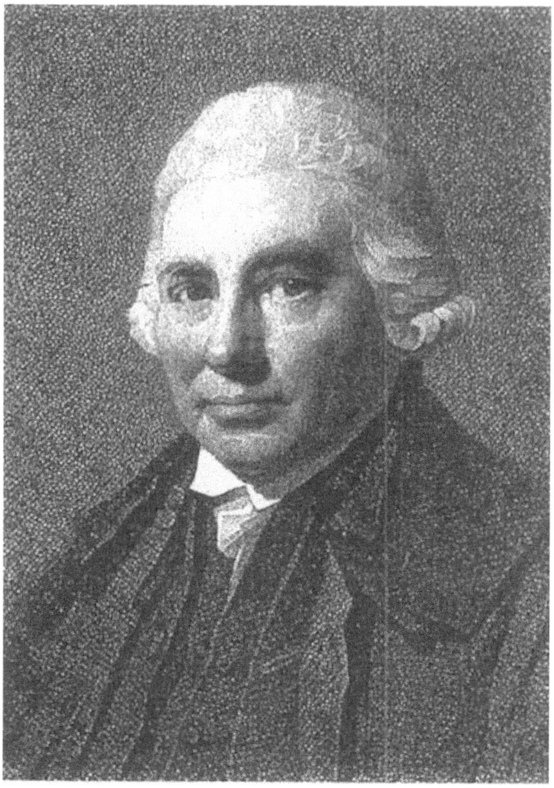

Figure 4–1. Engraving of Alexander Monro "Secundus" after a painting by H. Raeburn. From Ref. 4.

chair of clinical surgery, but Monro succeeded in blocking this proposal to remedy a major deficit in one of the greatest medical schools of the period until 1803.[7]

The other major black mark against Secundus is his manipulation of the succession of his son Alexander Tertius to his chair of anatomy, which he was to occupy till 1846. However, academic nepotism was rife at that time: Comrie[2] reported that eight out of ten appointments to medical chairs at the beginning of the nineteenth century went to the sons of professors. Charles Darwin (1809–1882), who came to Edinburgh to study medicine in 1825, wrote that the lectures of Monro Tertius on human anatomy were as dull as he was.[8] Another contemporary who gave up medical studies to become a distinguished scientist in marine biology, Edward Forbes (1815–1854), wrote of Tertius: "He was parsimonious in knowledge as in cash, although abounding in both."[9] Tertius did publish a pious volume of his father's unpublished theses and lectures, as well as his biography.[4]

Monro Secundus's general lectures had to await this posthumous publication in 1840 when his son Tertius was still in the habit of reading out his father's lectures to the students.[4] Secundus's first original book had been the splendidly illustrated quarto work of 1783: *Observations on the Structure and Functions of the Nervous System.*[10] This contained his unpublished much earlier work on the anatomy of the cerebral ventricles (see below). The clinical content was clearly influenced by Monro's senior colleague, the remarkable Robert Whytt (1714–1766), who had been professor both of the practice of medicine and of the institutes of medicine (physiology), as well as president of the College of Physicians of Edinburgh in 1763.

In 1764 Whytt and Monro had both attended a fatal case of hydrocephalus in a boy of age three. Whytt's description of the clinical features of hydrocephalus, *Observations of the Dropsy of the Brain—never before published,* was published posthumously by Whytt's son in 1768.[11] Whytt had earlier published the symptoms and signs of what, in retrospect, was probably tuberculous meningitis is children, and he had also performed some novel experiments on spinal reflexes in decapitated frogs. Whytt deserves recognition as one of the originators of the preeminence of the Edinburgh school later in that century; it attracted students from afar, including the future leaders of American medicine, by the quality of the teaching of Joseph Black (1728–1799) in chemistry, William Cullen (1710–1790) and John Gregory (1725–1773) in medicine, and of Monro Secundus in anatomy as well as in medicine. Monro Secundus ranged wide in his researches and discoveries: the anatomy of the eye and ear, of the testis, of bursae; the anatomy and function of the lymphatic system; thoracic paracentesis; the invention and use of the stomach tube; the nature of the nerve impulse.[2–4]

Alexander Monro Secundus led a highly successful and full professional life at Edinburgh, mixing with the leaders of the "Scottish Enlightenment"—the historian William Robertson, the philosopher David Hume, the economist Adam Smith, the chemist Joseph Black, the mathematician John Playfair—as well as his medical colleagues. He gardened at his Craiglockhart estate, enjoyed the theater, and was proud of having Mrs. Siddons as a patient; in addition, "he afforded . . . demonstrative evidence of the exhilarating powers of wine."[5]

He was married to Katherine Inglis, and they had seven children. His descendant (five generations on) Peter A. G. Monro, M.D. published Monro Primus's advice to Secundus's elder sister: *The Professor's Daughter; an essay on female conduct,*[6] which includes the Monro's distinguished family tree from 1609 to the present. Monro Secundus continued to teach until 1807; he failed after an apoplectic seizure in 1813, and died in his eighty-fifth year in 1817.

The title to Monro's lasting eponymous fame was documented by him rather belatedly, if obsessively. When he first published his classical description, *Observations on the Structure and Functions of the Nervous System,* in 1783,[10] he stated that he had first demonstrated the foramen (or, more correctly, the two foramina) 30 years earlier:

> So far back as the year 1753, soon after I began the study of anatomy, I discovered that the lateral ventricles of the human brain communicated with each other, and at the same place, with the Middle or Third ventricle . . . the four ventricles are in reality different parts of one cavity.

His age was 20 in 1753. He makes no mention in this context of his father or his other mentors. In this 1783 book he also quotes a letter written in 1762 in Latin by John Morgan (1735–1789) to Sir John Pringle (1707–1782) about Monro's demonstration of the foramen to him and other Edinburgh students; Morgan was to be the founder of the first American medical school in Philadephia.

The year 1764 saw the joint consultation with Robert Whytt and his own elder brother Donald Monro (1728–1802) on the three year old boy with hydrocephalus which was followed by autopsy. On 13 December of the same year Monro Secundus read a paper to the Edinburgh Philosophical Society, the forerunner of the Royal Society of Edinburgh, on the communications of the ventricles; he did not publish it in the society's Transactions, despite being the secretary of the society.

The 1783 book (Fig. 4–2) contains excellent and properly labeled drawings of the normal third ventricle, marking the site of the foramen, the anatomical relations, the vein from the lateral ventricle passing through the foramen into the third ventricle, to form posteriorly the vein of Galen. It also has a drawing "from memory" of a very dilated foramen from a case of hydrocephalus in a three year old child he had seen as early as 1753. Monro gave due credit to earlier anatomical descriptions of the cerebral ventricles which had indicated continuity of the four ventricles, particularly by Galen. The relevant quotation might have been Galen's:

> A passage opens out from the posterior ventricle which extends itself to the middle ventricle. Then you see how the two anterior ventricles open themselves discharging into the middle ventricle.[12]

Monro also referred to observations by Raymond de Vieussens, Jakob Benignus Winslow, and Joseph Lieutaud, but he was critical of their lack of anatomical detail, which he was the first to describe.

A major, and wrong, criticism of Albrecht von Haller's (1708–1777) account was Monro's denial of connection between the fourth ventricle and the spinal canal: the correct detailed description of the fourth ventricle foramina came from François Magendie (1825) and Hubert von Luschka (1859). Monro would not have known Leonardo da Vinci's drawings of wax casts of a continuous ventricular system.[13] Monro's other splendid quarto volume of 1797,[14] entitled *Three Treatises on the Brain, the Eye and the Ear,*[14] of which the first is *Observations on the Communications of the Ventricles of the Brain with each other and on the Internal Hydrocephalus,* repeats the 1783 descriptions, with further drawings of normal anatomy by A. Fyfe. Monro stated that since 1753 he had studied the bodies of 15 different persons who had died of internal hydrocephalus. He now also recorded his comparative anatomical studies in sheep, oxen, horses, and a whale, with similar findings regarding the cerebral ventricles.

The 1797 book starts with testimonials from his distinguished medical faculty colleagues Joseph Black, Andrew Duncan (1744–1828), John Gregory, Francis Home (1719–1813), and John Rutherford (1695–1779), saying that they concurred with Monro's observations. These were intended to confound the criticisms of unnamed teachers of anatomy in London who had remained skeptical—probably William Hunter and the Windmill Street anatomy school. Both Monro Primus and Monro Secundus had had longstanding professional disagreements about lymphatics and the like with William Hunter, despite their teacher–pupil–teacher relationships (see above).

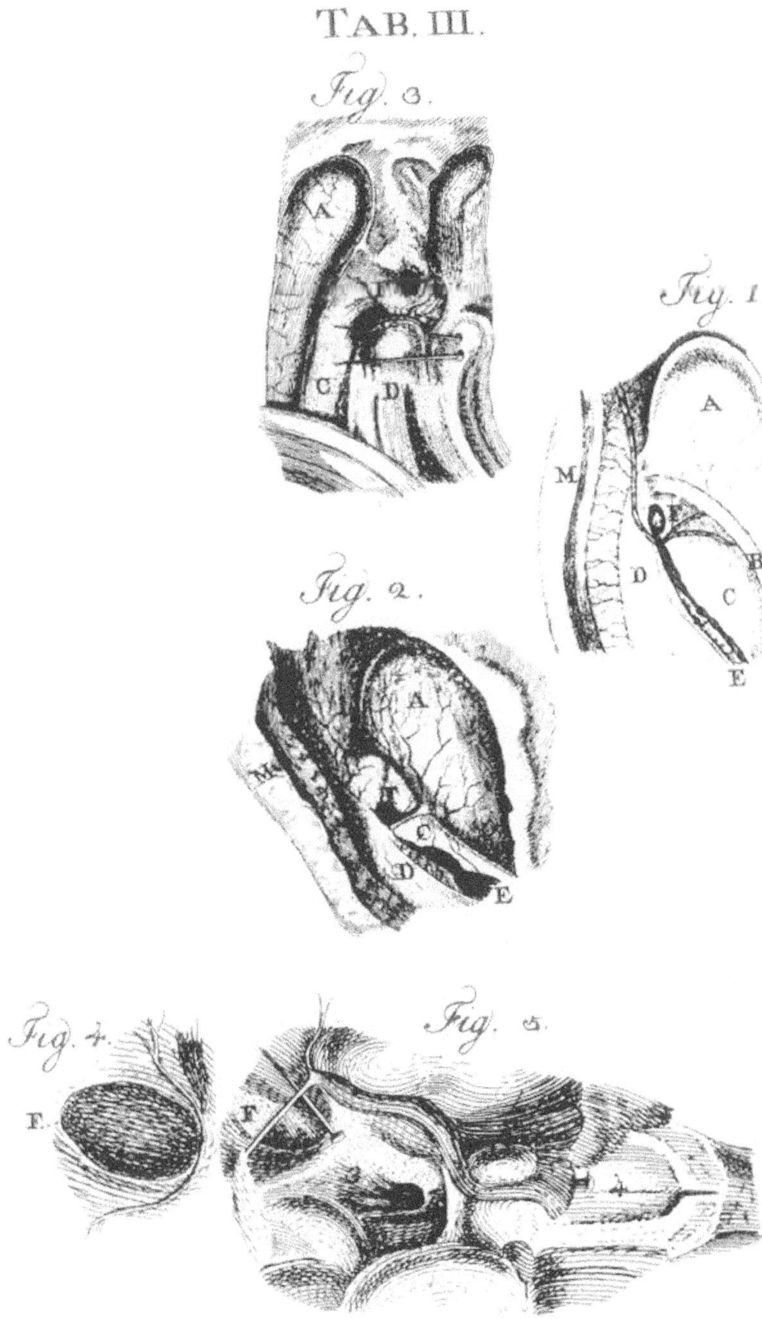

Figure 4–2. (a) *Drawing of foramen and its relations in the normal brain, together with dilated foramen in hydrocephalus (Monro's "Fig. 4").*

T A B L E III.

THE figures in this table reprefent the communication of the lateral ventricles of the human brain with each other, and with the third ventricle.

Figures I. and II. reprefent part of the bottom of the right lateral ventricle, with the fore part of the fornix, and a part of the feptum lucidum and corpus callofum. The anterior parts are turned towards the top of the table.

In both Figures,

A Reprefents the fore part of the right corpus ftriatum.

B Part of the centrum femicirculare geminum.

C The fore part of the right thalamus nervi optici.

D The fore part of the body of the fornix.

E The fore part of the right choroid plexus.

F A natural paffage by which the lateral ventricles communicate with each other and with the third ventricle. This paffage is bounded on the fore part by the anterior crura of the fornix; above, by the fore part of the body of the fornix, where it is about to form its anterior crura; behind by the meeting of the choroid plexufes of the two ventricles; below, by the thalami nervorum opticorum. Two veins, which are more conftant in their fituation than fuch fmall veins are generally, at this place, run into the choroid plexus; one of them comes from the fore part of the feptum lucidum, and is over the communication; the other is from the corpus ftriatum, and runs from it inwards and backwards to the choroid plexus.

M Reprefents a part of the corpus callofum, between the cut edge of which, and the body of the fornix D, a part of the feptum lucidum is feen,

Figure 4–2. (b) *Part of Monro's descriptive legend.* From Ref. 10.

In the 1797 text Monro discusses the symptoms and signs of both chronic and acute hydrocephalus, following Whytt's earlier teaching, and properly dismisses both medical and surgical treatment of hydrocephalus. As recently as 1925 Harvey Cushing had to agree with this negative attitude:

> Infants with hydrocephalus—for which a greater number of treatments have as yet been advocated (I have been guilty of advocating one or two myself) than successes recorded—if indeed there are any clear-cut successes recorded.[15]

They have come since, with the advent of tolerable plastic shunt tubing. Also, structural abnormalities at the foramen of Monro are often amenable to direct neurosurgical treatment.

The clinical significance of the interventricular foramen of Monro is based on disorders of the "third" circulation, that is, the circulation of the cerebrospinal fluid (CSF), as described by Magnus Gustav Retzius, Axel Key, Lewis Hill Weed, Harvey Cushing, and others. The CSF stems mainly from the choroid plexus in the lateral ventricles, passes through the foramen of Monro into the third, then through the aqueduct of Sylvius into the fourth ventricle, and on into the subarachnoid space via the foramina of Magendie and Luschka. The foramen of Monro is very narrow, liable to obstruction by any pathological process in, or near, the third ventricle. Such an obstruction will lead to dilatation of one or, more likely, both lateral ventricles, with symptoms of raised intracranial pressure: headache and vomiting, disorders of consciousness, eye movement and pupillary disorders, as described by Whytt and Monro.

Expanding lesions at this site are the various gliomas of the third ventricle; more chronic processes are upward extensions or pituitary tumors and craniopharyngiomas, which may cause pituitary or hypothalamic disorders en route, and rarely akinetic mutism, before leading to symptoms and signs of raised intracranial pressure. The most benign lesions are colloid cysts. It is ironic that one such cyst, 1 cm in diameter, was found postmortem in the third ventricle of Harvey Cushing, one of the pioneers of surgery in this territory.[16] A heavy smoker, Cushing died of vascular disease before the cyst had become large enough to obstruct his foramen of Monro.

References

1. Guthrie D. *A History of Medicine.* Edinburgh: Nelson; 1945.
2. Comrie JD. *History of Scottish Medicine.* London: Welcome Hist Med Museum; Baillière Tindall & Cox; 1932.
3. Simon SW. The influence of the Monro's on the practice of medicine. *Ann Hist Med (NY).* 1927;9:244–266.
4. Monro A. *Essays & Heads of Lectures on Anatomy, Physiology, Pathology & Surgery by the late A Monro Secundus with a memorial of his life by his son and successor.* Edinburgh: McLachlan Stewart & Co; 1840.
5. Moore N. Alexander Monro. *Dictionary of National Biography, 38.* London: Smith Elder & Co; 1894.
6. Monro PAG. The Professor's Daughter; an Essay on female Conduct by A Monro Primus. *Proc R Coll Physicians Edinb.* 1996;26 (suppl 2).
7. Simpson D. Chairs of Surgery at Edinburgh. *J R Coll Surg Edinb.* 1977;22:91–102.

8. Ashworth JR. Charles Darwin as a student at Edinburgh 1825–7. *Proc R Soc Edinb.* 1935;55: 97–113.
9. Campbell N, Smellie RMS. *The Royal Society of Edinburgh 1783–1983.* Edinburgh: Royal Society; 1983.
10. Monro A. *Observations on the Structure and Functions of the Nervous System.* London: Wm Creech; 1783.
11. Whytt R. *The Works of R. Whytt published by his son. Observations on the Dropsy of the Nervous System.* London: Becket & de Hondt; Edinburgh: Balfour; 1768:723–745.
12. Duckworth NLH, Lyons MC, Towers B. *Galen on Anatomical Procedures.* Cambridge: Cambridge University Press; 1962.
13. Clayton M. *Leonardo da Vinci: The Anatomy of Man.* Houston: Little Brown; 1997.
14. Monro A. *Three Treatises on the Brain, the Eye and the Ear illustrated by tables.* Edinburgh: Bell & Bradfute; 1797.
15. Cushing H. *Studies in Intracranial Physiology and Surgery.* London: Oxford University Press; 1926.
16. Fulton J. *Harvey Cushing.* Springfield, Ill: Charles C Thomas; 1946.

5

MEYNERT'S BASAL NUCLEUS

Franz Seitelberger

Theodor Meynert (1833–1892) was the first scientist to comprehend brain research as an independent interdisciplinary enterprise, demonstrated by his own fundamental contributions and the prospect of challenging research objectives. Meynert's important observations and intuitive visions foreshadow modern concepts and amazing recent results in the neurosciences.

Meynert was born in Dresden on 14 June 1833. His father was a historian, his mother an opera singer. The family moved to Vienna in 1841 and gathered a circle of renowned personalities of art and culture at their home. At school, Meynert showed great love of literature, music, and philosophy; at university after a crisis of maturity he became an enthusiastic student of medicine and developed an interest in the brain. As a student he worked with the excellent histologist Carl Wedl and in the laboratory of Carl von Rokitansky, the founder of modern pathology; the latter accepted him as assistant, furthering his work and professional career decisively. Meynert's first paper, "Lesions of the Pons and Midbrain with Report on Important New Methods of Preparation," appeared in 1861. On the basis of his thesis, "Structure and Function of the Brain and Spinal Cord and Their Significance in Disease," he was appointed Privatdozent in 1865 as well as director of the prosectorium of the State Psychiatric Hospital in Vienna. In fast succession he published pioneering discoveries and stimulating projects; his magnetic personality initiated close relations with several international representatives of the medical sciences and attracted colleagues and pupils both from Austrian monarchy and abroad, including Heinrich Obersteiner, Franz Chvostek, Sigmund Freud, Carl Wernicke, August Forel, Hubert Grashey, Moses Allen Starr, James Jackson Putnam, and Bernard Sachs. In 1870 he was appointed Extraordinarius of Psychiatry and Director of the First Psychiatric Clinic. Finally, Meynert switched to the Second Psychiatric Clinic, which was established for him at the General Hospital in 1874; there he opened a neurological

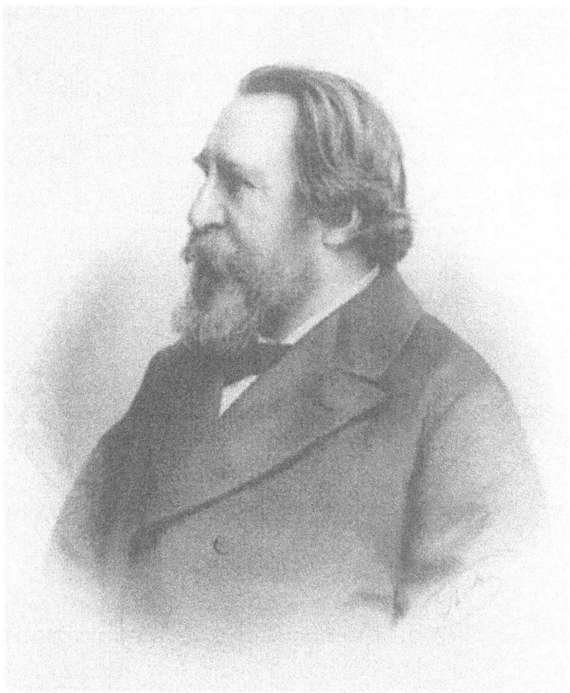

Figure 5–1. Theodor Meynert (1833–1892). From Institut für Geschichte der Medizin der Stadt Wien, Austria.

outpatient department in 1887. In the following years he enjoyed high official honors. In this period of his life, however, he was struck by tragic personal loss in his family and, at 59 years old, suffered an untimely death on 31 May 1892.

The intention of Meynert's primary research was the identification of the accurate course and caliber of efferent and afferent nerve fiber connections between gray matter (neuronal) brain areas, as well as the "projection fibers" from spinal cord to telencephalon.[1] He observed the fanlike radiation of the sensory fibers in the white matter of the postcentral and the origin of the motor fibers in the precentral gyrus of the cerebral cortex; furthermore, he traced the visual pathway from the retina to its termination in the occipital cerebral cortex in 1870.

Meynert undertook comparative studies on animals selected for their prominent faculties, for instance, jumping or climbing. The respective observations proved him one of the pioneers of comparative neuroanatomy. Meynert was the first to observe the central facts of the later "myelogenetic theory" of Paul Flechsig, and he tried to explain this phenomenon by means of the mechanistic inhibition theory of the philosopher Johann Friedrich Herbart.

The wealth of details that Meynert discovered using inadequate methods is truly amazing, as is the small number of erroneous statements. Numerous structures therefore carry his eponymous designation. Among them the structure of probably the highest importance is the nucleus basalis. Beside this structure, Meynert revealed the lamination of the cerebral cortex, the character of its cell types, and the regional differences of its cytoarchitecture.[2] He also confirmed that localized lesions of the cortex led to specific functional defects, revealing a cortical mosaic of conscious performances; for example, he first described the syndrome of sensory aphasia associated with a lesion in the posterior part of the superior temporal gyrus and the planum temporale in 1866. The eponym "Wernicke's aphasia" does not recognize Meynert's priority of its identification in 1874 (see Chapter 38).

Meynert had concentrated on methodical improvements of anatomical brain preparation. Thin serial sections were cut with a razor on a simple holder of the tissue block, fixed in alcohol and mostly stained with carmine or impregnated with gold. Last but not least Meynert also performed some quantitative neurohistological measurements.

This technique led to the publication of several novel results, such as the first description of the lamination and cellular diversity of the cerebral cortex, before the article "Vom Gehirn der Säugetiere" [About the brain of mammals] appeared in S. Stricker's *Handbook of Human and Animal Histology* in 1872.[3] In section 3 ("Die Hirnschenkelhaube und ihre Ganglien") a clearly extended ganglion underneath the fibers of the ansa peduncularis is identified, described as the second layer of substantia innominata, illustrated in his Fig. 245, and given the name "Ganglion der Hirnschenkelschlinge" (Fig. 5–2*a*). Its large spindlelike hyperchromatic nerve cells measured 15 μm in width to 50 μm in length. In view of this new constituent of the substantia innominata, Meynert distinguished four parts of the area: (1) ansa peduncularis; (2) nucleus (ganglion) of the ansa peduncularis; (3) inferior (ventral) peduncle of the thalamus; and (4) anterior part of the stratum zonale thalami.

In 1896, Meynert's linguistically difficult presentation of his discovery was elucidated by Albert Kölliker,[4] who also redesignated the ansa-ganglion as "Meynert's Basalganglion," that is, Meynert's basal nucleus (MBN). A short summary of Kölliker's still completely correct topohistological description of this nucleus follows:

> The central, nearly superficial part of the disclike formation of MBN is found in the basal forebrain parallel to the ventral basis of the nucleus lenticularis and underneath the commissura anterior from its lateral entrance onwards; laterally it reaches the amygdaloid complex; caudally it extends toward the tractus opticus; its oral part makes contact with substantia perforata anterior, the medial one reaches the tuber cinereum. (Fig. 5–2*b, c*)

Although additional histological details of the environment near the MBN, that is, the substantia innominata, were described in the following years, several authors did not mention it at all because of its unknown relevance. The term "Basal-kernkomplex" (coined by H. Brockhaus) relates to a widened extension of the substantia innominata in which three main magnocellular parts are distinguished.[5]

Remarkable progress in structural research methodology began in the 1960s with the invention of refined and novel preparative as well as selective qualitative procedures, including axonal transport techniques, and immunohisto- and immunocytochemical demonstration of cholinergic enzymes. Neuroanatomical studies in animals had shown that magnocellular forebrain nuclei, in particular MBN, receive afferents from the amygdala and several mes- and diencephalic structures, but from only a few neocortical areas, and in turn project to the amygdala but predominantly toward all parts of the neocortex.[6,7] It was also confirmed by retrograde nerve

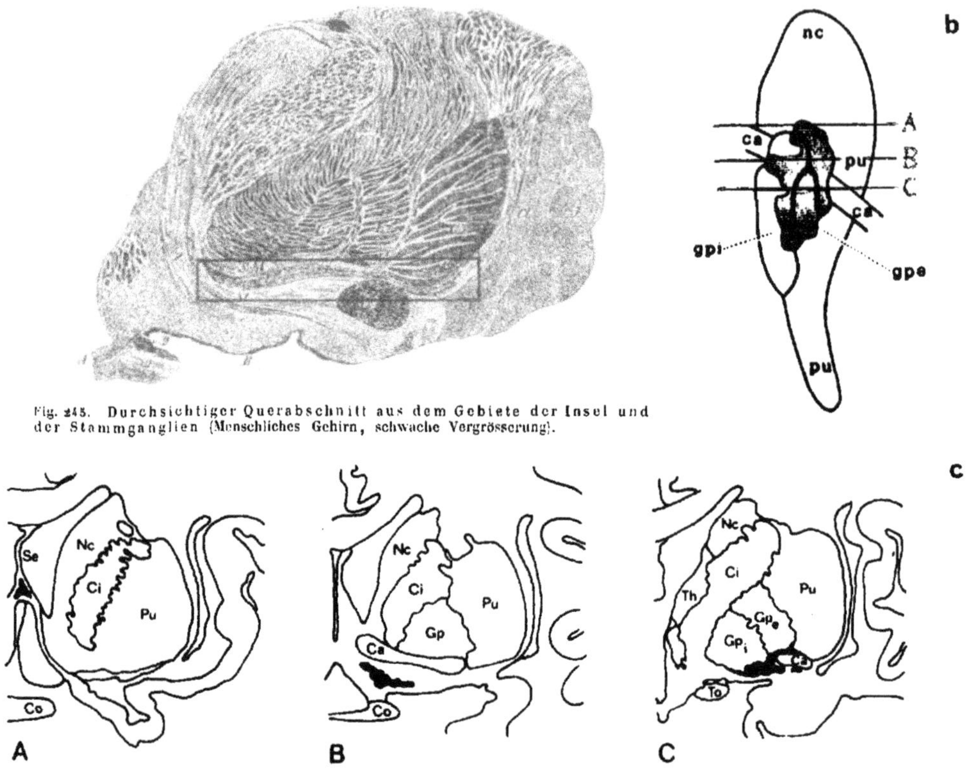

Figure 5–2. (a) *Frontal section of the basal forebrain, with MBN area marked.* From Ref. 3. (b) *Schematic horizontal sublenticular section through MBN. A, B, C: Positions of the frontal sections of part c.* From F. Tagliavini, Encyclopedia of Neurosciences vol. I, 1987, pp. 115–116, by courtesy of Birkhäuser Verlag, Basel, Switzerland. (c) *Schematic frontal sections through the forebrain.* From Ref. 5; by permission of Springer-Verlag, Berlin, Germany. *Abbreviations: Ca, commissura anterior; Ci, capsula interna; Co, chiasma opticum; Gp, globus pallidus; Gp_e, pallidum externum; Gp_i pallidum internum; Nc, nucleus caudatus; Pu, putamen; Se, septum; Th, thalamus; To, tractus opticus.*

cell loss in the MBN following lesions of the medial temporal lobe cortex in humans and monkeys. The relative size of the MBN progressively increases along mammalian evolution correlated to cerebralization,[8] indicating the important position of this nucleus among higher cortical brain functions of man.

Histochemistry and experimental immunocytochemistry in animals detected MBN and the horizontal limb of the diagonal band of Broca as the major cholinergic projection system to the neocortex, later also designated MBN-Ch4 complex.[9–11] This finding initiated intensive research. Nearly 90% of the magnocellular, hyperchromic, isodendritic MBN neurons are definitely positive for the cholinergic marker choline acetyltransferase (ChAT) and are rich in acetylcholinesterase (AchE) in the perikarya, axons, and dendrites. Likewise, the neocortical projection fields exhibit ChAT and AchE positivity. The cholinergic innervation of the primate and human neocortex is exclusively extrinsic.[12] The function of the above mentioned interstitial neurons of the MBN type is unknown.

The probable extension of the brainstem reticular formation and the connection with the basomedial limbic cortex might explain that arousal and memory are the main types of behavioral effects of the Ch4 neurons and that their cortical cholinergic projection also sustains the hippocampal theta rhythm. Limbic and paralimbic cortical projection areas are assumed to participate particularly in cognitive performances, attention, learning, and memory processes also by modifying the effect of emotional conditions on sensory events regarding their novelty and behavioral significance. Thus the cholinergic afferent system delineates a final common pathway mediating relevant factors of cognitive achievements.[13] Cholinomimetic drugs exert plain effects on learning and memory as well as other limbic functions such as mood, reward, and aggressiveness.

Recent experiments appear to demonstrate that cortical cholinergic innervation filters and allocates the conveyance of sensory information out of and into the limbic system concerning its behavioral relevance.

Neuropathological data were presented by autopsy human brain studies in Alzheimer's disease (AD) and senile dementia of the Alzheimer type (SDAT). Pronounced cell loss of the MBN in the frame of the pathohistological pattern of AD, including senile plaques, neurofibrillary tangles, granulovacuolar degeneration, and Lewy bodies in MBN neurons, were described as early as the 1950s (Fig. 5–3).[14] Later, casuistic studies in AD calculated the rather selective neuronal loss of the MBN at 80% and demonstrated it as a secondary sequel to cortical cholinergic damage.[15–17] MBN atrophy was found to be congruent with the demented state as well as with the neurochemical data of reduced concentration of ChAT and AchE in neocortical and hippocampal neurons without reduction of their number. Thus a relationship between neuronal disorders and dysfunctions of specific processing appears consistent with the findings. The "cholinergic hypothesis" of the cognitive implications of AD in later studies was also considered in relation to normal aging.

Furthermore, MBN and forebrain lesions similar to AD/SDAT in severity and pathological and chemical quality were found in several neurodegenerative processes associated with dementia, such as Parkinson's disease (already reported 1955 by Buttlar Brentano), Lewy body disease, ALS, Huntington's chorea, and Korsakoff's disease, indicating the involvement of responsible subpopulations of cholinergic cells in cognitive performances in degenerative disorders.

The presently available findings of structural and functional neuroscience indicate the prominent integrative role of the MBN in the afferent cholinergic forebrain—neocortex system, also demonstrated by severe retrograde changes in the MBN due to temporocortical lesions and inversely by selective changes in the neocortical concentration of MBN neurons.

In retrospect, one may state that Meynert's discovery of a small group of large neurons in the structural jungle of the nameless basal brain area, after an undisturbed anonymity of about a century, resurrected highly provocative questions to the neurosciences. Meynert's basal nucleus is found in that narrow, gatelike part of the

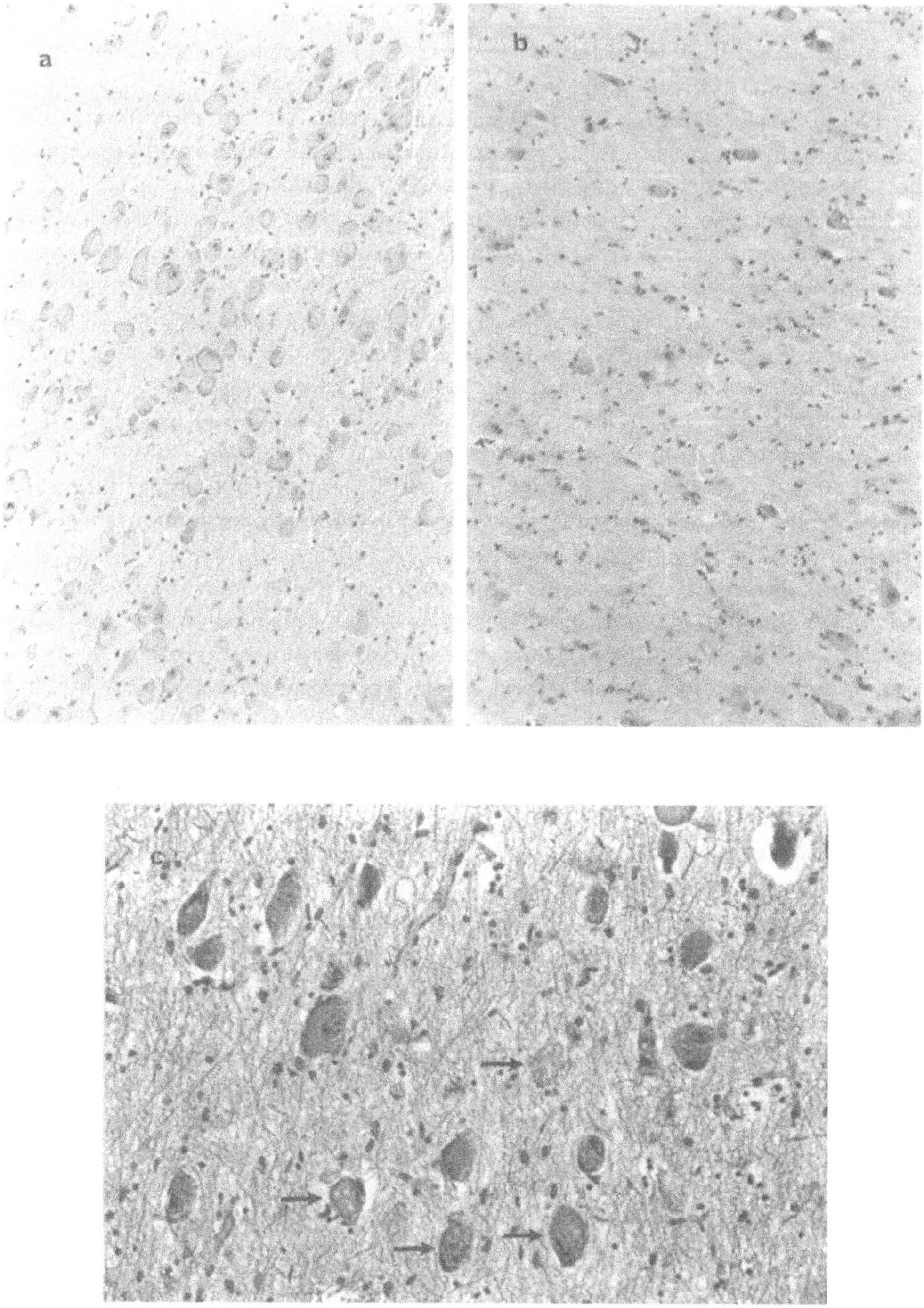

Figure 5–3. (a) *Nucleus basalis Meynert. Normal control. HE, ×100. Large, tightly packed neurons.* (b) *Nucleus basalis Meynert. Alzheimer's disease. HE, ×100. Severe loss of neurons; remaining exemplars atrophic, nuclei shrunken.* (c) *Nucleus basalis Meynert. Alzheimer's disease. HE, ×200. Reduced density of neurons; most show cytoplasmic changes: fibrillar inclusions, vacuoles, shadowlike degeneration.* By courtesy of Prof. Dr. H. Budka, Vienna.

forebrain which bridges the central, organized structures of the brainstem to the diversified structures of the telencephalon. In later scientific work, Meynert did not return explicitly to his solitaire: he could make no additional relevant findings because the methodical means of his time had been insufficient to disclose the functional potency of the nucleus.

Nevertheless, the relations and modes of cooperation between cerebral cortex and subcortical structures had been the central problem of his later investigations and conceptions. Let us glance at his overall concepts of brain functions.[18] Meynert carried morphological studies to their attainable limits and beyond by considering hypotheses fused into a coherent whole. He ascribed quasi personified functions to the anatomically and physiologically different brain regions. Thus he stated that the projection systems of the brain form the framework of the unconscious animal life, the "primary ego" or "the body as such." In contrast to this, he postulated an "ego-forming functional center of the brain" located in the cerebral cortex disposing of association and commissural systems; this "conscious secondary ego" depends on functioning cortical nerve cells. At this level, the objective sensory signals from the outer world are centrally integrated and subjectively interpreted. The cognitive processes also originate in association mechanisms. Meynert's association theory not only tries to explain learning and adaptation processes but also allocates the central position in cognition to its capacity of reaching conclusions. This faculty of reasoning based on material furnished by the sense organs and transmitted by afferent projections enables the brain to construct an image of the world. On the other hand the motor system operates in and on the environment. Among many factors controlling conscious movement is the "sensation of information" reflecting the memory of former body movements which are experienced as voluntary acts. This assumption of a sensory feedback anticipated the principle of cybernetic reafference.

Meynert's panoramic painting of the brain's universe in view of present knowledge undeniably needs some corrections. Nevertheless, many of his principal views and conjectures regarding structural and functional interconnections are proven and standing examples of functional neuroanatomy; for example, note his contributions to the theory of aphasia (see Chapter 38).

Finally, reading Meynert's striking comparison of nerve cell processes with tentacles and feeling threads of animals, one is reminded of the selective cognitive cholinergic network which was revealed by recent brain research in the area of MBN. Thus I feel induced to say that the cholinergic network in its remarkable structural complexity and in the unforeseen design of functional interconnectivity presents a classical example of a "Meynert-type pattern." In view of this, I find the eponym Meynert's basal nucleus not only appropriate but also intensely challenging to further searches in the realm of this structure for new discoveries.

References

1. Anton G. Theodor Meynert. Seine Person, sein Wirken und sein Werk. *Psychol Neurol.* 1930;40:256–281.

2. Seitelberger F. Theodor Meynert (1833–1892): pioneer and visionary of brain research. *J Hist Neurosci.* 1997;6:264–274.
3. Meynert T. Vom Gehirn der Säugetiere. In: Stricker S, ed. *Handbuch der Lehre von den Geweben der Menschen und Tiere.* Leipzig: Engelmann; 1872;2:694–808.
4. Kölliker A. Handbuch der Gewebelehre des Menschen. *Für Ärzte und Studierende. 2. Nervensystem des Menschen und der Thiere.* 6th ed. Leipzig: Engelmann; 1896.
5. Arendt T, Bigl V, Arendt A, Tennstedt A. Loss of neurons in the nucleus basalis of Meynert in Alzheimer's disease, paralysis agitans and Korsakoff's disease. *Acta Neuropathol (Berl).* 1983;61:101–108.
6. Hedreen JC, Struble RG, Whitehouse PJ, Price DL. Topography of the magnocellular basal forebrain system in human brain. *J Neuropathol Exp Neurol.* 1984;43:1–21.
7. Divac I. Magnocellular nuclei of the basal forebrain project to neocortex, brain stem, and olfactory bulb: review of some functional correlates. *Brain Res.* 1975;93:385–398.
8. Gorry JR. Studies on the comparative anatomy of the ganglion basale of Meynert. *Acta Anat.* 1963;55:51–104.
9. Davies P, Maloney AJ. Selective loss of central cholinergic neurons in Alzheimer's disease. *Lancet.* 1976;2:1403.
10. Mesulam M-M, van Hoesen GW. Acetylcholinesterase-rich projections from the basal forebrain of the rhesus monkey to neocortex. *Brain Res.* 1976;109:152–157.
11. Mesulam M-M, Mufson EJ, Lewey AI, Wainer BH. Cholinergic innervation of cortex by the basal forebrain: cytochemis-try and cortical connection of the septal area, diagonal-band nuclei, nucleus basalis (substantia innominata) and hypothalamus in the rhesus monkey. *J Comp Neurol.* 1983;214:170–197.
12. Mesulam M-M, Geula C. Nucleus basalis (Ch4) and cortical cholinergic innervation in the human brain: observations based on the distribution of acetylcholinesterase and choline acetyltransferase. *J Comp Neurol.* 1988;275:216–240.
13. Everitt BJ, Robbins TW. Central cholinergic systems and cognition. *Ann Rev Psychol.* 1997;48:649–684.
14. Perry E, Perry R, Blessed G, Tomlinson B. Necropsy evidence of central cholinergic deficits in senile dementia. *Lancet.* 1977;1:189.
15. Terry RD, Davies P. Dementia of the Alzheimer type. *Ann Rev Neurosci.* 1980;3:77–95
16. Whitehouse PJ, Price DL, Clark AW, Coyle JT, DeLong MR. Alzheimer disease: evidence for selective loss of cholinergic neurons in the nucleus basalis. *Ann Neurol.* 1981;10: 122–126.
17. Whitehouse PJ, Price DL, Struble RG, Clark AW, Coyle JT, DeLong MR. Alzheimer disease and senile dementia: loss of neurons in the basal forebrain. *Science.* 1982;215:1237–1239.
18. Meynert T. *Psychiatrie: Klinik der Erkrankungen des Vorderhirns begründet auf dessen Bau, Leistungen und Ernährung.* 1st half. Wien: Braumüller; 1884.

6

THE PURKINJE CELL

Jan Voogd

Jan Evangelista Purkinje (Purkyně) was born in 1787, in the castle of Libochovice, Bohemia, where his father acted as the estate manager. He received his first formal education at the Gymnasium connected to the monastery of the Fratres piarum scholarum, in Mikulov, South Moravia, and later joined this order. After completing his novitiate, he spent a year studying at the Piarist Philosophical Institute and was engaged with the tutoring of young people. In 1807 he left the order and moved to Prague, where he studied philosophy between 1808 and 1810 and earned his living as a tutor for the Hildprandt family, first in Prague, later in Blatná. Supported by one of his former employers, Baron Hildprandt, he started his medical studies in 1813 in Prague, where he received his M.D. in 1818. He was interested in the study of drugs and tested them on himself, believing that experiments on his own body provided better results. This practice was not rare in those days (see also Chapters 3 and 31). His thesis *Beiträge zur Kenntnis des Sehens in subjectiver Hinsicht* was published in 1819.

In 1823 he was appointed to the chair of physiology and pathology at the University of Breslau, in the Prussian province of Lower Silesia. The case of his appointment by the Prussian ministry of education received strong support from the Berlin anatomist Karl Asmund Rudolphi, whose daughter he later married, and possibly from Goethe, who was greatly interested in Purkinje's thesis studies in the domain of color vision. He remained in Breslau for 26 years, founding a physiological institute there. Two of Purkinje's children died of cholera in 1835 and only three years later his wife died during a typhoid epidemic.

Purkinje worked with several students who would become well known, including Gabriel Gustav Valentin (1810–1883). At the age of 63, in 1850, Purkinje was called to the chair of physiology at Prague, where he founded the first institute of physiology in the medical faculty of the Charles University. In an academic atmosphere, dominated by the German culture and language, he worked for the emancipation

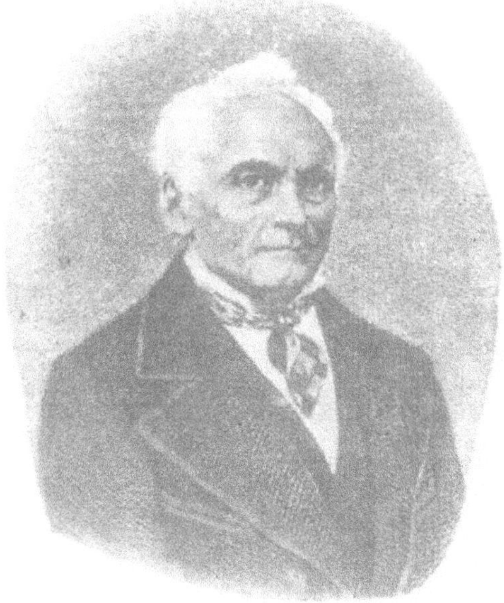

Figure 6–1. Jan Evangelista Purkinje (1787–1869). Courtesy Medizinhistorisches Institut, Zurich, Switzerland.

of the Czechs. He published and produced translations of the work of Schiller, Shakespeare, and Tasso in the Czech language, and he was one of the first to conduct his lectures in his native tongue. In Prague he became involved with politics and was elected to the Czech provincial parliament. He founded Czech journals and scientific and cultural societies, and he became an editor of one of the leading Czech daily newspapers. Purkinje died in Prague on 28 July 1869.

Purkinje's life and work were reviewed by Hirsch et al.,[1] Studnička,[2] and Bartelmez[3] and his position in the development of neuroscience was discussed by Clarke and O'Malley[4] and Jacobson,[5] to whom I am indebted for the data contained in this short biography. A list of publications of Purkinje and a bibliography on his life and work were published in his collected works.[6]

Purkinje's main scientific achievements date from his period at Breslau. His concept of physiology was wide-ranging; his lecture notes on general physiology cover anthropology, morphology and morphogenesis, mechanics, chemistry, general physiology or the philosophy of nature *(Naturphilosophie)*, and experimental and applied physiology.[2] His scientific contributions cover many of these fields. His thesis,[7] which he reedited and amplified during his early years in Breslau[8,9] and which contains the description of the Purkinje effect—the changes in apparent luminosity of colors in dim as opposed to bright daylight—is considered a major point in the emergence of experimental psychology. He published on vertigo, the physiology of speech, on (his discovery of) ciliary motion in hollow organs, on pharmacology, and on a variety of zoological subjects. Important parts of his work are the dissertations published by his students.

Purkinje's morphological studies were greatly facilitated by Lister's 1830[10] development of the achromatic objective for the compound microscope, which Purkinje acquired soon afterwards. There had been no important improvements in the fundamental structure of the microscope during the eighteenth century, and the instrument had fallen into disrepute because of the frequent artifacts that misled those who used it.[4] Ehrenberg,[11] Purkinje,[12] and Purkinje's student Valentin[13] were among the first to observe nerve corpuscles and the nerve fibers with this new instrument. Although their observations were accurate, they conceived of these corpuscles and fibers as anatomically separate structures, which, in some unknown way, were functionally related. Their observations should be seen in the perspective of the cell theory, conceived by Schwann a few years later,[14] and the development of the neuron theory, which had its beginnings in Remak's discovery of the unity of the ganglion cell and the nerve fiber in 1838.[15]

In September 1837 Purkinje read his paper on nerve and brain anatomy, entitled "Über die scheinbar kanalikulöse Beschaffenheit der elementaren Nervencylinder" [On the apparent canicular form of the elementary nerve cylinder] at a meeting of the Versammlung deutscher Naturforscher and Ärzte in Prague.[12] Only the first part of his lecture dealt with the concept of elementary nerve fibers as hollow tubes, a concept which Purkinje appears to discard. His lecture continued with two short excursions on the sympathetic plexus of the cerebral arteries and the structure of the choroid plexus and its role in the resorption of the cerebrospinal fluid, and then arrived at what we now consider his main topic: the ganglionlike constitution of certain parts of the brain. The analogy with peripheral ganglia refers to the presence of corpuscles, first observed in the ganglia by the Berlin professor of medicine Christian Gottfried Ehrenberg (1795–1876).[11] According to Purkinje, the ganglionic corpuscles are spherical or multipolar bodies, measuring 8 30/800 of a Viennese line (about .8 inch), with or without prolongations and containing a round, translucent nucleus, surrounded by a spherical envelope. The characteristic nucleolus of the nuclei of nerve cells is illustrated (Fig. 6–2), but it is not mentioned in the text of the proceedings of the meeting. The nucleus and the nucleolus of the ganglionic corpuscles earlier were identified, and the term "nucleolus" was introduced by Purkinje's student Valentin.[13] In the peripheral ganglia these corpuscles are surrounded by a cellular or fibrous capsule, but such a sheath is lacking around the ganglionic corpuscles of the brain. As yet, nothing definite could be concluded about the relation of these corpuscles to the nerve fibers. In the ganglia, nerve fibers wrap around the corpuscles, inside the capsule, without ever merging with them. In the brain the corpuscles generally lie embedded in a viscous, speckled substance, without fibers.

Purkinje proceeded to describe these corpuscles in thin, unstained sections of the substantia nigra, where they contained patches of dark brown pigment granules in the adult, though much less so in children, and where they were provided with daringly branching prolongations. Roundish, pigment-containing corpuscles were present in the locus coeruleus and the geniculate bodies. Similar corpuscles were observed in the Ammon's horn and the cerebral cortex,

> where they are elongated and fig-shaped, with prolongations at their fine tips. A great number of similar corpuscles, which surround the yellow substance [the granular layer] as a single layer, are present in all folia of the cerebellum. Each corpuscle faces the yellow substance with a blunt, rounded pole and contains the

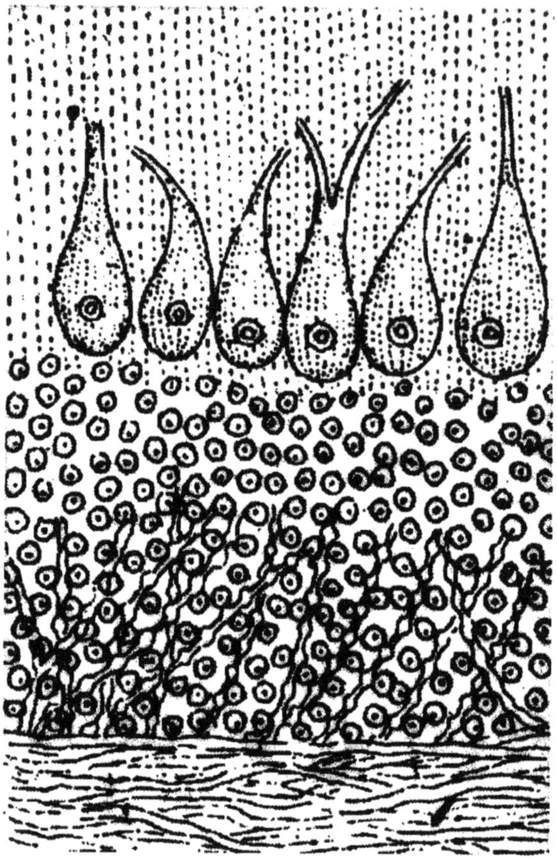

Figure 6–2. Drawing of the cerebellar cortex. Reproduced from Purkinje, 1838.[12]

> central nucleus within the space of its flasklike body; the other pole is taillike and directed outwards; its two prolongations get lost in the gray substance next to the meningeal surface. [Fig. 6–2][12]

Purkinje closed his address with some remarks on corpuscles in the dentate nucleus (rhomboid body), the inferior olive, and the pontine nuclei and he considered that ganglionic corpuscles are central structures, which are related to the nerve fibers as power centers to power lines, or as the peripheral ganglia to the peripheral nerves.

Purkinje's lecture, therefore, contains one of the first accurate descriptions of the somata and dendrites of nerve cells and the first account of the uniform structure of the cerebellar cortex with its single layer of large nerve cells, which have borne his name ever since.

The characteristic flattening of the Purkinje cell dendritic tree (Fig. 6–3) and the key position of these cells in the circuitry of the cerebellar cortex (Fig. 6–4) were discovered by the application of Golgi's chrome-silver impregnation or with methylene blue staining by Friedrich Gustav Jakob Henle,[16] Camillo Golgi,[17] and Santiago Ramón y Cajal[18] in the late nineteenth century and summarized by Cajal in his *Histologie du Système Nerveux.*[19] The ultrastructure of the Purkinje cells was first studied and later reviewed by Palay and Chan-Palay;[20] its basic electrophysiology was

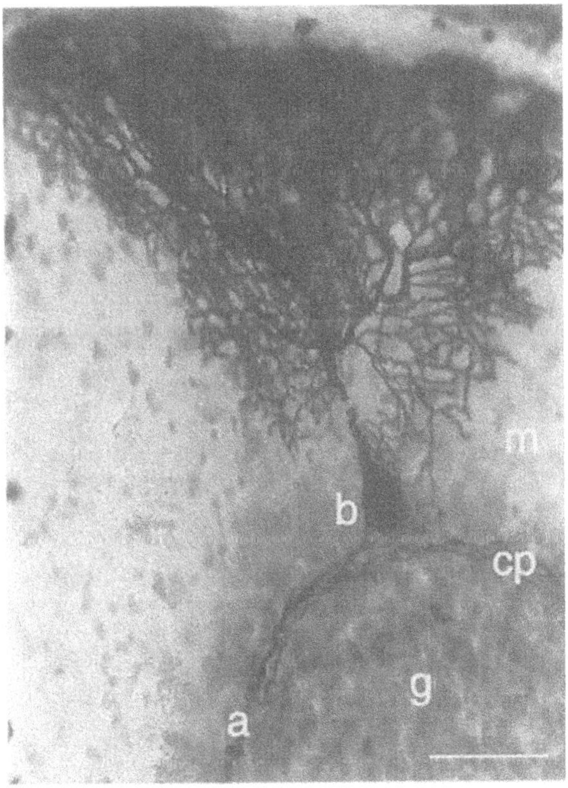

Figure 6–3. Profile of Purkinje cell of rat cerebellum. Intracellular injection with lucifer yellow and staining with anti–lucifer yellow antibody, counter-staining with cresyl violet. Note smooth proximal branches and distal spiny branchlets of the flattened dendritic tree, and the plexus of beaded axon collaterals. Abbreviations: a, axon of the Purkinje cell; b, cell body of the Purkinje cell; cp, collateral plexus of the Purkinje cell axon; g, granular layer; m, molecular layer. Bar = 50 µm. Courtesy of Dr. T.J.H. Ruigrok.

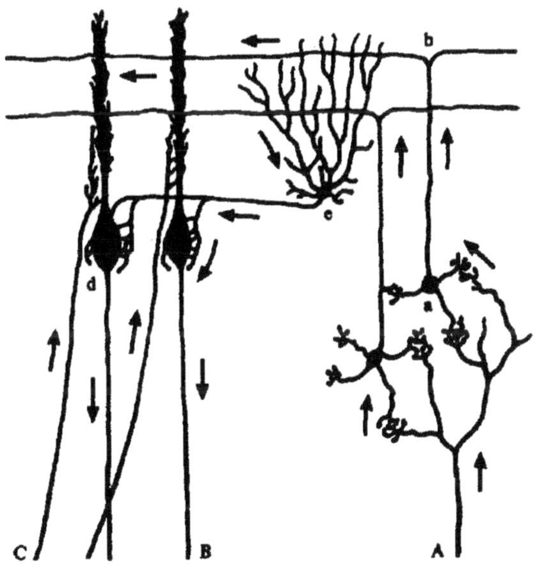

Figure 6–4. Diagram of the local circuitry and the flow of information (arrows) in the cerebellar cortex. The mossy fiber (A)*–parallel fiber* (*b*) *and the climbing fiber* (C) *afferent systems are shown. The flattened dendritic trees of the Purkinje cells are viewed en face. Axons from basket cells* (e) *form baskets surrounding the Purkinje cell somata; however, the main orientation of the basket cell axons should be perpendicular to the plane of this diagram.* Redrawn from Cajal[19] (1909/11) by Philip Wilson FMAA, AIMI. *Abbreviations: A, mossy fiber; a, granule cell; B, Purkinje cell axon; b, parallel fiber; C, climbing fiber; d, Purkinje cell soma with basket; e, basket cell.*

elucidated by Eccles, Ito, and Szentagothai.[21] More recent developments in the molecular physiology of these cells were considered by De Schutter and Bower in their papers on a membrane model of the cerebellar Purkinje cell.[22,23] The connections and the chemical anatomy of Purkinje cells recently were reviewed by Voogd.[24,25]

References

1. Hirsch A et al. *Biographisches Lexikon der hervorragenden Aerzte, 4.* Wien: Urban & Schwarzenberg, 1886.
2. Studnička FK. Jan Evangelista Purkyně (Purkinje) [1787–1869): his life and work. *Osiris.* 1936;2:464–483.
3. Bartelmez GW. Jan Purkyně (1787–1869). In: Haymaker W, Schiller F, eds. *The Founders of Neurology.* 2nd ed. Springfield, Ill: Charles C Thomas; 1970:254–258.
4. Clarke E, O'Malley CD. *The Human Brain and Spinal Cord: A Historical Study Illustrated by Writings from Antiquity to the Twentieth Century.* Berkeley: University of California Press; 1968.
5. Jacobson M. *Foundations of Neuroscience.* New York: Plenum; 1993.
6. Kruta V, Zapletal V. *Jan Evangelista Purkyně: Opera omnia, XIII.* 5th ed. Prague: Academia Nakladatelství Ceskolovenské Akademie; 1973.
7. Purkinje JE. *Beiträge zur Kenntniss des Sehens in subjectiver Hinsicht.* Prague: Vetterl; 1819.
8. Purkinje JE. *Beobachtungen und Versuche zur Physiologie der Sinne. 1. Beiträge zur Kenntnis des Sehens im subjectiver Hinsicht.* Prague: Calve; 1823.
9. Purkinje JE. Beobachtungen und Versuche zur Physiologie der Sinne, 2. Neue Beträge zur Kenntnis des Sehen in subjectiver Hinsicht. *Rust's Magazin Heilkunde.* 1825:3–83, 199–276, 391–429.
10. Lister J. Of the late Joseph Lister, with special reference to his labours in the improvement of the achromatic microscope. *Trans Microscop Soc Lond.* 1870;3:134–143.
11. Ehrenberg CG. Notwendigkeit einer feineren mechanische Zerlegung des Gehirns und der Nerven vor den chemischen, dargestellt aus Beobachtungen von C. G. Ehrenberg. *Ann Physik Chem (Poggendorff).* 1833;28:449–473.
12. Purkinje JE. Untersuchungen aus der Nerven und Hirnanatomie: Über die scheinbar kanalikulöse Beschaffenheit der elementaren Nervencylinder. Ber.üb. d. Versammlung deutscher Naturforscher und. Ärzte in Prague, September 1837, Prag 1838, S177–179. Cited from: Kruta V, ed. *Jan Evangelista Purkyně: Opera omnia.* 5th ed. Prague: Academia Nakladatelství Ceskolovenské Akademie; 1973;12:201–210.
13. Valentin GG. Ueber die Verlauf und die letzten Enden der Nerven. *Noca Acta Caes Leopoldina.* 1836;18:51–240, 541–543.
14. Schwann T. *Mikroskopische Untersuchungen über die Uebereinstimmung in der Struktur und dem Wachstum der Thiere und Pflanzen.* Berlin: GE Reimer; 1839.
15. Remak R. *Observationes anatomicae et microscopicae de systematis nervosi structura.* Berlin: G Reimer; 1838.
16. Henle FGJ. *Handbuch der systematischen Anatomie des Menschen,* no 3, pt 2. *Handbuch der Nervenlehre des Menschen.* 2nd ed. Braunschweig: Friedrich; 1879.
17. Golgi C. *Sulla fina anatomia degli organi centrali del sistema nervoso.* Milano: Hoepli; 1886.
18. Cajal, S. Ramón y. Estructura de los centros nerviosos de las aves, I: Cerebelo. *Revist Trimestr Histol Norm Patol* 1888;1:1–10.
19. Cajal, S. Ramón y. *Histologie du Système nerveux de l'homme et des vertebrés, I, II.* Paris: Maloine; 1909, 1911.
20. Palay SL, Chan-Palay V. *Cerebellar Cortex: Cytology and Organization.* New York: Springer Verlag; 1974.

21. Eccles JC, Ito M, Szentagothai J. *The Cerebellum as a Neuronal Machine.* New York: Springer Verlag; 1967.
22. De Schutter E, Bower JM. An active membrane model of the cerebellar Purkinje cell, I: Simulation of current clamps in slice. *J Neurophysiol.* 1994;71:357–400.
23. De Schutter E, Bower JM. An active membrane model of the cerebellar Purkinje cell, II: Simulation of synaptic responses. *J Neurophysiol.* 1994;71:401–419.
24. Voogd J, Jaarsma D, Marani E. The cerebellum: chemoarchitecture and anatomy. In: Swanson LW, Björklund A, Hökfelt T, eds. *Handbook of Chemical Neuroanatomy, Integrated systems of the CNS, 3. Cerebellum, Basal Ganglia, Olfactory System.* Amsterdam: Elsevier; 1996, 1–369.
25. Voogd J, Glickstein M. The anatomy of the cerebellum. *Trends Neurosci.* 1998;21:370–375.

7

THE SCHWANN CELL

Axel Karenberg

Medical eponyms often reflect a single outstanding discovery or a major contribution by the honored person to a particular field of the healing arts. The case of Theodor Schwann, however, represents a somewhat different situation. Given the widespread interests and the epoch-making discoveries of this scientist it seems almost an irony of history and terminology that he is remembered today mainly for his account of a minute, but very important structure of the peripheral nerve.

Theodor Schwann was born on 7 December 1810, in Neuss, a small provincial town in the Rhineland, which was a part of France during the Napoleonic era. His parents had wanted their talented son to become a theologian, and therefore sent him to a former Jesuit college at Cologne. After completing his final examination (*Abitur*) at the age of 18, however, young Schwann decided to study medicine, natural science, mathematics, and philosophy and attended the universities of Bonn and Würzburg. In Bonn he came in close contact with the famous anatomist and physiologist Johannes Müller and followed his academic mentor to Berlin. After receiving his M.D., he carried out postgraduate research at the Anatomical Museum, where he was Müller's favorite assistant.[4,13]

The succeeding years from 1834 to 1839 were Schwann's most productive period. Historians have analyzed the factors that influenced him at this early stage: his mentor's ability to create an inspiring academic milieu and to attract promising young researchers to his laboratory; the close contact with pioneer histologists in Berlin (such as Jakob Henle, Robert Remak, and Matthias Schleiden); the growing tendency in German-speaking Europe to replace vitalistic concepts of romantic philosophy *(Naturphilosophie)* with a purely empirical, reductionistic, and physical approach in the natural sciences; and, finally, the newly available achromatic microscopes of the early 1830s.[2,12]

Within this framework, Schwann conducted a series of epoch-making studies, each of which per se would have guaranteed him a prominent place in textbooks on

Figure 7–1. Theodor Schwann at the age of 56. Lithography by Ch. Soubre, reproduced from M. Florkin, and L.-E. Halkin, Chronique de l'Université de Liège. *Liège 1967.* Courtesy of Université de Liège, Bibliothèque générale, Centre d' Information et de Conservation des Bibliothèques.

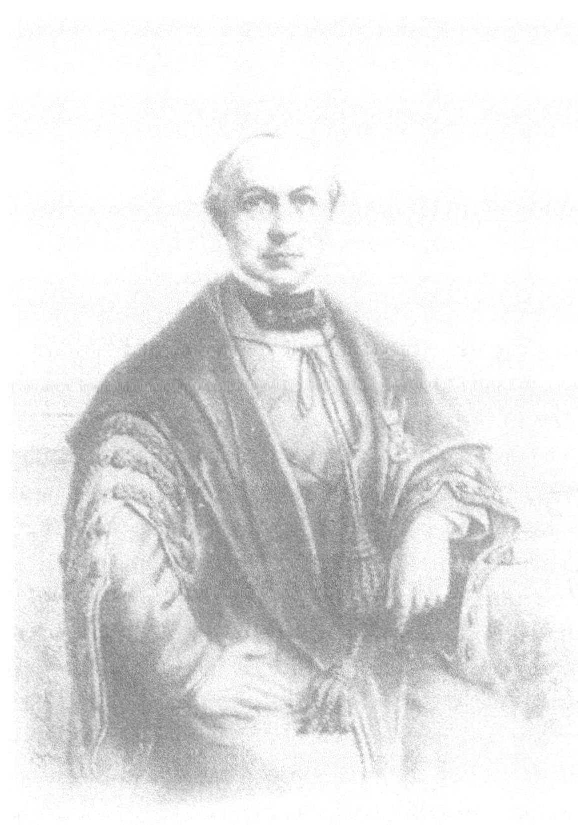

the history of science. As a forerunner of physiological chemistry he showed in his inaugural dissertation of 1834 that air is necessary for embryonic development. Applying the same idea to the problem of alcoholic and putrefactive fermentation, he proved in 1836 that these processes are associated with living organisms, which themselves are destroyed when the surrounding air is heated. He also discovered the organic nature of yeast and demonstrated that the yeast plant causes fermentation, which can be suppressed by heating the culture medium; in this respect, he can be regarded as a true harbinger of Pasteur's ideas in the 1850s. Furthermore, Schwann discovered the presence of pepsin in the gastric juice and demonstrated its power to break down nondiffusible albumens into peptones. As a physiologist he was the first to apply physical-mathematical methods to the investigation of the laws of muscle contraction. In his classic experiment, known as the *Fundamentalversuch,* he showed that the tension of a contracting muscle varies with its length. As an anatomist, finally, he described the striated muscle in the upper part of the esophagus as well as the fibrils in the dentinal tubes, the latter nowadays known as "Tomes's fibers."[6,7,13]

Generally, however, Schwann is remembered not for these contributions but for his pioneering work on cell theory, which also began in the mid-1830s and resulted in his famous 1839 monograph *Microscopical Researches into the Accordance in the Structure and Growth of Animals and Plants.*[10] The story of this landmark study has been told several times.[3,5,7] The year before its publication the botanist Matthias Schleiden demonstrated that plant tissues are composed of and developed from groups of cells. He considered the nucleus (or "cytoblast") to be the most important feature of these cells. Following a friendly after-dinner conversation with Schleiden in Berlin, Schwann, who had already observed nucleated cells in animal tissues, examined all the tissues known to him for the presence of cells and finally formulated one of the fundamental principles of modern science, the axiom of structural similarity in animal and plant tissues. To quote: "There is one common principle of development for the most diverse elementary parts of the organism, and that principle is the formation of cells."[11] He did not, however, insist on the cellular precursorship of all cellular progeny, which was later to be established by Robert Remak and Rudolf Virchow.[8]

In retrospect it is difficult to comprehend why the Prussian authorities were unable to offer a suitable academic position to a scientist of Schwann's caliber. But his explanation of alcoholic fermentation, in particular, had been subject to violent attacks by leading chemists, including Justus von Liebig, thus making it impossible for Schwann to pursue an academic career in the German states. In 1839 he left the Prussian capital to take the Chair of Anatomy at the Catholic University of Louvain in Belgium; in 1848 he moved to the neighboring University of Liège, where he occupied the same post until retirement. But his scientific enthusiasm and spirit of discovery was broken. As one of his biographers put it: "The scientist gave way to the professor, the inventor, and the theologian."[6] Schwann produced few original publications during his 40 years of academic life in Belgium. He developed a number of instruments, including a respiratory apparatus for mining workers, and gradually became a Catholic mystic, preoccupied with religious meditations. He never married and retired from academic life in 1880. While visiting one of his brothers in Cologne he died of an apoplectic attack at the age of 72 on 11 January 1882. The Schwann family tomb can be found in Cologne's old Melaten Cemetery, a short distance from the city center. His statue adorns the entrance of the Liège Zoological Institute, overlooking the Meuse River.

The first, though very brief reference to the cells and the sheath of the axis cylinder of nerves can be found in a three-part essay published in a Berlin journal of medicine and natural sciences, the *Neue Notizen aus dem Gebiet der Natur- und Heilkunde,* edited by Ludwig and Robert Froriep. In the January, February, and April issues of the 1838 volume, Schwann presented a sketchy outline of his findings and preliminary conclusions about the cell theory. A short enunciation concerning the nervous system, found on page 228 of the February issue, states:

> As yet I have carried out few studies on the origin of nerve fibers. Probably they too arise from the fusion of several cells. At least I have found cell nuclei in the nerve fibers of these [pig] embryos. It seems that the white sheath of the individual nerve fiber, which gives the whole nerve its white appearance, is at first lacking; the nerves therefore appear grey, and the individual fibers as seen under the microscope are also less sharply defined and without double contours.[10]

A full description of the myelinated nerve fiber, including what was later to be called the Schwann cell, appeared in the *Mikroskopische Untersuchungen* [Microscopical

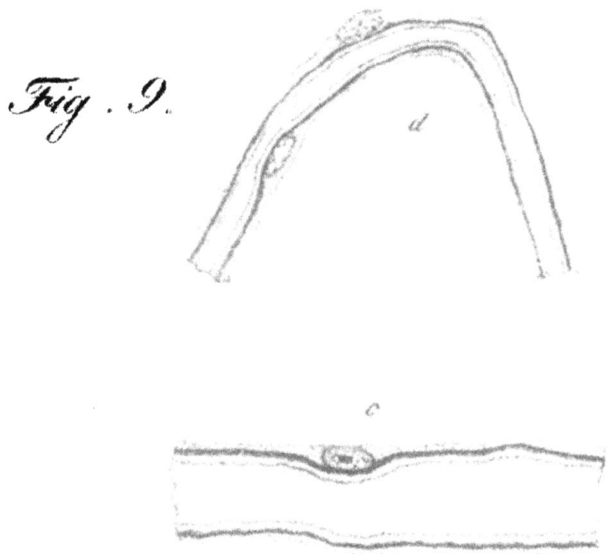

Figure 7–2. Part of a copperplate from Schwann's Mikroskopische Untersuchungen *(1839) "representing the vagus nerve of a calf. The reproduction clearly shows the nucleus and cytoplasm of the cell that bears Schwann's name.*

researches] of 1839. It runs, in a somewhat repetitive style, over ten pages and is accompanied by elegant engravings (Fig. 7–2). Schwann characterized the histological structure of the nerve fiber most clearly in the following passage:

> We remark . . . an external pale thin cell-membrane, having a granulated but not a fibrous aspect, the inner surface of which constantly exhibits cell-nuclei in the very early period of the development of nerve; but in the somewhat more advanced stage, when the white substance is developed, they are only occasionally found . . . The white, fat-like substance to which the peculiar appearance and the distinct outline of the nerves is chiefly referable, is deposited upon the inner surface of this cell-membrane . . . The rest of the cell cavity appears to be filled up by a firm substance, namely, the band discovered by Remak [axon].[11]

He states quite clearly that the external membrane is that of a separate cell. It was not, as believed by many other anatomists, a part of the *neurilemma,* as the connective tissue of the nerve was called in the terminology of Schwann's time.[9,12]

In contrast to this precise account, it is much more difficult to reconstruct Schwann's so-called cell chain theory in the development of peripheral nerve fibers. To grasp his basic concept it must be borne in mind that Schwann 's description of these fibers was mainly intended to serve as evidence for his theory of cellular primacy and universality for all forms of organic tissues.[3] At an initial stage, according to Schwann's theory, nerve fibers are laid down *in situ* by nucleated "primary nerve cells " which are part of the general mesenchymal structure and therefore visually indistinguishable from the surrounding cells. In a second step these primary nerve cells become arranged in rows and coalesce to form a syncytium in which the nerve fiber is then differentiated. At the end of this fusion process each nerve fiber should consist of one single "secondary nerve cell," which runs from the periphery to the central nervous system. Finally, Schwann discussed the question of how the white substance itself was formed. This process could, he argued, be explained in a threefold manner:

> It may take place, 1stly. By the white substance forming as a cortex, around each fiber, and in this manner enclosing it . . . 2ndly. The white substance might be regarded as a transformation and thickening of the cell-membrane of those fibers, or secondary nerve cells . . . 3dly. The white substance may be formed as a secondary deposit upon the inner surface of the cell-membrane, being chemically distinct from the latter.[11]

As pointed out above, he favored and supported the third view, but conceded that this should be regarded as a tentative explanation, which had to be proven by further research.

Can the discovery of the "Schwann cell" and the "sheath of Schwann" really be attributed to Theodor Schwann? In retrospect it is hardly possible to determine with any certainty who was actually the first to observe myelinated nerve fibers with the light microscope. As early as 1779 the Prague anatomist Georg Prochaska examined the sheath of the human ischiadic nerve and coined the term *vagina nervi.* He was followed, among others, by the Italian Felice Fontana, who described in 1781 a "marrowy component " of the peripheral nerves. Most likely both Prochaska and Fontana had observed the connective tissue enveloping the nerves and occurring within minor nerve stems—structures known nowadays as the *perineurium* and *endoneurium.* In 1816 Gottfried Reinhold Treviranus, a private scholar in Bremen, spoke of "skinny tubes which were filled with a tough matter, the nerve medulla itself, . . . held together in bundles by sheaths of cellular tissue." He thus introduced the term "nerve medulla," or myelin, by which, however, he denoted the content of the "nerve tubes."[2,9]

In the 1830s many investigators contributed to the elucidation of the morphological appearance of the minute structures of nervous tissue. The best description of nerve fibers was given by Schwann's colleague Robert Remak, who identified and described the central core of the myelinated fiber—soon to be known as the *band of Remak*—and who discovered the nonmyelinated, sympathetic fibers, which were also called *fibers of Remak.* In 1838—the year of Schwann's preliminary paper on cell theory—Remak mentioned in passing that these sympathetic fibers "are covered with small, oval or rounded, but more rarely irregular, corpuscles, which exhibit one or more nuclei, in size almost equal to the nuclei of the ganglion globules [nerve cells]," thus most likely referring to "Schwann cells" of nonmyelinated fibers.[2] Evidently both scientists had found the same type of cell in different kinds of nerve fibers at about the same time. But it was Schwann who called them "cells" and who provided in 1839 the above-mentioned detailed description as well as a theory of their development. From the historical point of view the eponym "Schwann cell" therefore seems perfectly justified.

On the other hand, it should be quite clear that the present-day concept of the peripheral nervous system has very little in common with Schwann's view of the nerve fiber. One of the most significant changes that occurred since the publication of the *Microscopical Researches* was the realization that Schwann cells are the glia of the peripheral nerve fibers and not neurons or "nerve cells"—a distinction, however, that did not exist in Schwann's time. Equally important was the discovery that the band of Remak—later called axon—was an outgrowth from the neuron and not the "proper cell-contents" of Schwann's secondary nerve cell. With the description of the nerve fiber constrictions, or nodes, by Louis Ranvier in the 1870s it also became clear that it was not a single cell that ensheathed the axon throughout its entire course; Schwann cells were longitudinally aligned, their nucleus being situated in the middle of a segment between two constrictions.

Electron microscopy and modern electrophysiological methods have shown that the myelin sheath, which plays a vital role in the conduction of impulses, consists of numerous spirally wrapped layers of the plasma membrane of the Schwann cell. Today we know that myelinated fibers are composed of single axons, whereas unmyelinated fibers consist of one or more smaller axons ensheathed by Schwann cell cytoplasmatic processes that do not form myelin.[1] We have also learned that Schwann cells play a vital role not only in myelination, but also in regeneration and neoplasia of peripheral nerves; occasionally, tumors originating from those cells have been called "Schwannomas." In present-day terminology myelin is regarded as an integral part of the Schwann cell. The term "sheath of Schwann" (*neurilemma*, or better, *neurolemma*), less used today, describes the thin outer layer of the Schwann cell cytoplasm which contains the nucleus as well as the thicker inner region that represents the myelin sheath. The progress made in the neurosciences during the past 160 years has thus dramatically changed the structural and functional interpretation of one of the basic cellular components of the nervous tissue, an element discovered by one of the most eminent scientists of the nineteenth century.

References

1. Bray GM. Schwann cell and axon relationship. In: Adelman G, ed. *Encyclopedia of Neuroscience, II*. Boston: Birkhäuser; 1987.
2. Clarke E, O'Malley CD. *The Human Brain and Spinal Cord*. Berkeley: University of California Press; 1968.
3. Causey G. *The Cell of Schwann*. Edinburgh: Livingstone; 1960.
4. Causey G. Theodor Schwann (1810–1882). In: Haymaker W, Schiller F, eds. *The Founders of Neurology*. Springfield, Ill: Charles C Thomas; 1970: 77–80.
5. Florkin M. *Naissance et déviation de la théorie cellulaire dans l'œuvre de Théodore Schwann*. Paris: Hermann; 1960.
6. Florkin M. Schwann, Theodor. In: *Dictionary of Scientific Biography*. New York: Charles Scribner's Sons; 1978;12:240–245.
7. Garrison FH. *An Introduction to the History of Medicine*. 4th ed. Philadelphia: Saunders; 1967.
8. Maulitz RC. Schwann's way: cells and crystals. *J Hist med.* 1971;26:422–437.
9. Münzer FT. The discovery of the cell of Schwann in 1839. *Q Rev Biol.* 1939;14:387–407.
10. Schwann T. [Three preliminary papers on cell theory]. *Neue Notizen aus dem Gebiet der Natur- und Heilkunde* 1838, no 91:34–36; no 103:225–229; no 112:21–23. English translation in:

Rather LJ, Rather P, Frerichs JB, eds. *Johannes Müller and the Nineteenth-Century Origins of Tumour Cell Theory.* Canton, Ohio: Science History Publications; 1986.

11. Schwann T. *Mikroskopische Untersuchungen über die Uebereinstimmung in der Struktur und dem Wachstum der Thiere und Pflanzen.* Berlin: GE Reimer; 1839. English translation: *Microscopical Researches into the Accordance in the Structure and Growth of Animals and Plants.* London: Sydenham Society, 1847. Reprint New York, 1969.
12. Watermann R. Theodor Schwanns Beitrag zur Neurologie. *Dtsch Z Nervenheilk.* 1960;181: 309–330.
13. Watermann R. *Theodor Schwann: Leben und Werk.* Düsseldorf: Schwann; 1960.

8

THE SYLVIAN FISSURE

Harm Beukers

Franciscus dele Boë, called Sylvius, was a descendant of a Protestant family from Cambrai, France.[1] For religious reasons the family moved to Germany, where Sylvius was born in Hanau in 1614. He studied medicine at the universities of Sedan and Leiden. He enrolled on 4 June 1632 at Leiden and held a disputation *Positiones variae medicae* under the presidency of Adolphus Vorstius in 1634. After a study tour to southern German universities, Sylvius became a doctor of medicine at the University of Basel on 16 March 1637, defending a thesis entitled *De animali motu ejusque laesionibus* under the presidency of Emanuel Stupanus.

Following a short period practicing medicine in his birthplace, Sylvius graduated again at Leiden University in November 1638. The second period in Leiden made him famous for his anatomy courses. In his funeral oration, it was said that "many students, and certainly not the worst ones, attended his courses, so that it seemed as if only he could understand and explain anatomy."[2] One of these students was Thomas Bartholinus, son of the famous Danish anatomist Caspar Bartholinus. Thomas's notes of the course in 1640–1641 were included in the 1641 edition of his father's well-known textbook *Institutiones anatomicae.* They were later published separately as *Dictata ad C. Bartholini Institutiones Anatomicas* in Sylvius's *Opera.* Physiology at the time was an integral part of anatomy. It was, therefore, not unusual that Sylvius demonstrated the circulation of the blood. He convinced the professors of the medical faculty of the truth of Harvey's theory. One of them, Johan Walaeus, became a fervent defender of Harvey's ideas, which Harvey used, describing crucial experiments supporting the circulation theory in his defense against Jean Riolan's criticism. The circulation concept was certainly not new to Sylvius; he had already defended lung circulation in his thesis of 1634—six years after Harvey's *De motu cordis.*

Since there was no prospect of a professorship in Leiden, Sylvius moved to Amsterdam in 1641. He practiced there for 17 years, spending his leisure hours

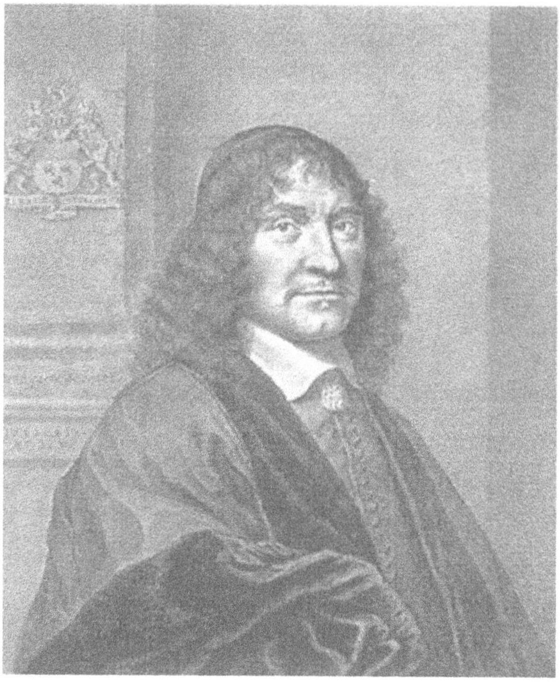

Figure 8–1. Franciscus dele Boë Sylvius (1614–1672). Courtesy of the Department of Metamedica, Medical Faculty, State University Leiden, The Netherlands.

studying anatomy and chemistry. He returned to Leiden in 1658, now as professor of medicine, officially accepting the chair with an inaugural address, *De Hominis Cognitione,* on 17 September. He devoted himself with great zeal to the task of teaching. His lectures were notably practical, usually about frequently occurring diseases. Students could grasp the practical implications of Sylvius's theoretical discussions in his bedside teaching during the daily visits to patients in the Caecilia Hospital. Using the Socratic method, he guided the students to the correct diagnosis, prognosis, and therapy. Finally, he demonstrated by postmortem the nature of the pathological changes underlying the clinically observed disease. We owe the first description of lung tubercles to these autopsies.

Clinical teaching in Leiden reached its pinnacle under Sylvius and attracted many students from outside as well as within the Netherlands. Sylvius's death, on 15 November 1672, put an end to a flourishing time of Leiden's medical faculty.

Sylvius's fame is also based on his involvement in iatrochemistry, that is, a system in which physiology, pathology, and therapy are described in chemical terms. Sylvius's basic concepts are summarized in the disputations held under his presidency, in particular the collection entitled *Disputationem medicarum decas* (1663), containing "the primary natural functions of the human body deduced from anatomical, practical, and chemical experiments." Sylvius's iatrochemistry was in fact a chemical humoral pathology. Fundamental to his system was the effervescence, that is, the vehement reaction between acid and alkaline secretions taking place, for instance, in the duodenum or the right heart ventricle.

Sylvius rejected the classical qualities and humors. From classical physiology he retained only the concept of the animal spirits. These spirits were isolated from blood transported by the carotid and cervical arteries in the capillaries on the brain surface in a process analogous to distillation. The most spiritual part of the blood passed the pores of capillaries, first in the gray matter and then in the white matter. During this process the aqueous parts were eliminated and "coagulated" to a fluid which moved through the ventricles. The animal spirit was the finest and purest body fluid. It resembled wine spirit, easily evaporating and expanding. It was partly used in the brain itself and partly transported through the nerves to the muscles. There, the unused animal spirit was resorbed by lymphatics and returned to the blood for reuse.

Sylvius published his pathology under the title *Praxeos medica idea nova.* Unfortunately, he could complete only the first volume (1671). The other volumes, including the appendix, were posthumously published by his former pupil Justus Schrader. Generally speaking, diseases were caused by abnormal effervescences due to abnormal secretions, which could be either sharp alkaline or sharp acidic. A defective animal spirit resulting from an accumulation of a volatile acid spirit, for instance, caused epilepsy. Therapy consisted of the prescription of alkaline salts, opposing the action of the excess of acid.

Little is known of Sylvius's family life. He married Anna de Lingne in 1649, when he was still living in Amsterdam. They had two children who died at a young age. Anna died in 1657, the year before Sylvius moved to Leiden. In December 1666 he married Magdalena L. Schletzer. One daughter was born from this marriage, but mother and daughter died during the plague of 1669, Magdalena at the age of 21. Sylvius suffered seriously from the plague but survived.

Anatomy was one of the pillars of Sylvius's medical system. His contributions to the anatomy of the brain were recognized by Thomas Bartholinus, who wrote in the revised edition of his father Caspar's anatomy textbook (1641) that "we cannot pass over in silence the very accurate anatomist D. Franciscus Sylvius [since] we borrow from his noble brain and ingenuity the admirable new structure of the brain."[3] Sylvius's "notae de cerebro" are clearly indicated by "F.S." in the textbook. According to his pupil Niels Stensen, he developed his own method of dissecting the brain, which was a combination of the traditional approach of Galen and that of Constanzo Varol.

The structures associated with Sylvius's name were, however, not described in these notes. Sylvius continued his anatomical research during the years in Amsterdam. The discoveries in neuroanatomy were published in the disputation *De spirituum animalium in cerebro, cerebelloque confectione, per nervos distributione, atque usu vario,* defended by the student Gabriel Ypelaer under Sylvius's supervision in February 1660 (Fig. 8–2). It was included as the fourth disputation in Sylvius's *Disputationem medicarum decas* (1663). The *fissura cerebri lateralis Sylvii* (Fig. 8–3) is described in paragraph nine of the thesis:

> The surface of the cerebrum is very deeply marked by twistings (gyri) which are somewhat similar to convolutions of the small intestine. Particularly noticeable is the deep fissure or hiatus which begins at the roots of the eyes (oculorum radices) . . . it runs posteriorly above the temples as far as the origin of the brain stem (medullae radices). It divides the cerebrum into an upper, larger part and a

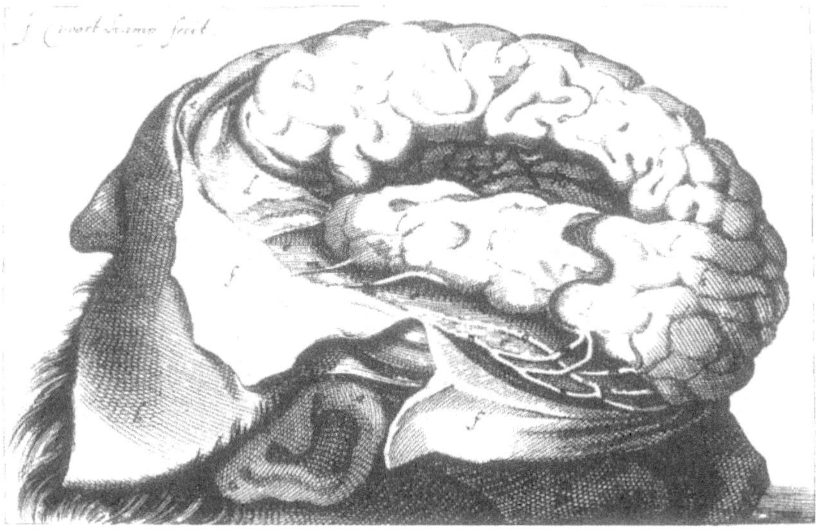

Figure 8–2. First page of Gabriel Ypelaer's De spirituum animalium in cerebro, cerebelloque consectione, per nervos distributione, atque usu vario, *published under Sylvius's supervision in February 1660. It was included in the fourth disputation in Sylvius's* Disputationem medicarum decas *(1663).*

> lower, smaller part. Twistings occur along the fissure's length and depth even with the origins of smaller convolutions at the most superior part of it.[4]

This is no doubt the first description of this structure, as is testified by Haller.[5] It derives from Sylvius's accurate study of the outer surface of the brain carried out as a consequence of his interest in the distribution of the vascular system on the brain surface and from his interest in the gray matter as far as it was related to the production of the animal spirits.

Other discussions concern another structure associated with Sylvius's name, the *aquaeductus Sylvii.*[6] The connection between the third and fourth ventricles had already been mentioned or supposed by Galen in *De usum partium* as a canal providing the only communication between the cerebrum and the cerebellum. Probably it was not the aqueduct, but the extension of the third ventricle to the subarachnoid space. Vesalius mentioned in the *Fabrica* (1543) an "anuslike orifice of the meatus which extends from the third to the fourth ventricle" below the quadrigeminal bodies. Vesalius's teacher and opponent, Jacob Sylvius, used the description of his former pupil. But this was not the source of the ascription of the aqueduct to Sylvius. The source undoubtedly was chapter 21 in the aforementioned disputation of Franciscus Sylvius. He described a *canalis vel aquae-ductus* between the conjointed roots of the spinal cord and under *pons Varoli* (our bridge) and the corpora quadrigemina. The aquaeduct was certainly known before Sylvius, and in that respect Haller[7] and Morgagni[8] were correct when they called attention to the impropriety of naming the aqueduct after Franciscus Sylvius. It seems that the attribution followed Thomas Bartholinus's words, a homage to his contribution to the anatomy of the cerebrum.

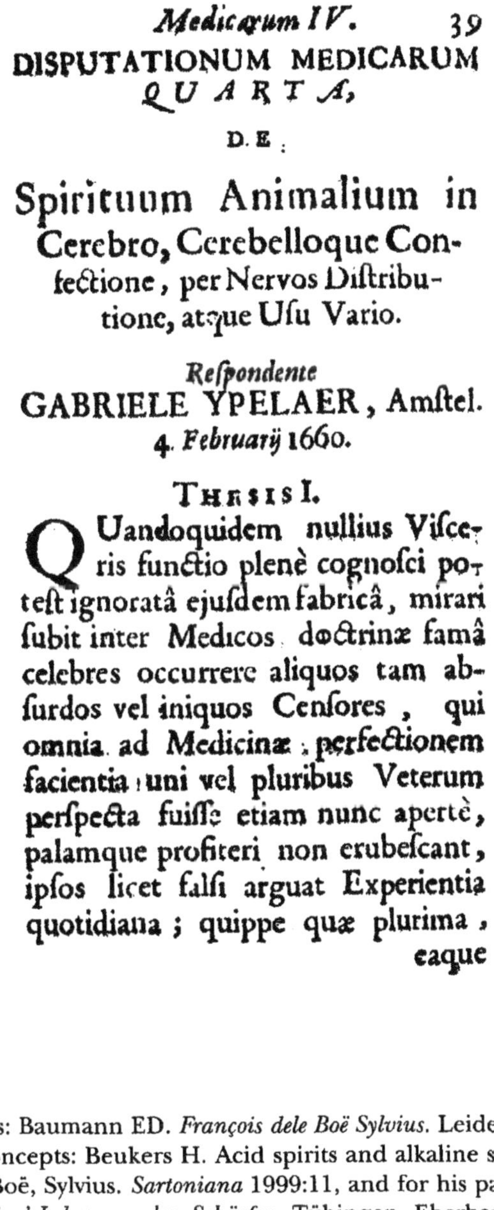

Medicarum IV. 39

DISPUTATIONUM MEDICARUM QUARTA,

DE

Spirituum Animalium in Cerebro, Cerebelloque Confectione, per Nervos Diſtributione, atque Uſu Vario.

Reſpondente

GABRIELE YPELAER, Amſtel.

4. Februarij 1660.

THESIS I.

QUandoquidem nullius Viſceris functio plenè cognoſci poteſt ignoratâ ejuſdem fabricâ, mirari ſubit inter Medicos doctrinæ famâ celebres occurrere aliquos tam abſurdos vel iniquos Cenſores, qui omnia ad Medicinæ perfectionem facientia uni vel pluribus Veterum perſpecta fuiſſe etiam nunc apertè, palamque profiteri non erubeſcant, ipſos licet falſi arguat Experientia quotidiana; quippe quæ plurima, eaque

Figure 8–3. Fissura Sylvii from Thomas Bartolinus's 1641 edition of his father Caspar Bartolinus's well-known book.[3]

References

1. The most detailed biography still is: Baumann ED. *François dele Boë Sylvius.* Leiden: Brill, 1949. Cf for Sylvius's physiology concepts: Beukers H. Acid spirits and alkaline salts: the iatrochemistry of Franciscus dele Boë, Sylvius. *Sartoniana* 1999:11, and for his pathology concepts: Leich H. *Franciscus Sylvius' Lehre von den Schärfen.* Tübingen, Eberhard-Karls-Universität, 1993 (thesis).
2. Schacht L. Oratio Funebris in Obitum Nobillissimi, Clarissimi, expertissimi D. Francisci dele Boë, Sylvii. In: dele Boë, Sylvius F. *Opera medica.* Amsterdam: Elsevier, 1679.
3. Bartholinus C. *Institutiones anatomicae.* Lugdunum Batavorum [Leiden],: Apud Franciscum Hackium, 1641.
4. Clarke E, O'Malley CD. *The Human Brain and Spinal Cord.* 2nd ed. San Francisco: Norman; 1996:43–44.
5. Haller A. *Bibliotheca anatomica.* Zürich, 1774;1:389.
6. Baker F. The two Sylviuses, an historical study. *Bull Johns Hopkins Hosp.* 1909;20:329–339.
7. Haller A. *Elementa physiologiae corporis humani.* Lausanne; Francisci Grasset, 1762;4:67.
8. Morgagni JB. *Epistolae anatomicae duae.* Leiden; Joannem à Kerkhem 1728:34.

9

THE CIRCLE OF WILLIS

Hansruedi E. Isler

Thomas Willis, born in 1621 the son of a farm overseer, entered the nearby Christ Church College, Oxford, as a student and house servant to one of its canons. Contemporary anecdotes depict Willis as a schoolboy on his way to Oxford, giving away his lunch to the needy, as a poor student, helping the wife of his canon in the preparation of medicines, and as a modest wandering doctor, reading and falling asleep on a shared horse on his way to Abingdon market. Studying arts and medicine in the second quarter of the seventeenth century gave him a full traditional Aristotelian and Galenic background.

Extracurricular influences became more important as his studies were interrupted by the Civil War and the siege of Oxford, where he served as a student volunteer with the Royalist army, while the growth of the New (experimental) Science in Oxford, and Harvey's new physiology, demonstrated in the university in a public experiment, encouraged independent research. Willis soon became a member of an informal group of experimental scientists, the Virtuosi. On the other hand, his practice grew from the saddlebags of a wandering doctor, inspecting urine samples in country marketplaces, to the most expensive medical practice in Oxford.[1] In the preface to *On fevers*[2] he described his method of medical research, based on careful notes on individual patients, as what we might term inductive generalization: he would sit down with his notes to compare his observations and adapt general notions from particular events.[3] This method was to be the common denominator of his clinical writings from 1659 to 1675.

Willis stood firmly by the High Church of England when Cromwell's government suppressed its rites. Clandestine services using the forbidden Common Prayer Book were held in his newly acquired house, Beam Hall, in the town of Oxford. This earned him a lasting place in official English history, as well as the friendship and protection of Gilbert Sheldon, Archbishop of Canterbury after the Restoration. It also secured him the academic post of Sedleian Professor of Natural History, where

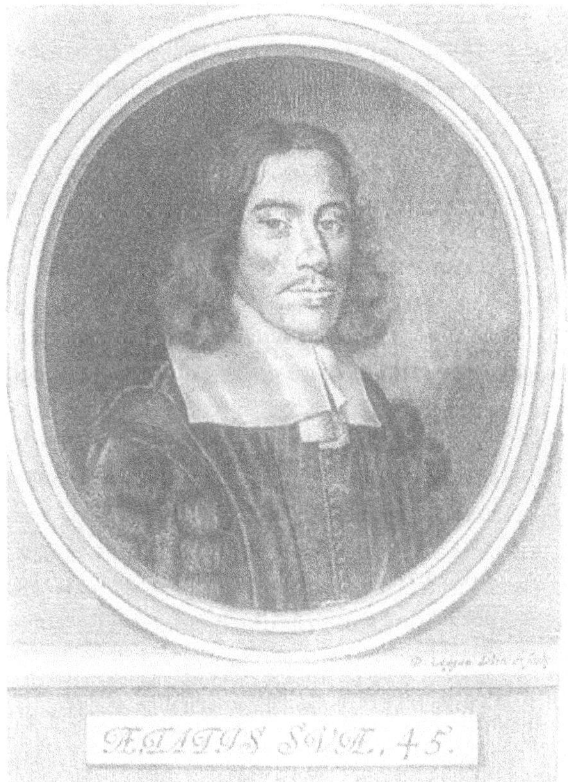

Figure 9–1. Thomas Willis (1621–1675), engraving by Loggan. From Ref. 13.

he was to read and comment on Aristotle's works on natural history, his *Physica, De Caelo,* the *Meteorologica,* the *Parva Naturalia, De Anima, Historia Animalum,* and *De partibus animalum.* Stimulated by the psychophysiological problems arising from Aristotle, he soon developed his own chemical, neuroanatomical, and neuropathological research, and he lectured about his results and their interpretation. He was still aware of Aristotle but even more of the "moderns" who strove to replace him, especially Pierre Gassendi, the Epicurean antagonist of Descartes. The philosopher John Locke, a medical student, took notes of Willis's lectures, which have been transcribed and edited by Kenneth Dewhurst.[4]

Willis kept his own chemical laboratory where he taught Robert Hooke, whom he later sent on to Robert Boyle, thus sending Hooke on the way to his later office of "curator of experiments" for the Royal Society, to be founded by the Virtuosi of Oxford and London. Willis investigated normal and pathological anatomy, first with Sir William Petty, the statistics expert for Ireland. The two anatomists revived the body of a young woman, Anne Green, who had been hanged for the murder of her child, and given to them for dissection. This event was immortalized in a broadsheet and echoed in Joyce's *Finnegans Wake.*[5] Together with (the later Sir) Christopher Wren, the architect of St. Paul's and many other London churches, they investigated blood circulation and the nervous system, using intravenous dye injections, comparative anatomy, and animal experiments.

Although collaborators changed, Willis kept his initial habit of working with teams. As most of their members later became famous in their own right, historians were often deceived, claiming that Willis, a mere fashionable physician, was not the true author of his works, which were rather those of his famous collaborators. It is necessary to know his work as a whole to see that there must have been one individual mind linking these divergent members, and connecting the different topics in one system of medicine, however complex. This cannot have been anybody but Willis himself since none of his collaborators encompassed that combination of vast clinical experience,[6] anatomical and pathological-anatomical knowledge, and biochemical convictions so typical of Willis's work.

In April 1657, Willis married Mary Fell and they had nine children. Willis was elected Fellow of the Royal Society in 1663; in 1666 he moved to London, where he lived as a practicing physician. After the death of his wife in 1670, he married Elizabeth Calley in 1672. Willis died of pneumonia in 1675 and was buried in Westminster Abbey.

His books were printed in Latin but they are now usually quoted from the posthumous 1681 English translation by a minor Restoration playwright, S. Pordage,[8] whose work is far from accurate. This is a serious source of misunderstandings since researchers of our time regularly mistake Pordage's translation for Willis's original.

Willis's best known work, *The Anatomy of the Brain* (1664),[9] is the source for the eponym the circle of Willis (Fig. 9–2). Its innovations include the concept of reflex action and the practice of interdisciplinary brain research by teams of investigators.

In this book Willis promised to complete his work on the brain with a section on "psychology," part of which was published in 1667 as a book. Convulsive diseases, seizures, hysteria, hypochondria, and extrapyramidal disorders are described as diseases of the brain. Willis describes what would come to be known as Jacksonian epilepsy, explaining the gradual progress of the convulsions as the result of accumulation of exploding animal spirits in the nerves originating in the brain. His theory of hysteria as a brain disease triggered a controversy with Nathaniel Highmore, the eponymist of the maxillary sinus, who believed that hysteria was a lung disorder.

In 1670 he published a second treatise on hysteria and hypochondria, again regarded as diseases of the brain, in reply to Highmore's critique. He appended a discourse on the warming of the blood, introducing the theory of internal combustion within the blood, with the help of oxygen absorbed from the lung. Oxygen had been described as *aer nitrosus* and shown to be indispensable for both combustion and respiration by several authors in Oxford and London. Another appended treatise, "of muscular motion," explained muscle contraction as an effect of explosions of the muscle, increasing its volume and shortening its length. The volume-increase was soon disproved by Francis Glisson in a simple experiment, but the idea was still accepted and used by Leibniz in the early eighteenth century.[10]

In 1672 the major part of the promised "psychology" was published in two parts: *De Anima Brutorum* [Of the soul of animals].[7] The first "physiological" part describes the activities of the animal soul which animates oysters and earthworms as well as higher animals, giving simple and complex nervous systems the power of sensation,

Figura I.ª

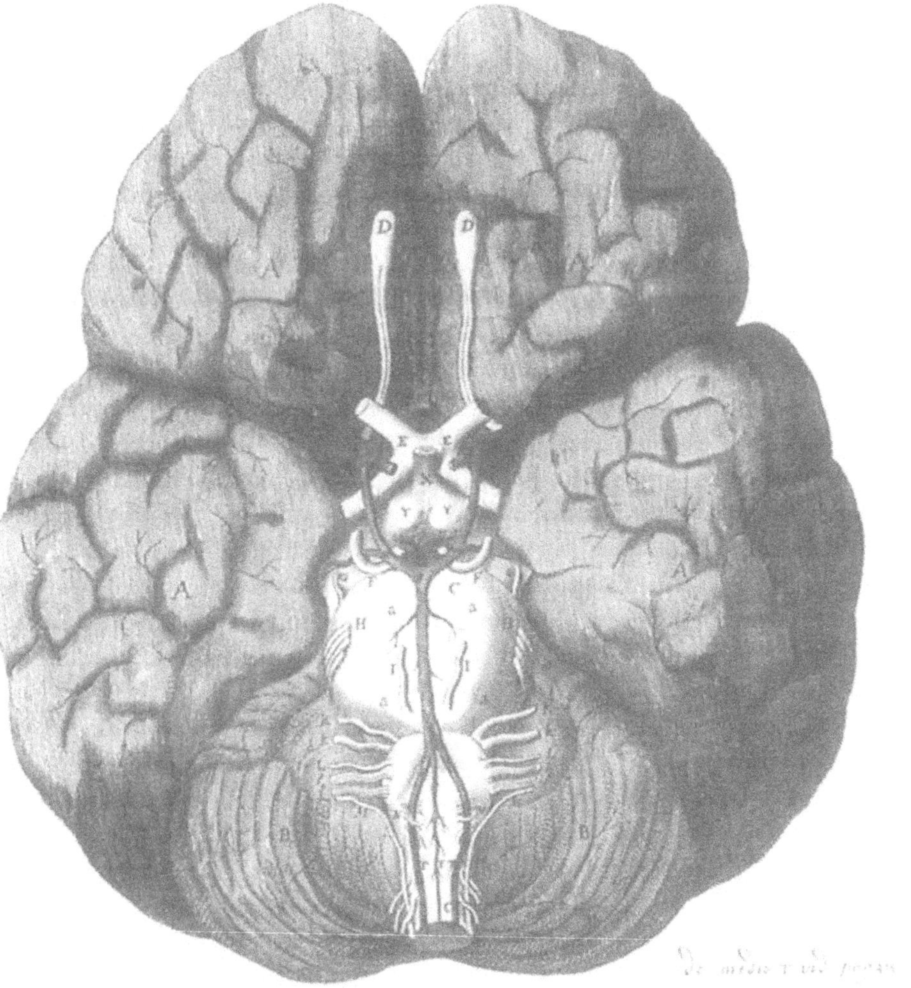

Figure 9–2. Circle of Willis. From Ref. 13, following p. 62.

locomotion, and simple mental functions. In man only this corporeal, material "sensitive soul" enables the immortal immaterial rational soul to interact with his body. The animal soul was supposed to consist of matter in a highly energetic form, comparable to fire and light. This was a non-Cartesian theory adopted from Descartes's antagonist Gassendi. The second, "pathological" part of the book was an early modern textbook of clinical neurology and psychiatry including a description of myasthenia gravis and a differentation of psychosis from feeblemindedness which remained popular until the nineteenth century. Willis also claimed that narcolepsy, which he described without using the term, was not a bad habit but a biochemical disease needing treatment. He thought that the body was able to produce its own narcotic substances, which we now know to be true; these are the endorphins, for which the body also has specific receptors.

Finally, Willis's *Rational Pharmaceutics* came out in 1674 and 1675, amounting to a complete textbook of internal medicine, including accurate descriptions of pulmonary tuberculosis and the first description of diabetes mellitus in European medicine.

The impact of Willis's works cannot be estimated on the strength of his early descriptions of diabetes, Jacksonian epilepsy, myasthenia, and other disorders. It can only be understood as the impact of a comprehensive system of medicine built up on the pattern of the Galenic humoral pathology deprived of its original content and modified to accommodate "modern" results such as Harvey's circulation of the blood and Willis's new reflex neurology and biochemical pathology. The system provided an infrastructure that supported "orphan" discoveries previously neglected, since they could now be placed in a context that apparently justified their importance. It met the urgent need for a new pathology after Harvey's discovery, and its influence in the last quarter of the seventeenth century can hardly be overestimated. But the system was so complicated that it was discarded in Britain after one generation, in favor of down-to-earth simplifications such as Sydenham's botanical nosology. The mainstays of the Willisian system, the reflex doctrine and the doctrine of pathways in the white matter, were finally reintroduced to Britain from Germany in the mid-nineteenth century by John Hughlings Jackson's teacher Thomas Laycock.[11] Even on the Continent where they survived in Johann August Unzer's research,[12] these doctrines had been severely criticized by the skeptic physiologist Albrecht von Haller.

The Anatomy of the Brain was the result of a first attempt to use what would now be called an interdisciplinary approach to unravel the secrets of the nervous system. Willis had previous experience of working in teams with Petty, other Oxford Virtuosi, but also with practicing physicians. He and his collaborators Richard Lower, (the later Sir) Thomas Millington, and (the later Sir) Christopher Wren used neuroanatomy, comparative neuroanatomy, animal experiments, pathological neuroanatomy, intravenous dye injections, and several new ways of preparing human and animal brains. Their descriptions and illustrations of the brain and its vessels and nerves were, as a whole, more accurate and complete than what had been given before:

> We have already shewn, that these Vessels are variously and very much ingrafted or inoculated among themselves, not only the Arteries with the Veins, but what is more rare and singular, Arteries with Arteries; to wit, the Carotidick Arteries of one side, in many places, are united with the Carotides of the other side; besides the Vertebrals of either side among themselves, and are also inoculated into the posterior branches of the Carotides before united. The joynings together of the Carotides, in most living Creatures, are made about the Basis of the Skull under the *Dura Mater.*[13(p82)]

Willis introduced the doctrine of the gray cortex as the source of cerebral activities, and the white matter as a mass of connections whose courses had to be traced. Accordingly, the team tried to follow tracts in the white matter, but their work was censured by skeptics, chiefly Nicolaus Steno, who believed that this was impossible. As their experimental animal died from lesions of the cerebellum, they mistook it for the center of the vital functions; they may have compromised brainstem centers by their relatively crude surgery. Wren drew the illustrations, and was given credit by Willis. It was Lower who followed the peripheral and autonomic nerves all along their course, achieving a more complete and accurate account and better illustrations than most previous works. Willis gave him credit for this, and coined the Greek term "neurologia." Even the term "psychology" entered the English language via the posthumous translation of Willis's *Anatomy of the Brain.*[3]

One principle was certainly more important than the circle of Willis: the doctrine of reflex action. "Actio est reflexa quae a sensione praevia incitata illico reflectetur"; an action is reflex when it is triggered by a previous sensation, and is immediately sent back. In *Cerebri Anatome* Willis gave the first complete account of reflex action.[14] The interpretation of stroke was another prominent feature of the book. Based on Willis's clinical and pathological-anatomical observations, the anastomoses of the cerebral vessels were understood as effective protection against ischemic accidents. The book introduced not only the term "neurology" but also much of the substance of this discipline.

Of course, the system of anastomoses at the base of the brain had been partly described previously by Gabriele Falloppio and others. References are listed in Trevor Hughes's book along with a careful account of Willis's contributions.[1] As Hughes writes, the Swiss physician Johann Jakob Wepfer of Schaffhausen "has priority" over Willis for the complete description of the circle in his 1658 book on stroke.[1(p65)] The arguments in favor of Willis are much stronger than that. Willis published the first complete illustration of the circle, probably drawn by Wren, with the help of the new method of taking the brain out of the skull developed by Willis's team. And the extent, quality, and profundity of Willis's brain researches enabled him to recognize the importance of this conformation, by the same expedient that enabled him to recognize the anterior commissure, the internal capsule, the stria terminalis, the inferior olives, the insensitivity of the brain to painful stimuli, the sensitivity of the meninges; and these qualities helped him to interpret various brain structures as brain organs serving distinct purposes. He was always able to allot a suitable place and function within his neurological context, however fantastic, to whatever structure or function he had found with his team. In the eighteenth century this impressed even Albrecht von Haller, a tough critic of medical research who rejected the first theory of electrical activity (by François Boissier de Sauvages de Lacroix of Montpellier) in the nerves for insufficient evidence and could not accept contemporary accounts of pathways in the white matter (as described by Johann August Unzer, a late follower of Willis's methods). Haller reviewed Willis's work and coined the eponym "circulus arteriosus Willisii."[15]

Haller, a Swiss physician, was quite aware of Wepfer's neurovascular work, and his verdict appears to have been well balanced. Willis's case of a man who died of a mesenteric tumor, having lived without any neurological deficit despite a nearly obliterated right carotid artery, probably with the help of the right vertebral artery, which was three times its normal size, shows that Willis was very much aware of the physiological importance of the circle.[1(p67),3(p104)] In his work, the original anatomical preparation, its correct illustration, and the interpretation within a coherent clinical, neuroanatomical, and neurophysiological context provide the full background and adequate setting for the eponym.

References

1. Hughes JT. *Thomas Willis (1621–1675): His Life and Work.* London: Royal Society of Medicine; 1991. Eponymists in Medicine.
2. Willis T. *Diatribae duae (De Fermentatione, de Febribus, de Urinis).* London: Ja Allestry, 1659.
3. Isler H. *Thomas Willis 1652–1675: Doctor and Scientist.* New York: Hafner Publishing Company; 1968.
4. Dewhurst K. *Willis' Oxford Lectures.* Oxford: Sandford Publications; 1980.
5. Joyce J. *Finnegans Wake.* New York: Viking Press; 1939:101–136.
6. Dewhurst K. *Willis' Oxford Casebook.* Oxford: Sandford Publications; 1981.
7. Willis T. *De Anima Brutorum, quae homines vitalis ac sensitiva est, exercitationes duae. Prior Physiologica . . . Altera Pathologica. . . .* Oxoniae: e theatro Sheldoniano; 1672. Quoted here from the Lyons edition (Lugduni: Huguetan; 1676: 63, ll 3–4).
8. Willis T. *Two Discourses concerning the Soul of Brutes, which is that of the Vital and Sensitive of Man. Englished by S. Pordage, Student in Physick.* London: Thomas Dring, Ch. Harper, and John Leigh; 1783. Gainesville, Fla: Scholar's Facsimiles & Reprints, 1971:46. (Usually quoted from the 1684 edition.)
9. Willis T. *Cerebri Anatome: Cui accessit Nervorum Descriptio et Usus.* Londini: types Jac. Flesher, Impensis Jo. Martyn & Ja Allestry, 1664. Oxoniae: e theatro Sheldoniano; 1672.
10. Stahl GE (with Leibniz GW). *Negotium Otiosum seu Skiamachia.* Halae: Litteris et Impensis Orphanotrophei; 1720.
11. Isler H. Laycock (1812–1876) as the source of Hughlings Jackson's reflex and evolutionary theories. In: Rose FC, ed. *A Short History of Neurology: The British Contribution 1660–1910.* Oxford: Butterworth-Heinemann; 1999:145–150.
12. Unzer JA. *Erste Gründe einer Physiologie der eigentlichen thierischen Naturthierischer Körper.* Leipzig: Weidmanns Erben und Reich; 1771.
13. Willis T. The anatomy of the brain and the nerves. In: Feindel W, ed. *Facsimile after the Englished edition by Samuel Pordage (1681), II,* Montreal: McGill University Press; 1965.
14. Canguilhem G. *La Formation du concept de réflexe aux XVIIe et XVIIIe siècles.* Paris: Presses universitaires de France; 1955.
15. See Keele KD. Physiology. In: Debus AG, ed. *Medicine in seventeenth century England.* Berkeley: University of California Press; 1974: 176; Haller A von. *Bibliotheca Anatomica.* Tiguri, 1774;1:475–477; and *Bibliotheca Medicinae Practicae.* Basileae, 1779;3:73–77.

10

WALLERIAN DEGENERATION

Alan H. Sykes

Augustus Volney Waller was born on 9 November 1816 at Elverton Farmhouse, Luddenham, near the town of Faversham in East Kent, England.[1–4] His ancestors had lived in that area for several generations. His father, William Waller (1773–1829), was a gentleman farmer; his mother, Jessie (Eaglestone), has not been traced. He was probably the eldest of seven children, but very few details of the family have survived; he is known mainly through the record of his published scientific papers. When he was young, a short time after the end of the Napoleonic war (1815), and travel through France again became possible, the family moved to Nice, then still a part of Savoy within the Kingdom of Sardinia. His father was said to be in the wine trade but he retained the farm in Kent and visited it frequently up to the time of his death, in December 1829, in Nice, where he was buried. As a result of his upbringing in France, Waller acquired a continental, rather than an English outlook, and in later years he lived and worked in several European countries.

Something of the character of Waller's father can be inferred from a number of anecdotal points from various sources. The name Volney, given to his son, honors the French intellectual republican Comte de Constantin Volney (1757–1820); he also expressed admiration for another French radical, the revolutionary thinker Comte de Mirabeau (1749–1791). Plainly Waller senior was concerned with the great reform movements of the times. He was friendly with the English liberal writer and politician William Cobbett (1763–1835) and he showed great sympathy toward the radical writer Richard Carlile (1790–1843), who was imprisoned for publishing seditious views on church and state. In this connection it is significant that Waller was not baptized until December 1833, when he was 17 years old. A younger brother, born in Nice in 1828, was not baptized until 1830. Both baptisms took place after the death of the father, suggesting a paternal opposition to religious practice which was not shared by his wife.

The family returned to England in 1832 possibly for financial reasons; his mother remarried and Waller was boarded for some time with an old friend of his father, Dr. William Lambe (1765–1847), physician with a practice in London. Lambe was an enthusiastic investigator who wrote several books on medicine, including an influential study of London drinking water obtained from the river Thames. He was a convinced vegetarian, a practice that had been adopted by his friend William Waller, who brought up his family on such a diet. It is not known whether young Waller remained a vegetarian; he never alluded to it. Thus Waller grew up in an intellectual environment, sharing English and French language and culture and exposed to novel ideas. Through his connection with Dr. Lambe he was in the company of an inquiring medical man, well-connected and at the top of his profession. These may have been formative influences in directing Waller into scientific medicine.

In 1834 Waller was awarded the Bachelier es Lettres from the Université de France, a qualification that allowed him to enter the medical school of Paris. There he studied under Alfred Donné (1801–1878), who introduced him to microscopy—of considerable significance for his later career—and under Adolphe Piorry (1794–1879), the doyen of the technique of percussion. His M.D. thesis of 1840 was devoted to topics in both of these fields. He returned to London, obtained the Licentiate of the Society of Apothecaries in 1841, and, with this additional English qualification, he set up practice in London at the age of 25.

During the next ten years, as a part-time amateur researcher, he laid the foundations of his future, eponymous, distinction. He became well-connected in scientific circles and, after publication of his seminal paper on degeneration, he was elected a Fellow of the Royal Society in 1851 when only aged 35. In 1844 he married Matilda Margaret Walls (1815–1888), the daughter of a London solicitor, and they had two children, Matilda Amelia (1845–1908) and Augustus Desiré (1856–1922). Augustus became a notable physiologist credited with the first recording of the human electrocardiogram.

In 1851 Waller gave up his practice to devote himself to full-time research. Appointments for physiologists in Britain at the time were very limited, so he went to Bonn, Germany, to work with the ophthalmologist Julius Budge (1811–1884). He moved from there in 1856 to the laboratory of Pierre Flourens (1794–1867) in Le Jardin des Plantes, Paris. During this period in mainland Europe he made important advances in understanding the pathways and the functions of the cervical autonomic nerves. With Budge, he contributed to the discovery of vasomotor nerves and they identified those segments of the spinal cord that controlled the operation of the ciliary muscles, which they termed the ciliospinal center. Waller was twice awarded the prestigious Prix Montyon of the French Académie des Sciences, once with Budge and once alone.

However, Waller was keen to return to England and in 1856 he applied for a post at University College, London, but had to withdraw because illness. He did succeed in being appointed professor of physiology at Queen's Collega Medical School, Birmingham, in 1858. This turned out not to be to his liking and, after failing to

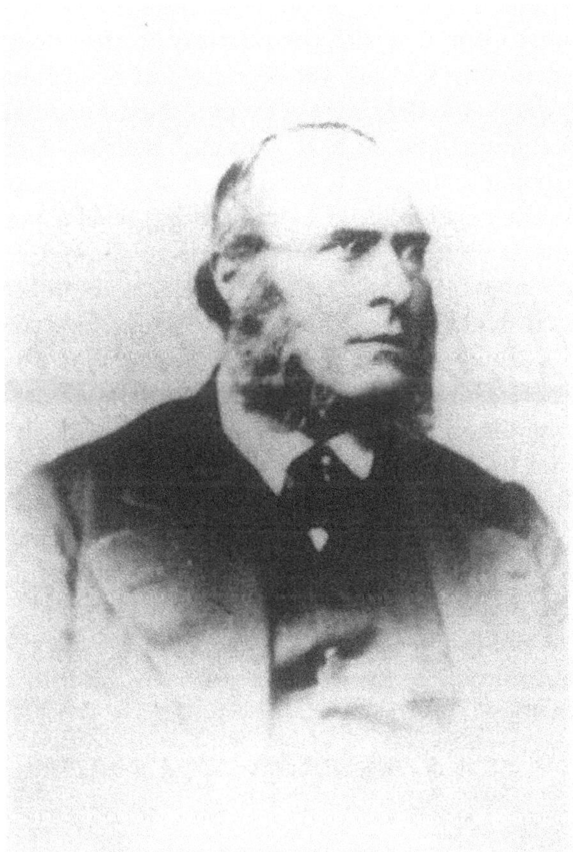

Figure 10–1. Augustus Volney Waller in later life. From *Mémoires de la Société de Physique et d'Histoire naturelle de Genève,* 1871, vol. 21, p. 1.

obtain the Linacre Chair of Anatomy and Physiology at Oxford, he retired in 1859 to live at St. Leonards-on-Sea, Sussex. Although still engaged in research (typically, he used his time at the seaside to study the sting of the sea anemone), he was without an established post. He therefore took up medicine again, first at Bruges, in 1862, and then in Vaud, Switzerland, in 1863. In 1868 he moved to Geneva, where he died on 18 September 1870 and where he was buried.

During this second period in mainland Europe Waller published a number of papers of somewhat ephemeral interest. His lasting contributions, however, belong to his time in London, Bonn, and Paris between 1849 and 1856; the most notable contribution was his work on degenerating nerve.

Waller became interested in the microscopy of the tongue during his student days when he conceived the idea of using the everted tongue of the frog as a preparation for directly examining nerves and blood vessels *in vivo.* He published several papers on his findings during the years up to 1849, incidentally observing, for the first time, the passage of leukocytes across the capillary wall (diapedesis).

He sought to establish the importance of the nerves supplying the tongue by sectioning them at different levels. In a short paper to the Royal Society in 1850 he described the changes brought about in the sectioned nerves.[5] The tissues were examined with the microscope after being teased apart; fixing, staining, and sectioning had not yet become part of histological technique. Waller found that proximal to the point of section the nerve retained its normal appearance save for a slight exudation at the cut end, later to be recognized as a consequence of axoplasmic transport. It became a point of principle with him that there was no retrograde degeneration, a view that has been somewhat modified subsequently. Below the section the whole of the nerve showed a consistent pattern of degenerative changes taking place over a period of about three weeks (Fig. 10-2). This, his seminal paper, was confined to the glossopharyngeal and hypoglossal nerves of the frog, but he later found the same sequence of events in other nerves and in other species including mammals. In his first experiments he cut the nerve on both sides but this quickly led to the death of the animal; unilateral section was well-tolerated and he realized that this also provided him with an unoperated side of the tongue to serve as a control.

Waller's now classic description of degeneration may be summarized as follows. There were no obvious changes during the first two days after sectioning but the nerve no longer became swollen when placed in water; it had lost its semipermeability. On the third and fourth days there was a slightly coagulated and turbid appearance of the myelin sheath. By the fifth or sixth day the changes were more distinct:

> a kind of coagulation or curdling of the medulla into separate particles of various sizes;

the neurilemma became loose and separated from the axon. By the seventh day

> the curdled particles became still more disconnected and in parts were removed by absorption. The tubular sheath was ruptured and disorganised. On the tenth day and upwards the coagulated particles lost their amorphous structure and assumed a granulated texture.

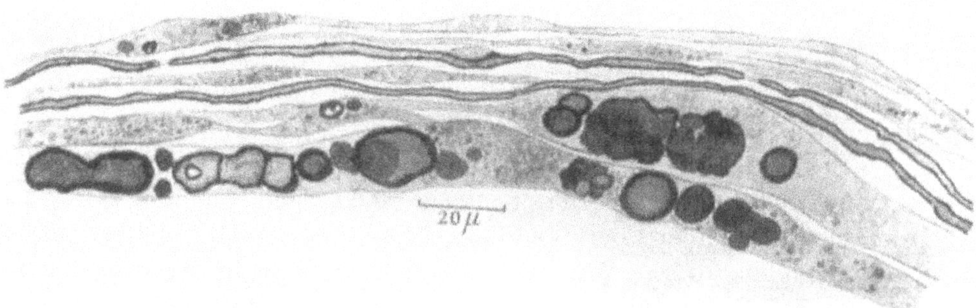

Figure 10–2. Degenerating fibers from a spinal nerve 17 days after section. The myelin has disintegrated into irregular droplets. Two fine medullated fibers remain intact above. From the author's collection.

By the twentieth day

> we find the presence of the nervous elements merely indicated by numerous black granules, generally arranged in a row like the beads on a necklace . . . they are still contained in the tubular membrane which is but very faintly distinguished.

His elementary histological technique did not allow him to observe cells, and so he missed seeing the proliferation of Schwann cells, which is a feature of Wallerian degeneration. These cells had already been recognized by Theodor Schwann (1810–1882; see Chapter 7) in his first description of the myelin sheath in 1839. Waller described what he saw but at first drew no conclusions beyond suggesting the relevance of his work to the study of nervous diseases. It was only later that he pointed out the physiological significance of his observations.[6,7]

First, he drew attention to the trophic function of the nerve cell; as he put it: "A nerve-cell would be to its efferent nerve what a fountain is to a rivulet which trickles from it—*a centre of nutritive energy.*" In so doing he added to the view that fiber and cell together constituted a single, whole cell and not separate elements, as was widely believed, a belief that was not finally overthrown until the advent of the neuron doctrine by Santiago Ramón y Cajal (1852–1934) long after Waller had died.

Second, he showed that, after sectioning, the whole of the distal portion underwent degeneration and had to be replaced; regeneration was not simply a matter of reuniting the cut ends of the nerves, as one might solder together a broken telegraph wire (an analogy he was able to use in the 1850s).

Third, he saw, brilliantly, that degeneration could serve as a vital marker; the dark-beaded nerve could be identified and traced along a mixed nerve trunk. He provided a graphic analogy:

> By it (i.e. degeneration) we could compel nature, as it were, to inject any nerve we wished with dark granular matter . . . equivalent to the injection of (blood) vessels; for a disorganised nerve fibre, when filled with its granular contents, is as easily traced under the microscope amongst sound fibres as a black sheep can be recognised among a flock of white ones.

This use of degeneration became known as the Wallerian method, which, he said, displaying a classical education, "Like the thread of Ariadne, conducts us to the unravelment of all the complicated anastomoses of the nerves of the head."

The value of the Wallerian method to neuroanatomy increased considerably after 1885 when Vittorio Marchi (1851–1908) introduced osmic acid, which, in the presence of potassium bichromate as a fixative, specifically stains degenerated myelin, making it much easier to trace. In the words of Liddell, "The method became a formidable research tool for the microscopist which affected histological technique enduringly."[8]

Although not the first to observe changes in degenerating nerve, Waller gave the fullest description of them and, above all, he was the first to recognize their wider significance. The 1850 paper is confined to morphology, but he was aware of the functional aspects of nerve. Later Waller showed that although an end organ could be paralyzed by cutting its nerve, the distal segment remained capable of transmitting impulses in response to a stimulus for a day or more, a finding confirmed by modern electrophysiological techniques.

The *Oxford English Dictionary* records the first appearance of the Waller eponym in 1876 and it has remained in use continually in books and paper to the present day. As a noun modifier it is sometimes written in the lower case, thus making it more a technical adjective than an obvious eponym. This is a measure of its widespread acceptance without reference to the original discoverer. It retains its value as a term which describes a well-established sequence of events following experimental section or accidental injury to a nerve, giving specificity to the common noun "degeneration." Furthermore, it serves to distinguish primary axonal degeneration, in which myelin degradation is secondary to axonal damage, from other forms of degeneration, such as segmental demyelination or experimental allergic neuritis, which initially leave the axon intact. Although an immense amount of detailed knowledge of degeneration and regeneration has accrued since Waller's day, the basic principles that he established have been upheld—the nutritive function of the cell body, the complete and simultaneous degeneration below the section as a prelude to regeneration, and the acceptability of the Wallerian method for mapping nerve pathways. The eponym surely has a future as important as its past.

References

1. Sykes AH. Steps in the career of A V Waller. *J Med Biog.* 1997;5:173–177.
2. Sykes AH. The physiological researches of A V Waller. *J Med Biog.* 1997;5:232–239.
3. Gertler-Samuel R. *Augustus Volney Waller (1816–1870) als Experimentalforscher.* Zurich: Juris-Verlag; 1965.
4. Denny-Brown D. Augustus Volney Waller (1816–1870). In: Haymaker W, Schiller F, eds. *The Founders of Neurology.* 2nd ed. Springfield, Ill: Charles C Thomas; 1970: 88–91.
5. Waller AV. Experiments on the section of the glossopharyngeal and hypoglossal nerves of the frog, and observations of the alterations produced thereby in the structure of their primitive fibres. *Philos Trans R Soc Lond B.* 1850;140:423–429.
6. Waller AV. A new method for the study of the nervous system. *Lond Med J.* 1852;4:609–625.
7. Waller AV. *The Nutrition and Reparation of Nerves.* London: Read, 1861.
8. Liddell EGT. *The Discovery of Reflexes.* Oxford: Oxford University Press; 1960:77.

II

Symptoms and Signs

11

CHEYNE–STOKES BREATHING

Peter J. Koehler and John B. Lyons

A frequently observed disorder of breathing, in which periods of apnea alternate with series of increasing and decreasing breathing, is named after two physicians who practiced in Dublin in the nineteenth century: John Cheyne and William Stokes. This type of respiratory disorder was possibly already described by Hippocrates, although his description is not complete. The text concerned deals with a certain Philicus, who suffered from a feverish disease, accompanied by black urine. He became confused after a few days, and subsequently he did not speak any more. The limbs were cold and livid. He died on the sixth day. During the last days "respiration [was] throughout like that of a man recollecting himself, and rare, and large."[1]

John Cheyne [2] was born in 1777, in Leith, Scotland, where his father John was a surgeon. He studied medicine at Edinburgh, where Alexander Monro (see Chapter 4), who gave his name to the interventricular foramen, was a teacher. Starting at the age of 13, he helped in his father's practice. Following graduation in 1795, Cheyne became assistant surgeon to the Royal Regiment of Artillery. In this capacity, he first arrived in Ireland, where the regiment was transferred to repress the uprising of 1798. He left the army in 1799, accepting an appointment at the Ordnance Hospital in Leith, and he combined this position with an assistantship in his father's practice. He became friendly with Charles Bell (1774–1842), who stimulated his interest in pathology. This friendship may have had an adverse effect on Cheyne's professional prospects in Scotland, as Charles's oldest brother John Bell (1763–1820), a brilliant surgeon and one of the best non-university teachers, had quarreled with James Gregory (1753–1821), an influential professor of medicine at Edinburgh. Cheyne left Scotland in 1809 and settled in Dublin. He was appointed physician to the Meath Hospital and professor of medicine at the College of Surgeons. Later he worked at the House of Industry Hospitals and became physician-general in the Irish army in 1820, thus achieving the highest medical rank in Ireland. "As my practice yielded

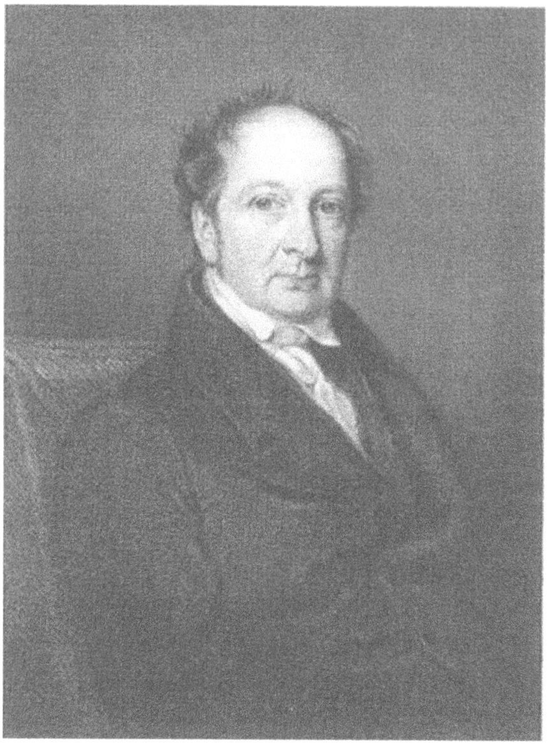

Figure 11–1. John Cheyne (1777–1836). Courtesy of the Wellcome Institute Library, London.

£5000, which was about its annual average during the next ten years, I felt that I had fully attained the object of my ambition."[1] He was one of the founders of the *Dublin Hospital Reports,* the journal in which he described the patient suffering from irregular respiration in 1818, as will be described below.[3] He published important work on croup in 1809.[4] Other publications by Cheyne were *An Essay on Hydrocephalus Acutus, or Dropsy in the Brain* and *Cases of Apoplexy and Lethargy.*[5,6] In the former, he referred to the classical work by Robert Whytt (1714–1766).[7] In the second book, among other things, he distinguished between subarachnoid and intracerebral hemorrhages. He is considered the first author to provide an illustration of subarachnoid hemorrhage.[2] Following the classical tradition, Cheyne still considered bloodletting an important treatment for apoplexy.

From about 1825, he was affected by endogenous depression. He wrote *Essays on Partial Derangement of the Mind in Supposed Connexion with Religion,*[8] published postumously, as a therapeutic exercise. After closing his practice, Cheyne lived with his son in Sherington, Buckinghamshire. He died in 1836.

In 1818, Cheyne described a 60-year-old man "of a sanguine temperament, circular chest, and full habit of body, for years had lived a very sedentary life, while he indulged habitually in the luxuries of the table," who had gone through a number of attacks of gout in the past. He had consulted Cheyne for palpitations and pain in the chest on the right side. He had fallen from a chair, but could not remember doing so. On examination, Cheyne found an "extremely irregular and unequal pulse," and the patient was confused. "I lost no time in having blood drawn from his arm to the amount of nearly a pound." Although the patient gradually regained consciousness, his heartbeat remained irregular and coughing increased, while his face became red. He complained of occipital headache. Following another bleeding and treatment of a cutaneous contusion by leeches, his condition improved. During the subsequent months, his heartbeat remained irregular and he was treated again for gout. Finally, he was found hemiplegic in his bed, unable to speak.

> The only peculiarity in the last period of his illness, which lasted eight or nine days, was in the state of the respiration. For several days his breathing was irregular; it would cease for a quarter of a minute, then it would become perceptible, though very low, then by degrees it became heaving and quick, and then it would gradually cease again: this revolution in the state of his breathing occupied about a minute, during which there were about thirty acts of respiration[1(p512)]

Cheyne regarded his patient as having died from apoplexy, which "must have depended upon increased action of the vessels of the head." At autopsy,

> some fluid between it [the arachnoid membrane] and the pia mater, and the vascularity of the latter increased, more particularly over the middle and posterior lobes of the cerebrum of the left side, where, in a large patch, it was thickened and of a deep red colour

The heart was about three times larger than normal. The inferior part of the right ventricular wall and almost the whole left ventricular wall had changed into a soft, fatty substance. The left ventricular cavity was markedly enlarged.[1] In a footnote, Cheyne wrote that he had observed a similar pattern of respiration in a family member of this patient, who had suffered from cardiac disease as well, but on whom autopsy had not been permitted.

William Stokes[1(pp301–303),9] was born in 1804. His father, Whitley Stokes, M.D. (1763–1845), a man of multiple interests, had submitted a thesis *On Respiration* (1793) to gain his medical degrees, and was the author of many other medical publications. Whitley Stokes also wrote *A Reply to Mr. Paine's Age of Reason* (1795) and *Observations on the Population and Resources of Ireland* (1821) directed against Thomas Robert Malthus (1766–1834). He held the chair of medicine in the Royal College of Surgeons in Ireland (RCSI) (1819–1828) and became Regius Professor of Physic at Dublin University in 1830.

Evidently he was a liberal father. William is said to have gone to school for one day only, during which he threw a slate at the teacher's head. Nevertheless, by private tutoring he managed to gather sufficient knowledge of Latin and other subjects to be able to study medicine in Dublin, Glasgow, and Edinburgh. He graduated in Edinburgh in 1825.

His first publication, in 1825, dealt with the stethoscope, invented by René Théophile Hyacinthe Laennec (1781–1826) seven years earlier. It was the first English publication about this instrument, which replaced the urine glass (uroscopy) to remain symbol of the medical profession ever since.[10] He was appointed physician to the Meath Hospital in Dublin in 1826. Here, in cooperation with Robert J. Graves

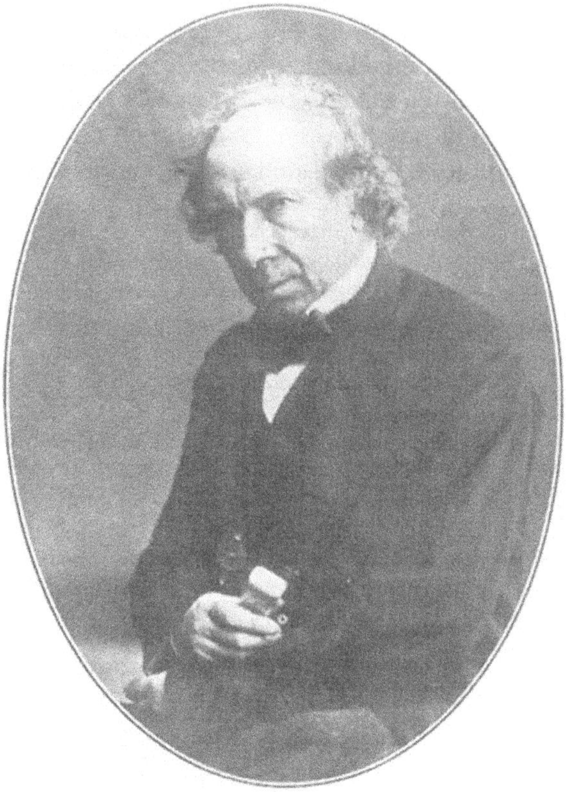

Figure 11–2. William Stokes (1804–1878). Courtesy of the Royal College of Physicians of Ireland.

(1796–1853), he established a new system of bedside teaching. He published on diseases of the chest, the heart, and the aorta, in influential books. He wrote about emphysema and distinguished bronchiectasis from phthisis. His description of paroxysmal tachycardia in *The Diseases of the Heart and the Aorta* (1854), published 13 years before Richard Payne Cotton's (1820–1877), is of great importance.[11] The book was translated into German, Italian, and French. Apart from the respiratory pattern described in this chapter, Stokes's name is also associated with Stokes–Adams syndrome, in which cardiac conduction block results in syncope.[12]

William Stokes married Mary Black of Glasgow in 1828; for a time they lived at his father's Harcourt Street house, moving to York Street, and finally to 5 Merrion Square. They had nine children, of whom the younger Whitley (1830–1909) became a distinguished Celtic scholar. Margaret (1832–1909) was an authority on archeology and author of *Notes on the Cross of Cong, Three Months in the Forests of France,* and other books. Sir William Stokes (1839–1900), Fellow of the RCSI, a pillar of the establishment, was surgeon-in-ordinary to Queen Victoria in Ireland and president of the RCSI in 1886; he died of enteric fever at Pietermaritzburg during the Boer War.

Henry Stokes, another of William and Mary Stokes's sons, joined the Indian Civil Service and gains entry to our chronicle as father of Henry and Adrian Stokes, surgeon and pathologist respectively. Henry Stokes (1879–1967), Fellow of the RCSI, was surgeon at the Meath, and possibly the first in Dublin to remove a parathyroid tumor. A pioneer in the techniques of blood tranfusion, he had acquired the requisite knowledge at the Western Front during World War I. Adrian Stokes was born in Lausanne on 9 February 1887 and educated at Trinity College. His interests, apart from sport, were exclusively scientific. He was both a Fellow of the RCSI and later a Member of the Royal College of Physicians, London. He, too, survived the Great War but died from yellow fever (1927) while working with a Rockefeller Research Unit in Africa.

William Stokes's commitments were time-consuming. "My father left me but one legacy," he said, "the blessed gift of rising early." He often arose at four or five o'clock in the morning to write until eight. Following breakfast, having a large practice, he saw patients. Then there were lectures and hospital duties. He took good care, however, not to exclude the lighter things of life, and a contemporary portrayed the doctor at leisure:

> In the evening he would either hear music—especially national Irish music—of which he was particularly fond . . . or on gala nights he would act in charades, when his curious solemn face and his wonderful wit, would elicit roars of laughter. He was particularly fond of acting the part of an old woman of the lower classes, though I have seen him appear even as a young lady in fashionable attire.[9]

He edited *Studies in Physiology and Medicine* by the late Robert J. Graves (1863), writing a biographical introduction, and he wrote the *Life and Labours* in *Art and Archaeology of George Petrie* (1868). These books were labors of love.

Stokes succeeded his father as Regius Professor of Medicine to Dublin in 1842. Several marks of honor were bestowed upon him, including those of the universities of Edinburgh, Oxford, and Cambridge. By recommendation of the English ambassador, he was decorated by the German emperor Wilhelm I with the Prussian order Pour le Mérite for his contributions to medicine. Originally the decoration was conferred only for military merits; from 1842 it was also given for achievements in the fields of art and science.[1,13] The closing phase of William Stokes's life was shadowed by ill-health. A widower, he lived in retirement, cared for by one of his daughters, at Carraig Breac, Howth, overlooking the sea. After some months of helplessness resulting from a stroke, he died on 7 January 1878.

In *The Diseases of the Heart and the Aorta,* well-known at that time, Stokes described a disorder of the pattern of respiration caused not by a lung condition but by an enfeebled heart, due to fatty degeneration of this organ or other causes.[1,12]

> The symptom in question was observed by Dr. Cheyne . . . It consists in the occurrence of a series of inspirations, increasing to a maximum, and then declining in force and length, until a state of apparent apnoea is established. In this condition the patient may remain for such a length of time as to make his attendants believe that he is dead, when a low inspiration, followed by one more decided, marks the commencement of a new ascending and then descending series of inspirations.

Stokes had observed the phenomenon particularly in patients who were to die a few weeks later. He also found that there were no signs of obstruction of the airways.

The eponym "Cheyne–Stokes" is still associated with the type of respiration described by Cheyne and Stokes. It is a disorder of respiratory control, mostly caused by intracranial conditions,[14,15] although it may result from other causes including lung edema, congestive heart failure, uremia, and hypoxemia. Sometimes, brief periods of Cheyne–Stokes breathing are observed in normal persons during sleep.[16] Usually, however, it is a matter of severe neurological or circulatory disorder. A literature search in Medline (1966–1998) produced 281 articles on "Cheyne–Stokes," mainly on congestive heart failure and neurological conditions. It is mentioned in most neurological textbooks.

References

1. Major R H. *Classic Descriptions of Disease.* Springfield, Ill: Charles C Thomas; 1932: 510–512.
2. Lyons J B. John Cheyne's classic monographs. *J Hist Neurosci.* 1995;4:27–35.
3. Cheyne J. A case of apoplexy in which the fleshy part of the heart was converted into fat. *Dublin Hosp Reps.* 1818;2:216–223.
4. Cheyne J. *The Pathology of the Membranes of the Larynx and Bronchia.* Edinburgh: Mundell, Doig & Stevenson; 1809.
5. Cheyne J. *An Essay on Hydrocephalus Acutus; or Dropsy in the Brain.* Edinburgh: Mundell, Doig & Stevenson; 1808.
6. Cheyne J. *Cases of Apoplexy and Lethargy.* London: Underwood; 1812.
7. Whytt R. *Observations on the Dropsy in the Brain.* Edinburgh: Balfour; 1768.
8. Cheyne J. *Essays on the Partial Derangement of the Mind.* Dublin: Curry; 1843.
9. Lyons J B. A great Dublin medical family. In: Proceedings of the 23rd Congress of the History of Medicine; 2–9 September 1972; London: 1010–1016.
10. Stokes W. *An Introduction to the Use of the Stethoscope.* Edinburgh: Maclachlan & Stewart; 1825.
11. Stokes W. *The Diseases of the Heart and the Aorta.* Dublin: Hodges & Smith; 1854:161.
12. Stokes W. Observations on some cases of permanently slow pulse. *Dublin Q J Med Sci.* 1846; 2:73–85.
13. Stokes W. *William Stokes: His Life and Works.* London: Unwin; 1898:220.
14. Brown H W, Plum F. The neurologic basis of Cheyne-Stokes respiration. *Am J Med.* 1961; 30:849–860.
15. North J B, Jennett S. Abnormal breathing patterns associated with acute brain damage. *Arch Neurol.* 1974;31:338–344.
16. Webb P. Periodic breathing during sleep. *J Appl Physiol.* 1974;37:899–903.

12

THE CUSHING REFLEX

H. August M. van Alphen

During his life, Harvey Williams Cushing (1869–1939) was considered the undisputed founder of modern neurosurgery.[1–5] It is not easy, however, to assess what this image was based on. Even as a boy, he was unbearable. His hotheadedness led his family to nickname him Pepper Pot. During his time at Yale University (1887–1891), his mother wrote to him: "Here is a little private word for my darling boy. May I say it without offence? You know that you have propensity to scold. Watch against it, my dear."[5(pp25–26)] During his stay in Europe as a junior surgeon (1900), his parochial haughtiness coaxed a smile from his hosts and teachers on several occasions. After returning to America, while at Johns Hopkins Hospital in Baltimore, he soon (1902) received a handwritten note from William Osler (1849–1919), to whom Cushing was very close, bearing the following text:

> You will not mind a reference to one point. The statement is current that you do not get on well with your surgical subordinates and colleagues. I heard of it last year and it was referred to by a strong admirer of yours in N.Y. The statement also is made that you have criticized before the students—the modes of dressings, operations etc. of members of the staff. This, I need scarcely say, would be absolutely fatal to your success here.[2(p205)]

In later years, he could still bully his co-workers in the operating theater and he often filled his secretaries with despair. One of his junior residents at Massachusetts General Hospital in Boston, where Cushing was appointed professor of surgery in 1912, confessed:

> As house officer I was his junior and suffered severely in that position for a year. He was an extremely hard man to work with, whether one was over him or under him, as his tremendous ambition for success made it impossible for him to allow anyone else to get any credit for work done.[2]

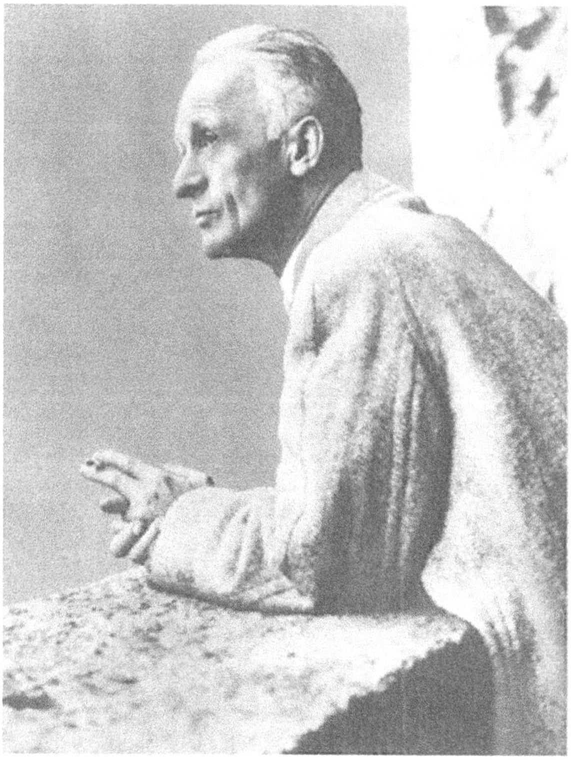

Figure 12–1. Harvey Williams Cushing (1869–1939). Permission of the American Association of Neurological Surgeons.

It was said of Cushing that his many books had been written with his residents' blood. One resident, Hugh Cairns, an Australian veteran of World War I and later a leading neurosurgeon in London and Oxford, wrote (1926) "that Gallipoli and the battle of the Marne were as nothing compared to the clinical stress of a year as Cushing's neurosurgical resident."[2(p539)]

Cushing was not particularly interested in people around him and he found it hard to listen to others. As a clinician he was an excellent observer and he could conduct a good neurological examination. He did not, however, pretend to be a prominent neurologist, and he made no essential contributions to neurology in his numerous publications. Like various other famous surgeons in those days, Cushing had a cast made of his hands and gave it an eye-catching position on the wall in his office. However, before his fame reached its peak, he had been surpassed as far as technical-surgical aspects were concerned by some of his pupils, including Walter Dandy and Gilbert Horrax. Furthermore, his scientific qualities were subject to criticism. The best-known eponym bearing his name, *Cushing's disease,* was attributed by him to *pituitary basophilism,* or a basophile pituitary adenoma (1932). Later it became clear that this syndrome was caused by hyperfunction of the adrenal cortex. Although Cushing published more than 50 papers on pituitary disorders, it was said that he had little knowledge of the function of the pituitary body.[6]

All these facts pale into insignificance compared to the recognition Cushing deserves for the development of neurosurgery and endocrinology. While working as a *house pupil* in the Massachusetts General Hospital (1896), he participated in the introduction of X-ray for clinical application. In the same year, he took this technique to Baltimore, where he built an X-ray unit in Johns Hopkins Hospital. A few years later (1901), he brought back from Italy Scipione Riva-Rocci's apparatus for determining blood pressure, He drew attention to the importance of measuring blood pressure in surgery and developed the first chart for registering blood pressure, pulse rate, and respiration during operations, while he himself gave the anesthesia. In imitation of Sidney Ringer (Norwich, England, 1835–1910) and the British physiologist F. S. Locke, Cushing demonstrated that solutions of saline administered to experimental animals should have a carefully balanced ionic content and he extended the use of Ringer's solution to surgical practice.

In Baltimore, he established the first experimental surgical laboratory "The Old Hunterian," according to the German model of practical teaching. Here junior residents could carry out surgical procedures on animals as part of their surgical training program (1905). This laboratory soon became a model, copied by many medical schools in the United States.

Furthermore, he had a very refined and precise style of surgery, a heritage from his teacher William Hallsted (1852–1922). By means of his very careful dissections and painstaking hemostasis, Cushing reduced the initial mortality in neurosurgery from 65% to less than 10%. In later years, hemostasis during surgery received his constant attention, as evidenced by the development of the silver hemoclip (1911) and the introduction of electrocoagulation evolved by the physicist W. Bovie (1926) into neurosurgery. In 1931 he operated on his two-thousandth verified brain tumor. A great deal of this material is incorporated in his numerous books and journal papers. He performed his last surgical procedure in August 1932, and in the same year he was appointed Doctor Honoris Causa in Medicine at the University of Amsterdam on the recommendation of the Dutch neurologist Bernard Brouwer (1881–1949). After his retirement he returned to his alma mater, Yale, in New Haven, where he was nominated Sterling Professor of Neurology (1933–1937) and later Director of Studies in the History of Medicine (1937–1939). Prior to this, he had declined an invitation to take a professorship in the history of medicine at Johns Hopkins University in Baltimore. Cushing also made a significant contribution in this branch of medicine, including his monumental biography *The Life of Sir William Osler* (1925), for which he was awarded the Pulitzer Price, and his *Bio-Bibliography of Andreas Vesalius.* His friend and executor of his literary testament, the neurophysiologist John Fulton (1943), published this after his death.

Although Cushing was never involved in traumatic brain injuries during his 30 year career as a neurosurgeon, he did contribute substantially to neurotraumatology by describing a phenomenon that still bears his name: the Cushing reflex. On completing his training in general surgery, Cushing spent a *Wanderjahr* in Europe (1900–1901) on the recommendation of William Osler, William Welch, and his father. This included a period in Professor Theodore Kocher's surgical department in

Berne, Switzerland. Kocher (1841–1917) was very interested in brain injuries and the concomitant changes in intracranial pressure and disturbance of blood circulation. He stimulated Cushing to do experimental work on this subject in different animals in Prof. Hugo Kronecker's physiological institute in Berne. Later that year, Cushing continued this research on dogs in Prof. Angelo Mosso's physiological laboratory in Turin, Italy, resulting in the following remarks by Kocher:

> Last winter, a study on intracranial pressure, which led to very useful results thanks to the author's extraordinary competence and unflagging zeal, was performed at my instigation by Dr. Cushing from Baltimore. It was carried out in Prof. Kronecker's physiological institute and later worked out further at Prof. Mosso's during a short period. I am very happy to have given the initial impetus to this work, and to have partly attended the experiments, because I consider the results of them decisive for the principles of intracranial pressure on essential points.[7] (Translation from German)

The experimental method was as follows. The animals had been lightly anesthetized with ether. Blood pressure was recorded through a catheter in the femoral artery. A large trephine opening was made in the midline of the skull. The dura was opened on one side of the longitudinal sinus, exposing part of the venous convolution and the pial vessels. A glass window enabled the cortical vessels to be observed throughout the experiment. Another, smaller, burrhole was made into which a precisely fitting metal canula was screwed. A rubber tube was attached to this, through which saline could be injected into the CSF space in order to elevate the intracranial pressure. A mercury manometer was connected to the tube to record the pressure. Respiration and time were also recorded.

Cushing described his observations in the following way:

> The accompanying charts demonstrate more plainly than can any description the striking regulatory phenomena on the part of the blood pressure, as controlled by the vasomotor center, which occurs during varying degrees of medullary compression. Until the intracranial tension (Hirndruck) exceeds that of the blood pressure, nothing more than the usual slight excitatory phenomena are seen; indeed if the fluid enters easily without compromising the sensitive dura this primary quickening of pulse and respiration may be absent. When, however, the pressure is increased until it exceeds that of the blood pressure and especially if this high intracranial tension has been rapidly produced, we may occasion momentarily the so-called major symptoms of compression with Kussmaul-Tenner spasms, evacuation of bladder and rectum, practical cessation of respiration, and pronounced vagus effect upon the heart often with a complete Stillstand lasting from 10 to 20 seconds. Then follows a release from this extreme vagus inhibition and the vasomotor centre begins to exert its striking influence.
>
> In the more simple condition when the pressure has been increased more slowly, these vagus symptoms are often avoided and the rise in blood pressure follows immediately upon the increase of Hirndruck to a level which temporarily exceeds it. Under these circumstances and when there has been no pronounced vagus effect, it can be seen that the rise in blood pressure is merely sufficient to carry it above the level of the compression fluid; in other words an arterial pressure is called out which suffices once more to carry blood to the centres in the medulla. If an unnecessary elevation of blood pressure has primarily been occasioned it will

> fall and continue along a line representing a level slightly above that of the compression. Should the intracranial tension be again increased the same phenomena will be again repeated, and in this way the blood pressure may be forced to a level considerably over 200 mm. of mercury before the vasomotor centre shows signs of giving way and fails to respond to the demands of an anemic medulla. Within reasonable limits of compression, however, this compensatory action may be indefinitely prolonged.[8]

Strictly speaking, therefore, the Cushing reflex has to be understood as a rise in systemic blood pressure as a reaction to an increase in intracranial pressure by active regulation of the vasomotor center in the medulla caused by a decrease in cerebral perfusion and subsequent hypoxia (Fig.12–2).

The results of these experiments were initially included in Theodore Kocher's book on cerebral concussion in 1901.[7] Later that same year, Cushing published the data as preliminary results in a paper entitled "Concerning a Definite Regulatory Mechanism of the Vasomotor Center which Controls Blood Pressure during Cerebral Compression".[8,9] In 1902 the experimental work was published in its ultimate form under the title "Physiologische und anatomische Beobachtungen über den Einfluss von Hirnkompression auf den intracraniellen Kreislauf und über einige hiermit verwandte Erscheinungen"[10] and as the Mutter Lecture, entitled "Some Experimental

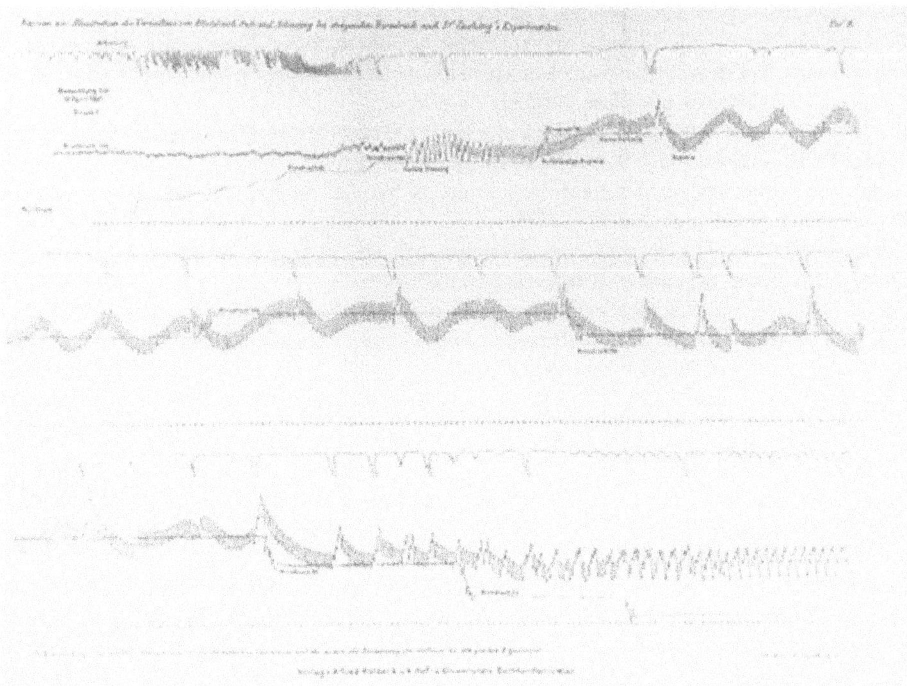

Figure 12–2. Progress of blood pressure in the experimental animal, if, under normal conditions, the intracranial pressure is elevated to 196 mm Hg. Chart from the first publication of the Cushing reflex in Theodore Kocher's 1901 book on cerebral concussion.[7]

and Clinical Observations Concerning States of Increased Intracranial Tension."[11] Some years later, Cushing again revised the material on W. W. Keen's request, as part of a chapter on surgery of the head in volume 3 of Keen's *Surgery*.[12] Since then, the Cushing reflex has been described several times, especially in the neurosurgical literature.[13] The phenomenon has not lost its significance, even in the modern concept of cerebral ischemia in severe head injury.[14]

References

1. Bucy P C, ed. *Neurosurgical Giants: Feets of Clay and Iron.* New York: Elsevier; 1985.
2. Fulton J. *Harvey Cushing: A Biography.* Springfield, Ill: Charles C Thomas; 1946.
3. Haymaker W, Schiller F, eds. *The Founders of Neurology.* Springfield, Ill: Charles C Thomas; 1970.
4. Kolle K, ed. *Grosse Nervenärzte, 1. Einundzwanzig Lebensbilder.* Stuttgart: Thieme; 1970.
5. Thomson EH. *Harvey Cushing: Surgeon, Author, Artist.* New York: Henry Schuman; 1950.
6. Jefferson Sir G. Harvey Cushing 1869–1939. In: Bucy P C, ed: *Neurosurgical Giants: Feets of Clay and Iron.* New York: Elsevier; 1985:51–65.
7. Kocher Th. *Hirnerschütterung, Hirndruck and Chirurgische Eingriffe bei Hirnkrankheiten.* Wien: Alfred Hölder; 1901:95–102.
8. Cushing H. Concerning a definite regulatory mechanism of the vasomotor center which controls blood pressure during cerebral compressure. *Bull Johns Hopkins Hosp.* 1901;12: 290–292.
9. Matson D D, German W J, eds. *Harvey Cushing: Selected Papers on Neurosurgery.* New Haven: Yale University Press; 1969:86–93.
10. Cushing H. Physiologische und anatomische Beobachtungen über den Einfluss von Hirnkompression auf den intracraniellen Kreislauf und über einige hiermit verwandte Erscheinungen. *Mitt Grenzgeb Med Chir.* 1902;9:773–808.
11. Cushing H. Some experimental and clinical observations concerning states of increased intracranial tension. *Am J Med Sci.* 1902;124:375–400.
12. Cushing H. Surgery of the head. In: Keen W W, ed. *Surgery, Its Principles and Practice.* Philadelphia: Saunders; 1908:17–276.
13. Northfield DWC. The intracranial pressure. In: *The Surgery of the Central Nervous System.* Oxford: Blackwell Scientific Publications; 1973:1–25.
14. Pacult A, Gudeman S K. Medical management of head injuries. In: Becker D P, Gudeman S K, eds. *Textbook of Head Injury.* Philadelphia: Saunders; 1989:192–220.

13

FROMENT'S SIGN

Frank Spaans

In the early part of the twentieth century, the boundaries between the various medical disciplines were much less sharply defined than they are now. Thus it is not surprising that although Jules Froment[1,2] was made professor of internal medicine at the University of Lyon (France) in 1928, he devoted most of his professional life to neurology.

Jules Froment was born in 1878, in a family without any medical tradition. His initial interest was in internal medicine, as is evident from his 1906 dissertation on abnormalities of the heart valve in Graves' disease. During World War I he was conscripted to work as a physician at the front, where he saw many nerve injuries caused by bullets. He studied the anatomy and function of the peripheral nervous system and was soon given a position in Paris with Joseph Babinski (1857–1932; see Chapter 18), whom he came to admire greatly. Even after having been appointed professor at Lyon, he kept up his contacts with Babinski and remained the most loyal defender of his views. At the time, the nosological position of hysteria was a regular cause of heated scientific debate. A case in point was the Babinski–Froment syndrome, a nervous disorder that resembled hysteria (or "pithiatism," as Babinski called it) but had to have an organic cause, since it was not susceptible to persuasion or suggestion. The cause was suspected to lie in the vegetative nervous system.[3]

Froment was also interested in the central control of the motor system, as is evident from his inaugural lecture, which was devoted to the erect human being, as well as from his publications on extrapyramidal disorders. One of the tests he described, referred to as Froment's maneuver, is sometimes applied to enhance rigidity in suspected Parkinson's syndrome. Froment found that rigidity as examined on the wrist joint would almost disappear if the patient is in complete rest and, in contrast, increase by active elevation of the free arm. He recorded these effects with electromyography and compared the maneuver with Jendrassik's maneuver (see Chapter 22) for enhancing tendon reflexes.[4]

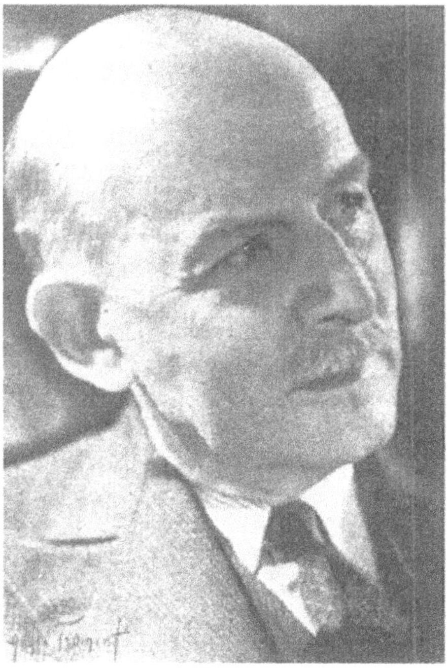

Figure 13–1. Jules Froment (1878–1946). Courtesy Archives of the University of Lyon.

In all of his studies on the motor system, he consulted *La Physiologie des Mouvements* by the eminent nineteenth-century clinician and founder of the electrodiagnosis of the neuromuscular system, Duchenne de Boulogne (1806–1875; see Chapter 46), for whom he had a boundless admiration. According to Froment, this book gave him the answers to innumerable questions.

Like many other physicians of his era, Froment was interested in a wide range of subjects, extensively studying, among other things, the various forms of aphasia and dysarthria. He was a respected member of the Société de Neurologie de Paris, but an active member of the Société de Philosophie de Lyon as well. Whereas several of his philosophical papers were of a markedly speculative nature, his publications on the diagnosis of peripheral nerve lesions were characterized by a high level of precision. In addition to the sign discussed here, he described numerous other tests for diagnosing peripheral nervous disorders,[2] but these have all fallen into disuse.

After an extremely industrious professional life, Froment retired in 1945 because of ill health. He died a year later.

In 1915, Froment's article *La préhension dans les paralysies du nerf cubital et le signe du pouce* [Prehension in paralysis of the cubital nerve and the thumb sign] appeared in the *Presse Médicale.*[5] The article, which runs to one closely printed page, provides an extremely detailed description and discussion of the sign. The figure included in the article shows why the sign is also known as *le signe du journal* (the newspaper sign; Fig. 13–2). In essence, the person being examined holds a sheet of paper between the extended thumb and the radial side of the palm and index finger, and then tries

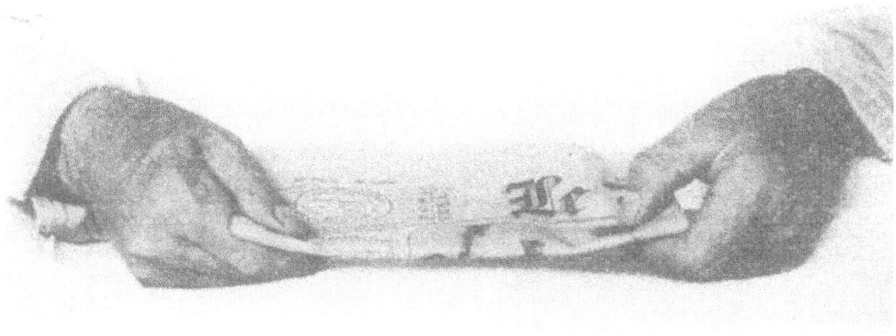

Figure 13–2. Illustration from Froment's original publication.[5]

to prevent its being pulled out of his hands. If the subject has a lesion of the ulnar nerve, resulting in a paresis of the adductor pollicis muscle, he will not be able to do so. At the same time, by way of compensation, the median innervated flexor pollicis longus will unconsciously be activated, leading to flexion of the terminal phalanx of the thumb.

> Clinically, of all the motor disturbances, which follow a lesion of the ulnar nerve, the most important is the change which is observed in the mechanism of prehension (due to the paralysis of the adductor of the thumb). It appeared therefore useful to call the attention of the neurologists to a new objective sign, which is found in such cases to rapidly detect the defect in this function and so appreciate its importance.[5]

Froment's sign is still used in the clinical diagnosis of ulnar neuropathies. According to Mumenthaler,[6] the sign is nearly always observed even in mild ulnar neuropathies, especially if a comparison can be made with a normal contralateral hand. Sunderland,[7] however, warns that the paresis of the adductor pollicis can be compensated not only by the flexor pollicis longus but also by the radial innervated extensor pollicis longus. This produces no flexion of the thumb, yielding a false-negative Froment's sign. This means that the examiner has to ensure that the extensor pollicis longus is not tightened during the test, by checking that the thumb is not placed in an unduly dorsal position. Mannerfeldt[8] has pointed out that the supplementary adductive function of the extensor pollicis longus can be suppressed by a slight flexing of the wrist.

Instead of a newspaper, a single sheet of paper is now used in the test.

References

1. Dechaume J, Girard P-F. Le Professeur Jules Froment. *J Méd Lyon.* 1946;27:745–751.
2. J. Froment. *Rev Neurol.* 1946;78:605–606. Obituary.
3. Babinski J, Froment J. Troubles nerveux d'ordre réflexe. Syndrome physiopathique. In: *Hysterie, pithiatisme et troubles nerveux d'ordre réflexe.* Paris: Masson; 1917.
4. Froment J C, Gardère H. La rigidité et la roue dentée parkinsonienne s'effacent au repos. Leur caractère dysstasique. *Rev Neurol.* 1926;1:52–53.

5. Froment J. La préhension dans les paralysies du nerf cubital et le signe du pouce. *Presse Méd.* 1915;23:409. English translation: Kaplan E B. Prehension and the sign of the thumb in paralysis of the ulnar nerve. *Bull Hosp Joint Dis.* 1972;33:193–196.
6. Mumenthaler M, Schliack H. *Lesionen peripherer Nerven.* 6th ed. Stuttgart: Thieme; 1993: 268–287.
7. Sunderland S. *Nerves and Nerve Injuries.* 2nd ed. Edinburgh: Churchill Livingstone; 1978: 768–769.
8. Mannerfeldt L. Studies on the hand in ulnar nerve paralysis. *Acta Orthop Scand.* 1966 (suppl 87).

14

GOWERS' SIGN

Nicolaas J. M. Arts

Gowers's classical paper on 220 personally examined cases of Duchenne's muscular dystrophy included the sign that bears his name.[1] He pointed out that the patient—usually a child—was seen to rise from the sitting position by first resting on his hands and knees and then "climbing up his legs" by straightening the legs, subsequently putting the hand on the knees, and finally straightening the trunk. It indicates a weakness of the muscles responsible for the extension of the knee and hip joints.

There is a double irony in this eponymic description: first, Gowers disliked eponyms (see later) and although few, if any, neurologists have made more original observations than Gowers, he was not the first to draw attention to the phenomenon.

William Richard Gowers was born on 20 March 1845 in Hackney, England.[2–7] His father, a cobbler, died when William was still a boy. Fortunately, this did not ruin his prospects, because he repeatedly received the help of benefactors who had developed a liking for the intelligent, industrious, and conscientious boy. William Gowers began his education at Christ Church School, Oxford, and was apprenticed at the age of 15 to doctor Thomas Simpson, a general practitioner at Coggeshall in Essex. At the time, apprenticeship in medicine at such a tender age was not unusual. After his two years' apprenticeship, the vicar of Coggeshall took him to London and introduced him to his old friend Sir William Jenner, physician at University College Hospital and president of the Royal College of Physicians. During his undergraduate years, William Gowers acted as Jenner's secretary and assistant. He qualified in 1862. At the university, Gowers won almost all of the postgraduate honors and was subsequently appointed assistant physician at University College Hospital (1872). Meanwhile he published several original articles on neurological topics and general medicine. He acquired the position of registrar or 'assistant to the physicians' at the National Hospital for the Paralysed and Epileptic at Queen Square, London, in 1870. This post had been specially created for him, possibly on

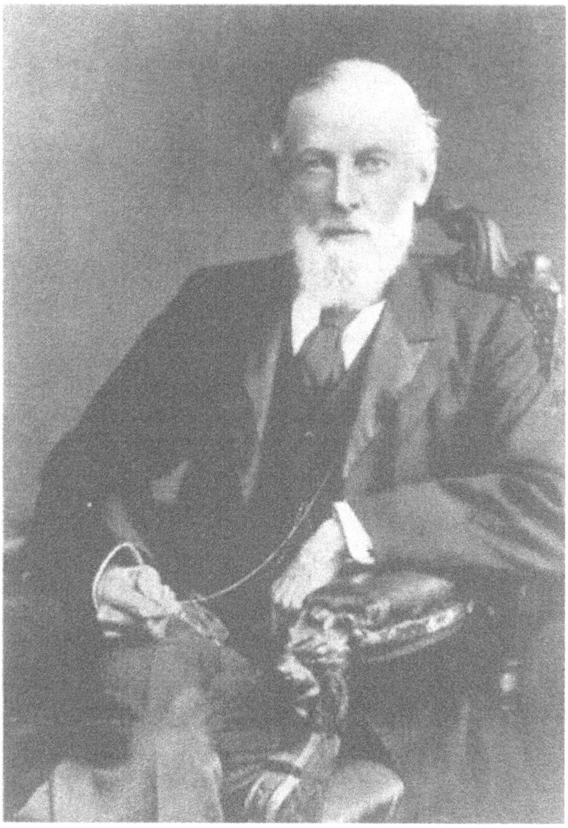

Figure 14–1. William Richard Gowers (1845–1915). Courtesy of the Institute of Neurology, National Hospital, Queen Square, London.

the advice of Russell Reynolds and Charlton Bastian, the men who had probably also aroused Gowers's interest in diseases of the nervous system. They were his teachers and colleagues at University College Hospital, but also physicians at the National Hospital. After four years as registrar, Gowers was elected assistant physician. He worked as a junior colleague to John Hughlings Jackson, who he frequently referred to later as "my master." Jackson was a physiologist and philosopher, a very sharp and original thinker, but a poor writer and uninspiring teacher. Gowers was less of a thinker, but a very talented writer, diagnostician, and teacher. Their personalities differed too. Jackson, as a shy but friendly man, was liked by almost everyone. Gowers was less popular; at times he was a difficult person and even cantankerous.

After a swift start, Gowers's further promotion at the National Hospital was exceptionally slow: it was not until 20 years later that he became full (or senior) physician. Meanwhile he had been appointed professor of clinical medicine and staff member at University College Hospital. In 1888, at the age of 43, Gowers suddenly retired from all his commitments at University College Hospital and devoted the rest of his working life to the study and instruction of neurology at the National Hospital.

For 20 years, week after week, Gowers examined and treated patients in a small and ill-equipped room. With his characteristic energy and thoroughness, he recorded in shorthand every symptom. In this way, he collected the enormous body of information and observations which formed the basis of his *Manual*.[8]

Gowers was so convinced of the value of shorthand—which at that time was called "phonography"—that he became one of the founding members of the Society of Medical Phonographers. After 1893, almost half of his papers were published in the periodical of this society, printed in the characters of Pitman's phonetic shorthand system and virtually inaccessible to the modern reader because this system faded into oblivion.

He became a famous lecturer throughout Europe and in the United States, and he attracted a large number of students and postgraduates. His accomplishments in no small way rendered the National Hospital at Queen Square the enjoyment of international reputation.

Testimony to his keen eye for technical details are his invention of a hemoglobinometer and improvement of the existing hemocytometer, which were used, in England at least, for more than 40 years. In addition, Gowers was well-versed in the art and techniques of drawing, etching, and painting. His works were regularly exhibited by the Royal Academy of Arts and he always illustrated his own books. In 1887 he was elected Fellow of the Royal Society and a knighthood was bestowed upon him in 1897. During the latter part of his life, he suffered from ill health, probably the result of generalized arteriosclerosis. He had to retire prematurely at the age of 62. He died in London on 4 May 1915.

Gowers made numerous important contributions to neurology. Usually, he would first publish his findings in papers, later uniting them in carefully edited and skillfully organized books. He was an outstanding writer with a remarkably concise style, always searching for "unimpeachable exactness" and rarely mistaking theories for facts. "We would be better doctors, better teachers, better writers, if we, from time to time read Gowers' [works] and thereby learn some of the art of perfect observation and perfect precise description, written in easy simple prose," Foster Kennedy stated.[4]

In his *Manual and Atlas of Medical Ophthalmoscopy*,[9] he described pathological changes of the fundus in ophthalmological, neurological, and general disease. One year later his *Diagnosis of Diseases of the Spinal Cord*[10] identified, for the first time, the relationship between the spinal segments and the vertebral bodies. In collaboration with a pupil, the neurosurgeon Victor Horsley, and based on dissection work, he discovered and demonstrated the dorsal spinocerebellar tract. This tract is now known as *Gowers' tract*, an eponym Gowers probably would not have approved of, for in 1884 he wrote:

> The direct pyramidal tract is also called the column of Türck; the postero-median column is called the column of Goll, and the postero-external column is called the column of Burdach. I have avoided the use of these terms. This system of nomenclature is full of inconvenience, increasing the difficulties of the student, and leading to frequent mistakes in scientific writings. There are very few observations in medicine regarding which it is not obvious that they would speedily have been made by some other than the actual observer; that it was very much of an accident that they were made by certain individuals. Scientific nomenclature should be itself

> scientific, not founded upon accidents. However anxious we may be to honour individuals, we have no right to do so at the expense of the convenience of all future generations of learners.[10]

These words seem to have had no effect at all. Besides the well-known sign and the above-mentioned tract, four other signs, three syndromes, and a chemical solution have been named after Gowers.[11]

In *Diagnosis of Diseases of the Spinal Cord*, Gowers introduced the term "knee-jerk" for the quadriceps reflex or patellar tendon reflex. Other words introduced by Gowers were amyotatic, abiotrophy, and fibrositis. Classical physical signs that were first recognized by Gowers are the nasal smile of myasthenics, fixation spasm, and pharyngolaryngeal nystagmus.

Gowers's *Epilepsy and Other Chronic Convulsive Diseases* (1881)[12] contains the first description of the tetanic nature of epileptic convulsions and the first description of the silent interval. The book also played a pivotal role in the transition from nineteenth century views on epilepsy to the widespread acceptance of John Hughlings Jackson's new ideas on this subject.

Descriptions of a multitude of new neurological conditions are given in Gowers's *Manual of Diseases of the Nervous System* (1886–1888).[8] This work rates among the truly great monuments of modern neurology and it was regarded as the "Bible of Neurology" for half a century. In it Gowers introduced the concepts upper motor neuron and lower motor neuron[13] and gave the first clear tracings (myograms) of the tremor patterns of alcoholic, hyperthyroid, Parkinsonian, and hysterical patients.[14]

The Border-Land of Epilepsy (1907), Gowers' last book, was one of his masterpieces.[15] It describes intermittent disorders, more or less resembling epilepsy, but without any known pathological substrate: faints, vagal attacks, vertigo, migraine, and sleep disorders.

Gowers's original description of the sign named after him appeared in the first installment of his paper on "pseudo-hypertrophic muscular paralysis,"[1] a verbatim report of a clinical demonstration of two boys with Duchenne muscular dystrophy (Gowers's designation was the anglicized form of Duchenne's *paralysie musculaire pseudohypertrophique*). After having demonstrated posture and gait of the first patient, a nine-year-old boy, Gowers continued:

> And now we will put him on the ground. You see that he is quite unable to rise without assistance. If a little aid be afforded him he helps himself in a very peculiar way—by putting his hands upon his knees, and then grasping his thighs higher and higher, and so by (as has been said) climbing up his thighs he apparently pushes his trunk up.

Gowers claimed no priority for his description of the phenomenon; he admitted that Duchenne had been the first to draw attention to it. At the same time he rejected Duchenne's claim of being the first to describe pseudohypertrophic muscular paralysis, because Edward Meryon had described it as a separate disease entity as early as in 1852, and the Italians Coste and Gioja had described several unequivocal cases another 15 years before (see Chapter 46).

Gowers accepted the common explanation for the phenomenon—that it was an attempt to help extension of the hip joint—but found it only partially satisfactory. He observed that there were two actions. First, the hands were placed on the knees and kept there; this was to assist extension of the knee joint. Only after that, the thigh was grasped and the hands moved alternately higher and higher, in order to assist extension of the hip joint. That these actions gave assistance to extension of the knee joint was proven, according to Gowers, by the fact that there is little extension of the hip joint when the hands are on the knees; the hands climb up and the hip joints are extended only after the knees have become fully extended. In some patients—and this is the second item of proof—only the first part of the phenomenon is seen; these patients, who can keep their knees extended, are able to bend their hips, touch the ground, and rise again, without any need to use their hands.

Gowers also described another expedient for effecting extension of the knee joint in cases of proximal weakness (see Fig. 14–2):

> In getting up they first put the hands on the ground (1), then stretch out the legs behind them far apart, and, the chief weight of the trunk resting on the hands, by keeping the toes on the ground and pushing the body backwards, they manage to get the knees extended, so that the trunk is supported by the hands and feet, all placed as widely as possible (2). Next the hands are moved alternately along the ground backwards, so as to bring a larger portion of the weight of the trunk over the legs. Then one hand is placed upon the knee (3), and a push with this and with the other hand on the ground is sufficient to enable the extensors of the hip to bring the trunk into the upright posture.

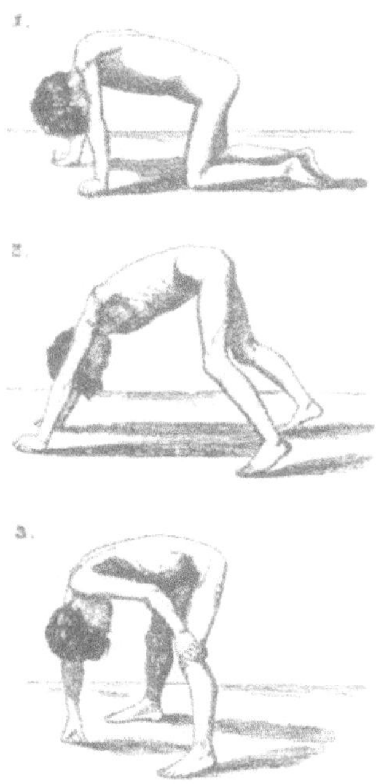

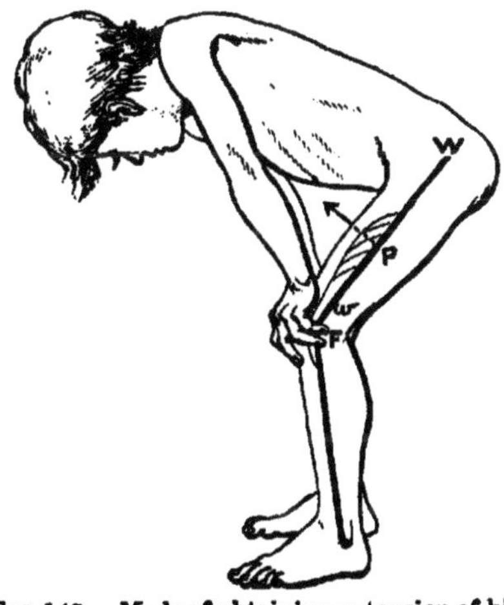

FIG. 142.—Mode of obtaining extension of hips in pseudo-hypertrophic paralysis. F, fulcrum of the lever formed by the femur. P, mean position at which the power is applied by contraction of the quadriceps femoris. W, position of weight in the ordinary mode of rising. w, the place to which part is transferred by putting hands on knees.

Figure 14–2. Gowers's illustrations of Gowers' sign. From Ref. 8.

In 1879 Gowers still thought that the sign was "practically pathognomic" for pseudohypertrophic paralysis: "I have never seen it absent in a case so long as the patient possessed the necessary muscular power. I have never seen it in another disease, and every doubtful case in which it was present ultimately proved to be an example of the effect." In the first volume of his *Manual*, published seven years later, he had changed his mind: "The mode of rising is not absolutely pathognomic, because it is present in other diseases which cause a gradual weakening of the extensors of the knee, but such gradual paralysis is exeedingly rare in early life, from any other cause." Since then, Gowers' sign has been described in other muscle diseases beginning with weakness in the pelvic girdle (especially Becker's type muscular dystrophy and limb-girdle dystrophy), in proximal ascending "pseudo-myopathic" diseases such as some spinal muscular atrophies, and in several subacute and chronic polymyositides. However, in the large majority of cases it indicates Duchenne's muscular dystrophy, and little of any fundamental importance has been added to Gowers's observations and explanations since.

Although Duchenne observed and described the phenomenon before him, Gowers was the first to give a full description of the sign and its variants, and the first to realize its diagnostic importance in other proximal myopathies. Moreover, Gowers was the first to note several important features of Duchenne's muscular dystrophy, for which Gowers' sign is so characteristic. He clearly described the predilection of males and noted that both parents were characteristically normal. He also noted that male relatives on the mother's side were affected with a similar illness.

Should one follow Gowers's advice then, and change this eponym for a descriptive term, for instance, the "leg-climbing sign"? Little would be gained. Leg-climbing sign would be as cryptic as Gowers' sign and have lost the implicit remembrance of one of the greatest clinicians in neurological history.

References

1. Gowers W R. Clinical lecture on pseudo-hypertrophic muscular paralysis. *Lancet.* 1879; 2:1–2, 37–39, 73–75, 113–116.
2. Critchley M. *Sir William Gowers 1845–1915; A Biographical Appreciation*. London: Heinemann; 1949.
3. Holmes G. Sir William Gowers at the National Hospital. *Br Med J.* 1951;2:1397–1399.
4. Kennedy F. William Gowers (1845–1915). In: Haymaker W, Schiller F, eds. *The Founders of Neurology.* 2nd ed. Springfield, Ill: Charles C Thomas; 1970.
5. Arts NJM. Introduction. In reprint of: Gowers W R. *The Border-Land of Epilepsy* (1907). Nijmegen: Arts & Boeve; 1995.
6. Mulholland R C. Sir William Gowers 1845–1915. *Spine.* 1996;21:1106–1110.
7. Sacks O W. Gowers' memory. *Neurology.* 1996;46:1467–1469.
8. Gowers W R. *A Manual of Diseases of the Nervous System.* London: Churchill; 1886–1888. Reprint: Nijmegen: Arts & Boeve; 1995.
9. Gowers W R. *A Manual and Atlas of Medical Ophthalmoscopy.* London: Churchill; 1879. Reprint of 3rd. ed. 1890: Nijmegen: Arts & Boeve; 1995.
10. Gowers W R. *The Diagnosis of Diseases of the Spinal Cord.* London: Churchill; 1880.
11. Pryse-Phillips W. *Companion to Clinical Neurology.* Boston: Little Brown, 1995.

12. Gowers W R. *Epilepsy and Other Chronic Convulsive Diseases.* London: Churchill; 1881. Reprint of US ed. 1885: Nijmegen: Arts & Boeve; 1994.
13. Phillips C G, Landau W M. Upper and lower motor neuron: the little old synecdoche that works. *Neurology.* 1990;40:884–886.
14. Fine E J, Soria E D, Paroski M W. Tremor studies in 1886 through 1889. *Arch Neurol.* 1990;47:337–340.
15. Gowers W R. *The Border-Land of Epilepsy.* London: Churchill; 1907. Reprint: Nijmegen: Arts & Boeve; 1995.

15

JACKSONIAN EPILEPSY

George K. York and Peter J. Koehler

The name of John Hughlings Jackson is associated with a form of focal seizure featuring the march of ictal movements through one side of the body, commonly beginning in the thumb. Hughlings Jackson also made important observations on aphasia and developed a theory of evolutionary neurophysiology which formed the basis of a practical model of bedside cerebral localization used in neurology and psychiatry.

John Hughlings Jackson was born in Green Hammerton, Yorkshire, on 4 April 1835, the youngest of five children. His father, Samuel Jackson, was a prosperous farmer and brewer who later suffered a severe financial crisis. His mother, Sarah Hughlings, was of Welsh descent. John Hughlings Jackson attended provincial schools in Green Hammerton and Nailsworth, Gloucestershire. At the age of 15 he was apprenticed to William Anderson, a physician in the city of York. After two years, he entered the York Medical School, where Anderson taught obstetrics.[1] Among his teachers was Thomas Laycock (1812–1876), who had an important influence on the young Jackson. Laycock had worked in France under the surgeon Alfred Armand Velpeau (1795–1867) and the pathologist Pierre Charles Alexandre Louis (1787–1872), inventor of the numerical method, or clinical statistics. In Göttingen he graduated summa cum laude in 1839. Laycock became professor in Edinburgh in 1855. He was an important connection between Hughlings Jackson and the French clinical–pathological method, and he kindled Hughlings Jackson's interest in neurophysiology.[2]

Jackson walked the wards at St. Bartholomew's Hospital in London in 1855, where he worked under the surgeon and pathologist James Paget (1814–1899). After qualifying as a Fellow of the Royal College of Surgeons and licentiate of the Royal College of Physicians and the Worshipful Society of Apothecaries, he returned to York to serve as resident medical officer at the York Dispensary until 1859.

In that year he returned to London and established his lifelong friendship with his fellow Yorkshireman Jonathan Hutchinson (1828–1913), who dissuaded Hughlings Jackson from abandoning his medical career for a life in literary philosophy and helped him to obtain his first hospital appointment at the Royal London Ophthalmic Hospital (Moorfields Eye Hospital), where both made important ophthalmological observations.[3]

In 1862 Hughlings Jackson was appointed to the National Hospital for the Paralysed and Epileptic, which had been established in 1859 and whose founding physicians were Jabez S. Ramskill (1825–1897) and Charles-Edouard Brown-Séquard (1817–1894).[4] Jackson was influenced by Brown-Séquard, who published extensively on epilepsy during this period and was among the first to treat it with bromide. Though there is no direct evidence that Brown-Séquard introduced into England the new ideas of his friend Paul Broca (1824–1880) on the localization of aphasia, he did teach Hughlings Jackson to distinguish between defects of articulation and language. An early case report attributed the following to Hughlings Jackson:

> But then, as was frequently pointed out at this Hospital by Dr. Brown-Séquard the defect is not one of talking, but rather of language . . . In some extreme cases Dr. Brown-Séquard used to point out that the patient had lost altogether the power of expression, not by oral language only, but even by making signs.[5]

In 1865 Hughlings Jackson married his cousin Elizabeth Dade Jackson, author of children's stories. In May 1876 she died childless of an illness characterized by partial seizures, possibly septic cerebral thrombophlebitis, complicating pregnancy.

Edward Farquhar Buzzard (1871–1945) depicted Jackson as follows:

> I remember him in those days as the generous, kind-hearted but rather grave family friend or pseudo-uncle whose mind seemed to be in a state of constant conflict between his desire to give pleasure and his fear of being bored or bound.[6]

Others portray him as quiet, modest, serious, and shy. He did not like physical exercise. Being of restless disposition, he could not endure boredom. He rarely stayed until the end of a dinner, left the theater at the end of the first act of a play, and entered medical lectures when the discussion started. He suffered from migraine, vertigo, and deafness. He died of pneumonia on 7 October 1911 and is buried at Highgate Cemetery in London.

Hughlings Jackson was an early advocate of evolutionary neurophysiology. His evolutionary principles were originally derived from the Estonian embryologist Karl Ernst von Baer (1792–1876), who characterized ontogeny as a progression from a homogeneous, simple, unspecialized state to a heterogeneous, complex, specialized state. The English popular philosopher Herbert Spencer (1820–1903) recast von Baer's embryological law as a general scientific principle applicable to biology, psychology, and sociology. He postulated that organs, living beings, and societies share a hierarchical organization with simple and homogeneous structures evolving into complex, heterogeneous, and interconnected structures. Hughlings Jackson, in turn, applied these principles to clinical neurology, expressing the

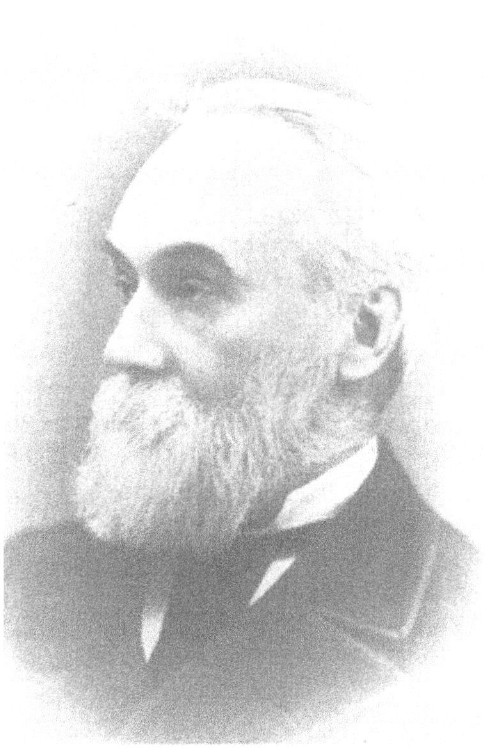

Figure 15–1. John Hughlings Jackson (1835–1911). From J. Hughlings Jackson, Neurological Fragments, Oxford: Oxford Univ. Press, 1925.

pathophysiology of the nervous system as the reverse of evolution, which he termed dissolution. He wrote:

> The doctrine of evolution daily gains new adherents. It is not simply synonymous with Darwinism. Herbert Spencer applies it to all orders of phenomena . . . I have long thought that we shall be very much helped in our investigations of diseases of the nervous system by considering them as reversals of evolution, that is, dissolution. Dissolution is a term I take from Spencer as a name for the reverse of the process of evolution.[7]

Hughlings Jackson was, above all, a practical physician, and he developed clinically useful methods of bedside cerebral localization. He regarded the nervous system as an exclusively sensorimotor hierarchy composed of three evolutionary levels. The lowest level was assumed to be located in the spinal cord, medulla oblongata, and pons, representing the most simple movements. The middle level was situated in the cerebral cortex and possibly also the corpus striatum, re-representing the movements of the lower level in more complex patterns. The highest level, located in the prefrontal cortex, "re-re-represents" movements, which are most complex at this level. Each element, or center, of each level contains a complete representation of the next lower level, but each center is uniquely related to a particular body part. The function of each center follows Spencerian evolutionary principles in being more organized, voluntary, complex, differentiated, and specialized than the function of a lower center. People with dissolution of the nervous system exhibit symptoms which are less complex, less specialized, and less voluntary than normal subjects. Patients with diseases of higher centers develop two types of symptoms, negative symptoms due to the loss of function of the controlling superior center and positive symptoms due to the emergence of lower centers. Positive symptoms are simpler and less differentiated than the negative symptoms, which they replace.[8]

The utility of Jacksonian cerebral localization can be seen in his theory of epilepsy.[9] According to Hughlings Jackson, epileptic discharges can have their origin at any evolutionary level. Discharges at the lowest level resulted, among other things, in spinal attacks, including the attacks that Brown-Séquard elicited in his experimental animals.[10] The discharges may spread vertically to other levels, or horizontally to other centers at the same level. Attacks in which partial discharges march horizontally across the middle level, which we now consider the primary motor cortex, bear the eponym "Jacksonian epilepsy."

The work for which Hughlings Jackson's name is immortalized was published between December 1867 and December 1868. In the 21 December 1867 edition of the *Medical Times and Gazette* he wrote:

> Then in unilateral convulsions the "aura" nearly always begins in the hand; sometimes, however, in the side of the face, and rarely in the leg. So the speculation is that, although each movement is everywhere represented, there are points where particular movements are specially represented.[11]

In August 1868 he claimed that this somatotopic representation occurred in the corpus striatum and thalamus. His description and interpretation of the Jacksonian march was published 19 December 1868:

> I think the mode of beginning makes a great difference as to the march of the fit. When the fit begins in the face, the convulsion in involving the arm may *go down* the limb . . . When the fit begins in the leg, the convulsion marches up; when the leg is affected after the arm, the convulsion marches *down* the leg.[12]

In his 1870 *Study of Convulsions,* he proposed that the Jacksonian march suggested somatotopic representation on the cortex in the region of the corpus striatum.[13] His observations were dramatically validated by the 1870 experiments of Gustav Theodor Fritsch (1838–1891) and Eduard Hitzig (1838–1907), which demonstrated that focal galvanic stimulation of different parts of the cortex in dogs evoked movement in different parts of the body. The later work of David Ferrier (1843–1929) confirmed the existence of somatotopic representation in the cortex.

The importance of the Jacksonian march to clinical neurophysiology lies in its unambiguous demonstration of the somatotopic representation of the body in the brain. Hemiparesis and unilateral convulsions can be considered reciprocal processes, the first caused by destroying (negative), the second by discharging (positive) lesions of the same tissue. The march of ictal movements through the body recapitulates the sequence that parts of the body are represented in both the corpus striatum and the cortex. The Jacksonian march disproved the theory that all parts of the nervous system are functionally equipotential and validated the clinical concept that analysis of the temporal development of a focal neurological deficit is diagnostically useful. The knowledge of somatotopic representation allowed the astute neurologist to predict the presence of focal pathology in the nervous system with tolerably consistent accuracy.

The term "Jacksonian epilepsy" was first used by Jean-Martin Charcot (1825–1893). Charcot noted that Louis-François Bravais (1801–1842) had described the phenomenon in 1827, a priority which Hughlings Jackson accepted.[14] Charcot wrote:

> Mais dans ces derniers temps, un savant anglais, Mr. Jackson de Londres, est revenu sur ce sujet et il a traité la question d'une façon si particulière qu'il m'est arrivé quelquefois d'appeler cette affection l'épilepsie Jacksonienne et le nom lui en est resté . . . l'étude de Mr. Jackson est si importante que véritablement il méritait bien d'attacher son nom à cette découverte.[15]

[But lately, an English scholar, Mr. Jackson of London, came back on this subject, and he discussed the issue in a way so particular that it sometimes happened to me to call that disorder Jacksonian epilepsy and the name remained associated ever since . . . Mr. Jackson's study is so important that he really deserves his name to remain connected with this discovery.]

Charcot proposed the eponym "Bravais–Jackson" be used as an alternative: "*ce sera plus juste; il est vrai que ce serait un peu long!*"[15] [It will be more fair; it is true that it would be somewhat long!]. Posterity, however, has settled on the eponym "Jacksonian epilepsy." Richard Bright (1789–1858) and Robert Bentley Todd (1809–1860) had also described patients with a march of focal seizures prior to Hughlings Jackson.[16,17]

Hughlings Jackson made other important observations about epilepsy. He described the epileptic discharge as an "occasional, sudden, excessive, rapid, and local discharge of grey matter." Using this concept of the epileptic discharge, he demonstrated that the mechanisms of focal and generalized seizures were not essentially different. Although many of Hughlings Jackson's contemporaries did not consider partial seizures to be epileptic, he maintained that all epileptic seizures were the result of discharges originating in pathologically changed tissue in the central nervous system. He rejected the generally accepted theory that generalized epilepsy was a reflex from the medulla oblongata, evoked by certain peripheral stimuli, or "unfelt irritations."

The use of the eponym Jacksonian epilepsy to denote the march of ictal movements through the rolandic cortex is widespread throughout the English-speaking world. The 1981 International Classification of Epileptic Seizures lists Jacksonian seizures as a type of partial simple seizure.[18] Twentieth-century textbooks of neurology use the eponym to describe the same phenomenon that Hughlings Jackson observed, and they attribute to it the same significance, making the eponym a deserving tribute to a seminal neurologist. The eponym *Epilepsie Jacksonienne,* Jacksonian epilepsy, applied by Charcot for the first time, is still frequently used, in a deserving tribute to a distinguished neuroscientist.

References

1. Critchley M, Critchley E A. *John Hughlings Jackson: Father of English Neurology.* Oxford: Oxford University Press; 1998.

2. Greenblatt S H. The major influences on the early life and work of John Hughlings Jackson. *Bull Hist Med.* 1965;39:346–376.
3. Hutchinson J. Obituary. John Hughlings Jackson, M.D., F.R.C.P., F.R.S. *Br Med J.* 1911;2:952.
4. Holmes G. *The National Hospital Queen Square: 1860–1948.* Edinburgh: Livingstone; 1954.
5. Hughlings Jackson J. Clinical remarks on hemiplegia, with loss of speech in its association with valvular disease of the heart. *Medical Times and Gazette.* 1864;1:123.
6. Buzzard E F. Hughlings Jackson and his influence on neurology. *Lancet.* 1934;2:909–913.
7. Hughlings Jackson J. Evolution and dissolution of the nervous system. Croonian Lectures delivered at the Royal College of Physicians, March 1884. *Lancet.* 1884;1:555–558, 649–652, 739–744.
8. York G K, Steinberg D A. Hughlings Jackson's theory of cerebral localization. *J Hist Neurosci.* 1993:3:153–168.
9. Temkin O. *The Falling Sickness: A history of Epilepsy from the Greeks to the Beginnings of Modern Neurology.* 2nd ed, rev. Baltimore: Johns Hopkins University Press; 1971.
10. Koehler P J. Brown-Séquard's spinal epilepsy. *Med Hist.* 1994;38:189–203.
11. Hughlings Jackson J. Remarks on the disorderly movements of chorea and convulsion. *Medical Times and Gazette.* 1867;2:669–670.
12. Hughlings Jackson J. Notes on the physiology and pathology of the nervous system. *Medical Times and Gazette.* 1868;2:696.
13. Hughlings Jackson J. *A study of convulsions.* London: John Churchill and Sons; 1870: 162–204. (St. Andrews Medical Graduates' Association. Transactions, 1869)
14. Bravais L.-F. *Recherches sur les symptômes et le traitment de l'épilepsie hémiplégique.* Paris: Didot le Jeune; 1827. Thèse de Paris no. 118.
15. Charcot J M. *Leçons du mardi à la Salpêtrière.* Paris: Delahaye & Lecrosnier; 1887:15.
16. Bright R. *Reports of Medical Cases.* P 2. London: Longman; 1831;2:538.
17. Todd R B. *Clinical Lectures on Paralysis, Certain Diseases of the Brain, and Other Affections of the Nervous System.* London: Churchill; 1856:395.
18. Commission on Classification and Terminology of the International League against Epilepsy. Proposal for revised clinical and electroencephalographic classification of epileptic seizures. *Epilepsia.* 1981;22:489.

16

TODD'S PARALYSIS

John B. Lyons

Robert Bentley Todd was born in Dublin on 9 April 1809. His immediate ancestors had settled in the west of Ireland. His paternal grandfather was a surgeon and apothecary in Sligo, from which coastal town his father, Charles Hawkes Todd, moved to Dublin for apprenticeship in 1797, obtaining the Letters Testimonial, or license, of the Royal College of Surgeons in Ireland (RCSI) in 1803. Charles remained in the Irish capital and married Elizabeth Bentley. They had 15 children, all of whom survived to adult life. There were nine sons and six daughters; four of the former entered the medical profession; three became clergymen; one a barrister-at-law; one a solicitor.

Charles and Elizabeth's second son's name incorporated the maternal surname, Bentley. Todd père was surgeon to the House of Industry Hospitals, an editor of the *Dublin Hospital Reports,* and professor of anatomy and surgery in the RCSI, where he held the office of president in 1821. He died on 19 March 1826, at the early age of 44, by which time Robert was reading for the bar.[1]

After his father's death, Todd was advised to change to medicine, because of straitened family circumstances. He entered the RCSI (where he was charged no fees) and graduated LRCSI (licentiate) in 1831. Without delay he moved to London but, as he boasted in later years, he was "without a sixpence to help himself."[2] He managed to complete a couple of terms at Oxford University, and was granted its M.B. in 1833. A bright future lay ahead: a lectureship in anatomy and physiology at the Aldersgate Medical School was followed by his appointment to the chair of physiology and morbid anatomy at King's College, with an intervening period of two years teaching at the Westminster Medical School. In addition to academic excellence—he was B.A., Trinity College, Dublin (1829); LRCSI (1831); M.A. (1832) and D.M. (1836) Oxon; Fellow, Royal College of Physicians (1837); Fellow of the Royal Society (1838); Fellow, Royal College of Surgeons (1844)—he displayed a flair and capacity for administration. He held clinical appointments at the Western Dispensary and the

Royal Hospital for Children, and he was physician to King's College Hospital (1839–1859), of which he was one of the founders. The massive *Cyclopaedia of Anatomy and Physiology,* which he edited, was said to have done a great deal to encourage and advance the study of contemporary physiology and comparative and microscopic anatomy.

Todd was concerned, too, about low nursing standards. The problem, he decided, must be attacked at its roots. Education and clinical training under residential conditions were required, and with this in mind he planned the Training Institution for Nurses for Hospitals, Families and Sick Poor, a name shortened to St. John's House at its foundation in July 1848.

This gifted man was fated to die suddenly, his life swept away in his Brook Street consulting room by a torrential gastric hemorrhage secondary to hepatic cirrhosis, on 20 January 1860. He was survived by his widow, to whom he left about £14,000, the residue to be divided equally by their son and three daughters.[3] He was buried in Kensal Green Cemetery, London.

James Collier (1870–1935), physician to the National Hospital, Queen Square, judged him to be the United Kingdom's greatest clinical neurologist prior to Hughlings Jackson.[4] The terms "afferent" and "efferent" were coined by Todd in the *Cyclopedia of Anatomy and Physiology,* which also contains what Sir William Gowers (1845–1915; see Chapter 14) regarded as the first account of tabes dorsalis. The phenomenon of post-ictal paralysis observed by Todd is spoken of as "Todd's paralysis."

Figure 16–1. Robert Bentley Todd (1809–1860). Courtesy Royal College of Surgeons in Ireland.

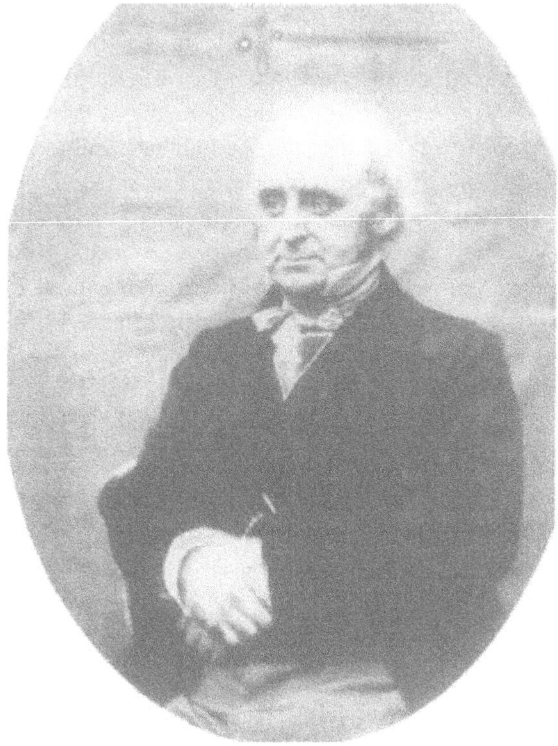

We find the original description of postictal paralysis in Todd's Lumleian Lectures delivered before the Royal College of Physicians in 1849. He spoke on convulsive disorders, under which rubric he discussed chorea, tetanus, and epilepsy.[5]

He saw epilepsy as a disease

> characterized mainly by the occurrence at intervals sometimes remarkably uniform in duration, of attacks of loss of consciousness, frequently sudden, often preceded by some kind of warning. These attacks last for a longer or shorter interval, when the patient recovers, as if awaking from sleep, but continues in a drowsy state for a variable term.

He described auras, including the olfactory aura "in the case mentioned by Heberden, where a smell of musk ushered in the attack." The fit is usually generalized but may predominate, or be confined to, one or the other side. Fits sometimes cease spontaneously, and Todd points out that many so-called remedies for epilepsy have acquired the credit of curing the disease, through being given in a case in which the spontaneous tendency to recovery was effective:

> A paralytic state [he wrote] remains sometimes after the epileptic convulsion. This is more particularly the case when the convulsion has affected only one side or one limb: that limb or limbs will remain paralytic for some hours, or even days, after the cessation of the paroxysm, *but it will ultimately perfectly recover.*[5(p668)] (Emphasis added)

Illustrative examples are not given, but what became known as "Todd's paralysis" is discussed more fully in his *Clinical Lectures.* The cases of "epileptic hemiplegia" presented at King's College Hospital in the early 1850s include a 10-year-old boy, a 26-year-old laborer, a 29-year-old woman, and several others. The boy's fits were confined to the right side, "and after each, the patient was distinctly paralysed on that side, with relaxed muscles . . . The paralysis was of motion only, and was not complete, a slight amount of power remaining."[6(p782)]

Mary A. Goodbody, aged 29, developed a left-sided weakness and the paralyzed parts "had their sentient power very much diminished." She left hospital perfectly well seven weeks later. Ellen Biddlecomb, aged 24, had convulsions followed by paralysis of the left arm with pain in the affected limb. It recovered in two days. Detailed protocols in the *Clinical Lectures* reveal that recovery was not infrequently imperfect.

The laborer's right-sided weakness had not improved for 18 months prior to his admission, "but became worse after each fit and recovered to a certain point before the next." Todd states: "In that form of hemiplegia which is associated with *epileptic fits,* the prognosis is not in general satisfactory."[6(p783)]

Alexander Robertson of Glasgow reported (1869) some cases of unilateral convulsions followed by paralysis and observed:

> I am inclined to think that the late Dr Todd was correct in supposing that severe and protracted convulsions may themselves, in some instances, be causative of palsy of a few hours' or days' duration through simply the exhausting influence exerted on the cells of the central ganglia, without much, if any, appreciable change of tissue.[7]

One of Robertson's cases displayed severe infantile hemiplegia with a shriveled, useless arm; the only patient submitted by him to autopsy had severe traumatic epilepsy, but the extent of the cerebral pathology went unrecognized.

Writing in the *West Riding Lunatic Asylum Medical Reports* (1876) John Hughlings Jackson stated:

> When the discharge has ceased and the convulsion is over, we very often find paralysis . . . For example after a convulsion beginning unilaterally, there is very often hemiplegia. Hemiplegia so occurring was called Epileptic Hemiplegia by Dr Todd.[8]

Jackson attributed the paralysis to "temporary exhaustion . . . of the nervous centres in which the discharge began," an explanation which he designated "Todd and Robertson's Hypothesis."

Jackson said:

> It is understood, of course, that we are speaking of paralysis following seizures which we may call chronic . . . We speak of cases such as those in which a small tumour or other "foreign body" in the mid-cortical region of the brain leads to instability of cells near it—leads to what I have called a "discharging lesion;" the cells rendered unstable occasionally "explode" or liberate much energy, or, in other words, discharge excessively, and all of them much more nearly simultaneously than the comparatively stable cells do in health. After their excessive discharge has ceased, as signified by cessation of spasm, there often is paralysis, and that paralysis is temporary."[9]

Gowers said:

> Loss of motor power, paralysis, may succeed a fit of epileptic type—post convulsive paralysis . . . It is most distinct after unilateral convulsions (and constitutes the "epileptic hemiplegia of Todd"), but the general prostration after a bilateral convulsion is probably analogous. After a severe fit it may be due to exhaustion of the nerve-elements, but the transient palsy that succeeds a very slight fit must be ascribed to inhibition of the motor centres.[10]

Despite the eponym's long-established currency, it is pardonable to ask "What is Todd's paralysis?" Wilson believed that differing opinions were held "in regard to its frequency, nature and importance."[11] I have, therefore, collected descriptions from the modern literature. They are typified by the account given by Lord Brain:

> Jacksonian convulsions are usually associated with permanent weakness of the part of the body which is the focus of the fit, but after each convulsion there is often a temporary extension of this weakness to other parts (Todd's paralysis).[12]

Houston Merritt wrote:

> Transient hemiparesis (Todd's paralysis) following a jacksonian, local or generalized seizure is more common in patients with a tumour than in those having convulsive seizures caused by any other condition.[13]

Gastaut and Broughton stressed the importance of distinguishing transient postictal paralysis (Todd's paralysis) from unilateral atonic seizures and from somatic inhibitory seizures.[14] O'Donohoe mentions "a short-lived hemiparesis (Todd's paralysis)," which he appears to associate with partial epilepsy. "Its resolution may be followed by the persistence of minimal neurological signs on the affected side."[15(p96)] Adams and Victor refer to unilateral seizures followed by "a Todd's paralysis lasting several hours to days" and to the increased weakness seen postictally in infantile hemiplegia.[16]

One should perhaps ask if some of Todd's cases of "hemiplegic epilepsy" were not really examples of transient cerebral ischemia. This suspicion is supported by Meyer and Portnoy, who write: "We wish to emphasize . . . that impaired circulation of the brain predisposes the individual to postepileptic paralysis."[17] Todd had argued to the contrary, holding that

> many of the cases of sudden loss of consciousness, followed by hemiplegia, which are popularly and even medically described as "apoplectic fits" are of the epileptic nature.[18(p789)]

Case CCIX, however, is described by Todd with rare equivocation: "In this case the attacks, although not strictly epileptic in nature, were undoubtedly of that character."

An investigative study of postictal paralysis in nine patients with experimental data from monkeys has shown that the phenomenon results from temporary neuronal anoxia.[17(p184)] This claims to be a more specific confirmation of Todd's own conclusion: the exaltation of the nervous force causing the fit is followed by "a state of depression or exhaustion, not only in the parts primarily affected, but in parts of the brain in connection with them."[18(p791)] More recently Robert Effron has questioned the acceptability of Meyer and Portnoy's evidence. He argues that Todd's paralysis is inhibitory rather than due to postictal exhaustion, an explanation originally offered by Gowers.[19]

Those modern authors who associate postictal paralysis with partial epilepsy, possibly accompanied by some slight permanent impairment of motor function, appear to give a faithful representation of Todd's clinical viewpoint as represented in the *Clinical Lectures.* Jackson wished to ensure that the results of structural lesions were not confused with the manifestations of disordered neurophysiology. It is difficult, however, to accept either inhibition or exhaustion lasting for weeks or months.

That vasospasm may account for "the milder and transient postictal hemiparesis" and occlusion of cerebral arteries resulting in irreversible postictal hemiplegia has been recently suggested by O'Donohoe.[15(p60)]

In a recent Japanese study, technetium-99m-hexamethylpropylene-amineoxime single-photon emission computed tomography was performed in two patients with Todd's paralysis following prolonged hemiconvulsions. Cerebral hyperperfusion was noted.[20]

Recalling that Bravais described epileptic hemiplegia in a thesis submitted in 1827 to the University of Paris, Goldblatt[21] questions Todd's priority, but Jefferson has long since tipped the scales in Todd's favor by his comments on Bravais's work:

> It is clear [Jefferson wrote] that he [Bravais] has no conception of any physiological basis for the epileptic seizures . . . His intention, indeed, was to define a variety of epilepsy which he thought to be more curable . . . than the generalized sort, and

his method of cure was by the use of vesiculatory applications (especially cantharides) circularly around the distal portion of the limb that led in the attack.[22]

References

1. Cameron Sir C. *History of the Royal College of Surgeons in Ireland.* Dublin: Fannin; 1916:437.
2. Lyons J B. Some contributions of Robert Bentley Todd. *J Hist Neurosci.* 1998;7:11–26.
3. McIntyre N. Robert Bentley Todd. *King's Coll Gazette.* 1956;35:79–91, 184–198.
4. Collier J. Inventions and the outlook in neurology. *Lancet.* 1934;2:855–859.
5. Todd R B. On the pathology and treatment of convulsive diseases. *London Medical Gazette.* 1849;8:661–671, 724–729, 766–772, 815–822, 837–846.
6. Todd R B. *Clinical Lectures.* 2nd ed. London: Churchill; 1861.
7. Robertson A. On unilateral convulsions, localizations, etc. *Edinb Med J.* 1869;15:513–523.
8. Jackson J H. On epilepsies and on the after effects of epileptic discharges. *West Riding Lunatic Hospital Reports.* 1876;6:266–309.
9. Jackson, J H. On temporary paralysis after epileptiform and epileptic discharges. *Brain.* 1881;3:433–451.
10. Gowers W R. *A Manual of Diseases of the Nervous System.* London: Churchill; 1893:743.
11. Wilson SAK. *Neurology.* London: Butterworth; 1955;3:1624.
12. Brain W R. *Diseases of the Nervous System.* London: Oxford University Press; 1955:258.
13. Merritt H. *Textbook of Neurology.* London: Kimpton; 1963:231.
14. Gastaut H. Broughton R. *Epileptic Seizures.* Springfield, Ill: Charles C Thomas; 1972:238.
15. O'Donohoe N V. *Epilepsies of Childhood.* London: Butterworth; 1979.
16. Adams R, Victor M. *Principles of Neurology.* New York: McGraw-Hill; 1985:246.
17. Meyer J S Portnoy H D. Postepileptic paralysis. *Brain.* 1959;82:162–185.
18. Todd R B. *Clinical Lectures.* London: Churchill; 1860.
19. Efron R. Post-epileptic paralysis. *Brain.* 1961;84:381–394.
20. Kimura M, Sejima H, Ozasa H, Yamaguchi, S. Technetium-99m-HMPAO SPECT in patients with hemiconvulsions followed by Todd's paralysis. *Pediatr Radiol.* 1998;28:92–94.
21. Goldblatt D. Great names of our profession. *Semin Neurol.* 1986;6:332–335.
22. Jefferson G. Jacksonian epilepsy. *Post-Grad Med.* 1935;11:150–162.

17

LHERMITTE'S SIGN

Jos A. M. Frederiks

Lhermitte's sign consists of the sensation of a lightning discharge of electrically experienced paresthesias running down the spine into the legs and less often also into the arms; it is provoked by bending the neck. Lhermitte described his sign in patients with multiple sclerosis in 1924. History teaches, however, that Lhermitte's sign is not pathognomic for multiple sclerosis. Moreover, it had been described earlier by other investigators. In fact, Lhermitte's sign was "décrite par Pierre Marie et baptisée par Babinski"[1] [described by Pierre Marie and baptised by Babinski]. Basically, the phenomenon is not really a "sign" but a symptom, an experience, expressed as a characteristic complaint of the patient.

Jean Lhermitte was born in Mont-Saint-Père, a village near Château-Thierry, France, on 20 January 1877. Following his primary education in St. Étienne, he studied medicine in Paris. Maurice Klippel (1858–1942), Fulgence Raymond (1844–1910), Georges Hayem (1841–1933), and Pierre Marie (1853–1940) were among his teachers.[2,3] Jean Lhermitte was rather short, always well-groomed, and charming. His colleagues and his students knew him as a warm-hearted and friendly man. Notwithstanding his loquacity, he was an attentive listener. Conversations with Lhermitte were always enriched by his profound knowledge of many fields of science and art. His marriage was blessed with a son and a daughter. He died, peacefully, in his sleep, in 1959.[2–4]

Following his graduation in 1907, he soon became well-known as a prominent clinician and thorough neuropathological investigator in France and abroad. He was clinical director of the Salpêtrière and one of the founders of modern neuropsychology together with well-known pupils such as Julian de Ajuriaguerra and Henry Hécaen. His well-known son was the Paris neurologist François Lhermitte, who died in 1998. Jean Lhermitte wrote many papers and books. He wrote authoritatively on the frontiers of psychiatry, psychology, and even mysticism (partly inspired by his

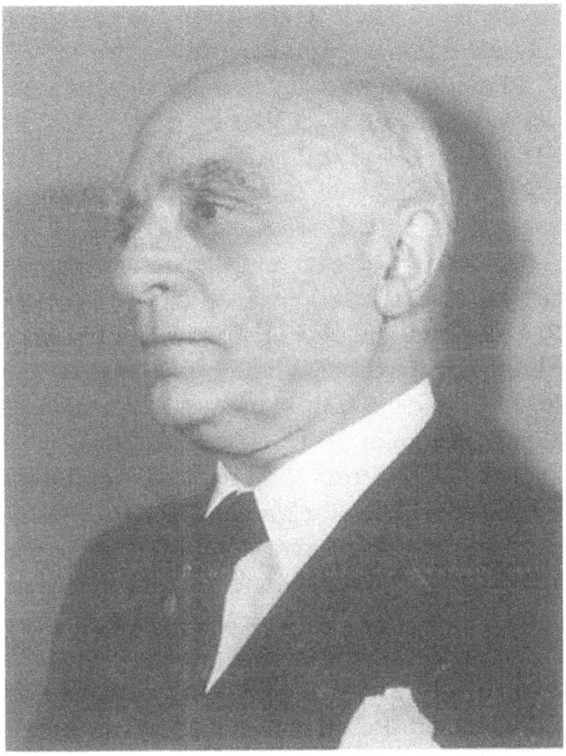

Figure 17–1. Jean Lhermitte (1877–1959). Courtesy of the late Prof. François Lhermitte.

deeply religious conviction). "If there was ever such an entity as neuropsychiatry, Jean Lhermitte was its High Priest."[4]

One of his first well-known works (originally published as his thesis) was *La Section totale de la Moelle dorsale* (1919). Many neurological, neuropsychiatric, and neuropsychological publications followed. Some of the most important monographs are *Paraplégie des Vieillards, Les Psychonévroses de Guerre* (with Gustave Roussy) (1917), *Les Blessures de la Moelle et de la Queue de Cheval* (1918), *Les Fondements biologiques de la Psychologie* (1925), *Le Sommeil* (1928), *Les Mécanismes du Cerveau* (1938), *L'Image de nôtre Corps* (1939), *La Psychopathologie de la Vision* (with de Ajuriaguerra) (1941), *Les Rêves* (1941), *Le Cerveau et la Pensée* (1951), *Les Hallucinations* (1951), *Mystiques et faux Mystiques* (1952), *Vrais et faux Possédés* (1956), and *Le Problème des Miracles* (1956).

Although well-known by the eponymous symptom, his name is also associated with the syndrome of anterior internuclear ophthalmoplegia (Lhermitte's syndrome) and with Lhermitte–Duclos disease (dysplastic cerebellar gangliocytoma).

Lhermitte described his sign in three patients suffering from multiple sclerosis in 1924 and 1927.[5,6] One of these patients gave the following description:

> Lorsque je baissais la tête, je ressentais une secousse violente dans la nuque et une douleur ressemblant à celle que produit un courant électrique me parcourait tout le corps, depuis la nuque jusqu'aux pieds, en suivant la colonne vertébrale.

[When I bent the head, I felt a violent shock in the neck and a pain like an electric current running through the whole body, from the neck down the vertebral column into the feet.] The occurrence of the sign does not depend on the position of the body and it may be experienced by active as well as passive bending of the neck.[7]

Lhermitte was not the first investigator writing on the subject. The very first description, by Marie and Chatelin in 1917, describes it in patients with head injury.[7] In 1918, Babinski and Dubois mentioned the phenomenon in patients suffering neck injury.[8] In fact, Bereil and Devic (1918) were the first authors describing the phenomenon in multiple sclerosis.[9]

Guided by Babinski and Lhermitte, Jean Ribeton published a thesis (1919) on the symptom following neck injury in 13 patients.[10] However, not until Lhermitte's 1924 paper did the phenomenon become recognized as an important manifestation of multiple sclerosis.[5] Although the association with multiple sclerosis still exists—it may be one of the early symptoms—Lhermitte's sign may be present in a number of other afflictions of the cervical spinal cord.

The phenomenon soon became important in neurological practice and was associated with Lhermitte's name around 1930. A new eponym was born! The publications by Alajouanine[1] and McAlpine[11] broadened the reputation of the sign. Today, Lhermitte's sign is mentioned in practically all neurological textbooks and handbooks, in specific publications on multiple sclerosis, and in oncological literature.

Lhermitte's sign was first reported in patients with traumatic cervical cord disorders. Alajouanine et al. concluded that Lhermitte's sign is not pathognomic for multiple sclerosis and presented case histories of its occurrence in atlantoaxial subluxation, tumor, disc hernia, and arachnoiditis.[1] Lhermitte pointed to the possibility of causes other than multiple sclerosis, but the sign has often been described as occurring in multiple sclerosis.[5,9,11–14] Less frequently, the sign has been described in the following conditions: subacute combined degeneration of the spinal cord (vitamin B_{12} deficiency), cervical injury, cervical radiation myelopathy, cervical cisplatin myelopathy.[15] And the sign is sporadically mentioned in cervical (sporadically thoracal) disc hernia, cervical spondylosis, cervical (sporadically thoracal) tumor, herpes zoster, arachnoiditis, pyridoxine intoxication, cystinuria, bone marrow transplantation, Behçet's disease, nitrous oxide intoxication, and chemotherapy with docetaxel. A disorder of the cervical spinal cord, including demyelination of the dorsal columns, is present in most of these disorders.[15] The lesion is mostly located at the cervical, rarely at the thoracic level.[16–19] Demyelination of the posterior column is always present.[12]

Lhermitte's sign is often seen in patients with multiple sclerosis. The occurrence of Lhermitte's sign in young people without a history of cervical injury, chemotherapy, or radiation therapy raises the suspicion of multiple sclerosis.[12] The symptom may occur early in the disease when no other signs are present. For this reason, Lhermitte's sign has great diagnostic significance.

The striking similarity of the descriptions given by all patients who experience Lhermitte's sign strongly suggests a common genesis. The patients always describe the symptom as lightning and "electrical" ("electric shock"), lasting at most two seconds.[12]

From the beginning, Lhermitte presented clinicoanatomical arguments for his thesis that the phenomenon has its anatomical origin in the cervical *dorsal columns.*[4]

This view was confirmed later by clinicoanatomical studies in multiple sclerosis and other diseases;[1,12,20,21] electrophysiological and MRI data;[21,22] and demonstration of ipsilateral electric sensations elicited by direct mechanical stimulation of the dorsal columns during surgery under local anesthesia.[1]

Provocation of Lhermitte's sign by bending the neck—including bending of the neck involuntarily during laughing, coughing, sneezing, and bending the body—is characteristic.[12] But what is the significance of flexion of the neck in Lhermitte's sign? The cervical part of the spine is its most mobile part. When the neck is bent, the cervical part of the spine may elongate a few centimeters.[23] This causes *stretching* of the ligamenta denticulata and of the posterior columns.[1] Demyelination of dorsal column fibers probably produces enhanced excitability of the sensory nerves, making them sensitive to mechanical influences such as local pressure or stretch.[5,12,22–24] Demyelinated fibers "exhibit ectopic impulse generation, increased mechanosensitivity, abnormal interactions between fibers (cross-talk), and impulse reflection."[25] This increased excitability is not a negative symptom but must be considered a positive symptom.[23,26] It is in concurrence with the observation that Lhermitte's sign is not influenced by analgesics but is relieved by antiepileptic drugs including phenytoin and carbamazepine.[27,28]

It is understandable that Lhermitte's sign is often compared with Hoffmann–Tinel's sign (see Chapter 21) in lesions of peripheral nerves and with phosphenes elicited by eye movements in optic neuritis.[12]

Further use of the term "Lhermitte's sign" is deserved and justified. The eponym is now widely accepted, and the sign, "one of the best-known and most commonly used eponyms in the neurological literature,"[29] has—as an outstanding symptom of damage to cervical dorsal columns—appeared to be an important and welcome addition to neurological practice.[1,30]

References

1. Alajouanine T, Thurel R, Papaïoanou C. La douleur à type de décharge électrique, provoquée par la flexion de la tête et parcourant le corps de haut en bas. *Rev Neurol.* 1949;81: 89–87.
2. Mollaret P. Jean Lhermitte (1877–1959). *Rev Neurol.* 1959;100:131–132.
3. Pearce JMS. Jean Lhermitte 1877–1959. *J Neurol Neurosurg Psychiatry.* 1994;57:846.
4. Critchley, M. *The Ventricle of Memory: Personal Recollections of Some Neurologists.* New York: Raven Press; 1990.
5. Lhermitte J, Bollack J, Nicolas M. Les douleurs à type de décharge électrique consécutives à la flexion céphalique dans la sclérose en plaques. Un cas de forme sensitive de la sclérose multiple. *Rev Neurol.* 1924;31:56–62.
6. Lhermitte J, Levy G, Nicolas M. Les sensations de décharge électrique symptôme précoce de la sclérose en plaques. Clinique et pathogénie. *Presse Méd.* 1927;39:610–613.
7. Marie P, Chatelin C. Sur certains symptômes vraisemblablement d'origine radiculaire chez les blessés du crâne. *Rev Neurol.* 1917;31:336.
8. Babinski J, Dubois R. Douleurs à forme de décharge électrique consécutives aux traumatismes de la nuque. *Presse Méd.* 1918;26:64.
9. Bereil T, Devic E. Sur un cas de douleurs à type de décharge dans la sclérose en plaques. *Lyon Méd.* 1918;141:559.

10. Ribeton J. *Étude clinique des douleurs à forme de décharge électrique consécutives aux traumatismes de la nuque.* Paris: Faculté de Médicine; 1919. Thesis.
11. McAlpine D, Lumsden C E, Acheson E D. *Multiple Sclerosis: A Reappraisal.* Edinburgh: Livingstone; 1965:104.
12. Kanchandani R, Howe J G. Lhermitte's sign in multiple sclerosis: a clinical survey and review of the literature. *J Neurol Neurosurg Psychiatry.* 1982;45:308–312.
13. Lhermitte J. Multiple sclerosis: the sensation of an electrical discharge as an early symptom. *Arch Neurol Psychiatry.* 1929;22:5–8.
14. Poser C M. Onset symptoms of multiple sclerosis. *J Neurol Neurosurg Psychiatry.* 1995;58: 253–254.
15. Frederiks JAM. Het teken van Lhermitte. In: Koehler P J, Bruyn G W, Arts NJM, eds. *Het neurologisch Onderzoek in Eponiemen.* Nijmegen: Arts & Boeve; 1995:242–245; 292–294.
16. Jamieson DRS, Ballantyne J P. Unique presentation of a prolapsed thoracic disk: Lhermitte's symptom in a golf player. *Neurology.* 1995;45:1219–1921.
17. Ventafridda V, Caraceni A, Martini C, Sbanotto A, De Conno F. On the significance of Lhermitte's sign in oncology. *J Neuro-Oncol.* 1991;10:133–137.
18. Baldwin R N, Chadwick D. Lhermitte's "sign" due to thoracic cord compression. *J Neurol Neurosurg Psychiatry.* 1986;49:840–841.
19. Ongerboer de Visser B W. Het teken van Lhermitte bij thoracale wervelaandoeningen. *Ned Tijdschr Geneeskd.* 1980;124:390–392.
20. Gautier-Smith P C. Lhermitte's sign in subacute combined degeneration of the cord. *J Neurol Neurosurg Psychiatry.* 1973;36:861–863.
21. Gutrecht J A, Zamani A A, Salgado E D. Anatomic-radiologic basis of Lhermitte's sign in multiple sclerosis. *Arch Neurol.* 1993;50:849–851.
22. Nordin M, Nyström B, Wallin U, Hagbarth K E. Ectopic sensory discharges and paresthesiae in patients with disorders of peripheral nerves, dorsal roots and dorsal columns. *Pain.* 1984;20:231–245.
23. Smith K J, McDonald W I. Spontaneous and mechanically evoked activity due to central demyelinating lesion. *Nature.* 1980;286:154–155.
24. Waxman S G. Membranes, myelin, and the pathophysiology of multiple sclerosis. *N Engl J Med.* 1982;306:1529–1533.
25. Kocsis, J D. Waxman, S G. Demyelination: causes and mechanisms of clinical abnormality and functional recovery. In: Koetsier J C, ed. *Handbook of Clinical Neurology,* 47. *Demyelinating Diseases.* Amsterdam: Elsevier Science Publishers; 1985: ch 2.
26. Smith K J. Conduction properties of central demyelinated and remyelinated axons, and their relation to symptom production in demyelinating disorders. *Eye.* 1994;8:224–237.
27. Cambier J. Le signe de Lhermitte. *Presse Méd.* 1993;22:1611–1614.
28. Ekbom, K. Carbamazepine: a new symptomatic treatment for the paraesthesiae associated with Lhermitte's sign. *Z Neurol.* 1971;200:341–344.
29. Gutrecht J A. Lhermitte's sign: from observation to eponym. *Arch Neurol.* 1989;46:557–558.
30. Wilkins R H, Brody I A. Lhermitte's sign. In: *Neurological Classics.* New York: Johnson Reprint Corporation; 1973:111–113.

III

Reflexes and Other Tests

18

BABINSKI'S SIGN

Jan van Gijn

Europe was in turmoil in 1848. Revolts were rife. In Poland, nationalists fought against the foreign tyranny of Russia and Austria. Defeat upon defeat led a steady stream of refugees to Paris, at that time the hub of political and intellectual freedom. One of them was the engineer Alexandre Babinski. A few years later he married a compatriot, Henriette Weren. They were blessed with two children: in 1855 Henri, and in 1857 Joseph, the main hero of this essay. From 1862 Alexandre worked as a construction engineer in Peru. In 1870 he came back to enlist in the army of his adopted country in the war against Germany. From then on his health deteriorated—he suffered from Parkinson's disease—and it fell upon Henri, a mining engineer, to go abroad and support his parents and fund the medical education of his younger brother.

In the period of his residencies (1879–1885), Joseph performed morphological and microscopical studies, for the first and only time in his life. This work resulted in an article about the muscle spindle[1] and a thesis on multiple sclerosis.[2] In 1885, by a stroke of luck he became Jean-Martin Charcot's *chef de clinique,* without ever having served under him as a resident. He had submitted his thesis in a competition of the Paris hospitals, just missed the gold medal, but instead was offered the post as a kind of second prize. In those times, Charcot was deeply engaged in the study of hysteria. He regarded it as a localized, albeit functional disorder of the central nervous system. In Babinski's work, hysteria would also be a leading theme, though his approach was rather different. Charcot mainly used the case history as the key instrument in making a diagnosis, whereas Babinski came to rely more and more on assessment of the nervous system by means of extensive physical examination, an art he helped to develop.

Near the end of the 1880s, Joseph generated enough income to take his turn in supporting the family and to move to a more spacious apartment on the Boulevard

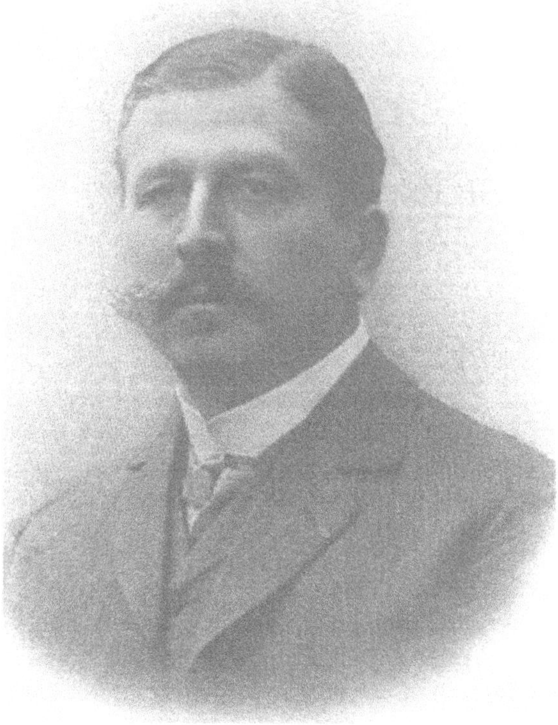

Figure 18–1. Joseph Babinski (1857–1932). Source: Académie de Médecine, Paris, France.

Hausmann. Henri returned from his foreign travels and gradually assumed the role of housekeeper. After the death of their parents (the mother in 1897 and the father in 1899), the two brothers would continue to inhabit the same apartment for another 30 years, in a close and harmonious relationship. Henri would serve as secretary, driver, and, above all, cook. Under the pseudonym Ali-Bab he published a tome on gastronomy that was as authoritative as it was weighty; it went through several editions.[3]

In 1892, Joseph failed in the competition for the rank of assistant professor (*professeur agrégé*). The examination was traditionally riddled with protection and intrigue, but in that year it developed into an outright scandal. The main culprit was Charles Bouchard (1837–1915), a former pupil of Charcot, now full professor and chairman of the jury. Bouchard, said to be consumed by ambition and envy, contrived to include all three pupils of his own among the five candidates who passed (from a total of 16). Neither a series of incensed articles in the *Progrès Médical* nor a petition to the responsible minister could reverse the outcome. Babinski never tried again; he became reconciled to the notion that an academic career was beyond his reach. Meanwhile (from 1890) he had left Charcot's Salpêtrière and started to practice in La Pitié, where he was nominated chief in 1895 and stayed until his retirement.

As was usual in those times, Babinski spent only mornings at the hospital; in the afternoon he would see private patients. He was tall, with steel blue eyes, thoughtful and deliberate in his words and gestures. The traditional ward round did not suit him—he preferred to have the patients brought in to him. Patients were already undressed on entering. The history was limited to a few laconic questions, soon followed by the most important part of the encounter—the neurological examination. It was especially objective signs he sought, elicited with pin, patella hammer, and electrical stimulator. All this took place in silence, occasionally interrupted by a brief comment. Then, rather abruptly, he would summon the next patient.

In 1922 Babinski retired, at the age of 65. Meanwhile he had been awarded many distinctions, especially from abroad. His successor, L. H. Vaquez (1860–1936), enabled him to continue a weekly clinical demonstration. He also continued to attend the monthly meeting of the French Neurological Society, which he had helped to found in 1899. In 1930 it became more difficult for him to move around; after Henri had died, in the autumn of 1931, he lost interest in life. He died on 29 October 1932. His friends and admirers buried him at the Polish cemetery in Montmorency.

The plantar reflex had been known to physicians since 1868, but only as a flexion synergy of the entire leg. Subsequently this flexion synergy was rediscovered a number of times, each time under a different name.[4] Sometimes movements of the toes were noted as part of the synergy, in one direction or another. The authors in question attached little importance to these observations, yet some later analysts would pass these off as prior discoveries.[5,6]

Babinski was the first to study the responses of the toes in a systematic fashion. His initial report was made in 1896, as an oral communication before the Société de Biologie (the Société de Neurologic would not be founded until three years later). Babinski's text is so concise and clear that it can be reproduced in full.

Sur le réflexe cutané plantaire dans certaines affections organiques du système nerveux central.

J'ai observé dans un certain nombre de cas d'hémiplégie ou de monoplégie crurale liée à une affection organique du système nerveux central une perturbation dans le réflexe cutané plantaire dont voici en quelques mots la description.

Du coté sain la piqûre de la plante du pied provoque, comme cela a lieu d'habitude à l'état normal, une flexion de la cuisse sur le bassin, de la jambe sur la cuisse, du pied sur la jambe et des orteils sur le métatarse.

Du côté paralysé une excitation semblable donne lieu aussi à une flexion de la cuisse sur le bassin, de la jambe sur la cuisse et du pied sur la jambe, *mais les orteils, au lieu de se fléchir, exécutent un mouvement d'extension sur le métatarse.* Il m'a été donné d'observer ce trouble dans des cas d'hémiplégie récente remontant à quelques jours seulement, ainsi que dans des cas d'hémiplégie spasmodique de plusieurs mois de durée; je l'ai constaté chez des malades qui étaient incapable de mouvoir volontairement les orteils, comme aussi sur des sujets qui pouvaient encore exécuter aux orteils des mouvements volontaires; mais je dois ajouter que ce trouble n'est pas constant.

J'ai aussi observé dans plusieurs cas de paraplégie crurale due à une lésion organique de la moelle un mouvement d'extension des orteils à la suite de la piqûre de la plante du pied, mais, comme en pareil cas, il n'y a pas chez le malade même de point de comparaison, la réalité d'un trouble est moins manifeste.

En résumé, le mouvement réflexe consécutif à la piqûre de la plante du pied peut subir dans les paralysies crurales reconnaissant pour cause une affection organique du système nerveux central non seulement, comme on le sait, une modification dans son intensité, mais aussi une perturbation dans sa forme.

On the cutaneous plantar reflex in certain organic disorders of the central nervous system. I have observed that in a certain number of cases of hemiplegia or lower limb monoplegia, related to an organic disorder of the central nervous system, there is a disturbance of the cutaneous plantar reflex which I shall describe in a few words.

On the healthy side, pricking of the sole provokes, as is usual in normal subjects, flexion of the thigh on the pelvis, of the leg on the thigh, of the foot on the leg, and of the toes upon the metatarsus.

On the paralyzed side a similar excitation also results in flexion of the thigh on the pelvis, of the leg on the thigh, and of the foot on the leg, *but the toes, instead of flexing, execute a movement of extension upon the metatarsus.* I have had the occasion to observe this trouble in cases of recent hemiplegia, the onset having been only a few days before, as well as in cases of spastic hemiplegia of several months' duration; I have found it in patients who were incapable of moving their toes voluntarily, as well as in subjects who could still make some voluntary movements with the toes; but I should add that this trouble is not constant.

I have also observed that in several cases of paraplegia of the lower limbs due to an organic lesion of the spinal cord an extensor movement of the toes occurs following a pin-prick in the sole of the foot, but, as there is no mode of comparison within the same patient, the true existence of an abnormality is less obvious.

In summary, the reflex movements following a pin-prick in the sole of the foot may, in paralysis of the lower limbs attributable to an organic disorder of the central nervous system, undergo not only, as is well known, a change in intensity, but also a disturbance in its form.

The discovery of the "toe phenomenon" was not a chance observation. Babinski had devoted himself to a systematic study of hemiplegic patients, with the aim of finding objective signs that were characteristic of organic disease and thereby could help in distinguishing this from hysterical hemiplegia. These efforts resulted in a large series of signs, of which the toe reflex was only one, though by far the most important. He first found the organic contracture of the hand.[7] The "toe phenomenon" was followed by papers describing hypotonia of the arm,[8] weakness of the platysma muscle,[9] involuntary hip flexion on rising from a supine position,[9] involuntary pronation of the arm,[10] and abnormal passive movements of the arm during movements of the trunk.[11]

In 1897, Babinski no longer associated the toe phenomenon with general disorders of the central nervous system, but more specifically with dysfunction of the pyramidal tract.[12] At the same time he drew a parallel with the plantar reflex in the newborn, in whom the pyramidal system was not yet fully developed. After another year he added a few clinical details to his original observations, this time in an article structured as a clinical demonstration.[13] First, he pointed out that in normal subjects the toes can remain *immobile* after stimulation of the sole of the foot. Second, it turned out that reflex extension of the toes was most easily elicited from the outer side of the sole, whereas it was the other way round for the normal flexor response of the toes. Finally, he had observed the abnormal response also in metabolic disorders (epilepsy, intoxication with strychnine) and in meningitis. In 1903, Babinski described abduction of the smaller toes on stimulation of the sole; the phenomenon was often but not always associated with pathological toe extension, but it could also be found in normal subjects.[14] The term *signe de l'éventail* (fan sign) was neither coined nor liked by Babinski.[15] And whoever it was who launched the myth that only the combination of an upward movement of the big toe and abduction of the other toes constitutes a pathological toe response in its classical form, most certainly it was not Babinski.

The term "Babinski sign" was first used in 1898, by the Belgian neurologist Arthur van Gehuchten (1861–1914). This tribute was part of a very courteous response to Babinski, who had been slightly piqued by an allusion van Gehuchten had made to the relationship between the sign and the pyramidal system.[16] The term "plantar reflex according to von Strümpell" is now used only by elderly Dutch neurologists, to designate the normal toe response. Adolf Strümpell never had anything to do with the plantar reflex, and neither he nor any of his compatriots ever claimed such a thing. It is an authentically Dutch misconception, which could flourish for a few decades in splendid isolation.[4,17]

The pathophysiology of the phenomenon is slightly different from that first supposed by Babinski because the normal (downward) plantar response is not part of the flexion synergy of the leg. Paradoxically, it is the toe extensors that form part of the flexion synergy in dogs or other mammals, and also in neonates: in a physiological sense the toe extensors (anatomical term) are flexors, as they shorten the limb on contracting.[18] As the pyramidal tract becomes fully myelinated, between the first and second year of life, two functional changes occur with it. First, the influence of the pyramidal tract is strongest on distal muscles and—in the leg—in flexors. By that influence the upgoing movement of the big toe becomes excluded from the flexion synergy of the leg. This suppression clears the way for the normal (downward) response of the toes. That response is not part of a more complex pattern but a monosegmental skin response, very similar to the abdominal reflexes. With lesions of the pyramidal system the "neonatal" state of affairs may return if two other conditions are fulfilled: (1) at least a trace of the former flexion synergy should be retained, and (2) the involved part of the pyramidal tract should project on motor neurons of the foot.[19]

The great acclaim that greeted the Babinski sign has caused many epigones to stake their claims.[4] In the pursuit of everlasting fame all eyes were on the toes alone, and many lost sight of the pathological toe response being part of a complex synergy. At the efferent side many flexor muscles of the leg are involved, and at the afferent side the synergy can be elicited from as many skin sites. Also in the practical interpretation of toe responses it is useful to take account of the flexion synergy of the leg.[20]

References

1. Babinski J. Sur la présence dans les muscles striés de l'homme d'un système spécial constitué par des groupes de petites fibres musculaires entourées d'une gaine lamelleuse. *C R Séances Soc. Biol.* 1886;3:629–631.
2. Babinski J. *Étude anatomique et clinique sur la sclérose en plaques.* Paris: Masson; 1885.
3. Ali-Bab. *Gastronomie pratique: études culinaires, suivies du traitement de l'obésité des gourmands.* 9th ed. Paris: Flammarion; 1928.

4. van Gijn J. *The Babinski Sign: A Centenary.* Utrecht: Universiteit Utrecht; 1996.
5. Ritter G. Historische Bemerkungen zum sogenannten Babinskischen Phänomen. *J Neurol Sci.* 1967;5:1–7.
6. Pearce JMS Remak, father and son. *Lancet.* 1996;347:1669–1670.
7. Babinski J. Contractures organique et hystérique. *Bull Soc Méd Hôp.* 1893;3:327–343.
8. Babinski J. Relachement des muscles dans l'hémiplégie organique. *C R Séances Soc Biol.* 1896;48:471–472.
9. Babinski J. Diagnostic différentiel de l'hémiplégie organique et de l'hémiplégie hystérique. *Gaz Hôp.* 1900;73:521–577.
10. Babinski J. De la pronation de la main dans l'hémiplégie organique. *Rev Neurol (Paris).* 1907;15:755.
11. Babinski J. Monoplégie brachiale organique (mouvements actifs et mouvements passifs). *Rev Neurol (Paris).* 1909;17:218–220.
12. Babinski J. Discussion. Congrès International de Neurologie. *Bull méd.* 1897;11:896.
13. Babinski J. Du phénomène des orteils et de sa valeur sémiologique. *Sem méd.* 1898;18: 321–322.
14. Babinski J. De l'abduction des orteils. *Rev Neurol (Paris).* 1903;11:728–729.
15. Babinski J. De l'abduction des orteils (signe de l'éventail). *Rev Neurol (Paris).* 1903;11: 1205–1206.
16. van Gehuchten A. A propos du phénomène des orteils. *J Neurol.* 1898;3:284–286.
17. van Gijn J. [Strümpell or Babinski? History of plantar reflex] Strümpell of Babinski? De geschiedenis van de voetzoolreflex. *Ned Tijdschr Geneeskd.* 1975;119:1700–1707.
18. Marie P, Foix Ch. Les réflexes d'automatisme médullaire et le phénomène des raccourcisseurs; leur valeur sémiologique, leur signification physiologique. *Rev Neurol (Paris).* 1912;23: 657–676.
19. van Gijn J. The Babinski sign and the pyramidal syndrome. *J Neurol Neurosurg Psychiatry.* 1978;41:865–873.
20. van Gijn J. Equivocal plantar responses: a clinical and electromyographic study. *J Neurol Neurosurg Psychiatry.* 1976;39:275–282.

19

THE BARRÉ AND MINGAZZINI TESTS

Peter J. Koehler

Routine neurological examination often is comprised of the performance of the Barré test and, less often, the Mingazzini test, in order to find a latent pyramidal paresis of the arms or of the legs. Some physicians perform the Barré test by having the patient stretch the arms, the forearm in supination, the wrists and fingers in extension. With a pyramidal tract lesion, one observes the fingers or wrist drift downward, and if the pyramidal syndrome is more severe, the arm goes down on one side. Sensory and cerebellar disturbances may also show on this test, but with a different pattern of movement. Other physicians test with extended elbows and supinated forearms, while watching whether the patient pronates one of the forearms. One wonders which of these two methods was originally described by Barré. A similar test exists for examining the legs for latent paresis. For this purpose the Mingazzini test is often used: the patient, in supine position, is asked to bend his legs at the hips and knees, while the eyes are closed. The physician observes whether one of the legs moves downward. In this essay I discuss how Barré and Mingazzini originally performed the tests.

A biographical sketch of Jean-Alexandre Barré (1880–1967) is provided in Chapter 34 on the Guillain-Barré syndrome.

Giovanni Mingazzini was born in Ancona, Italy, on 15 February 1859.[1,2] After finishing his medical studies, he worked at the Istituto di Fisiologica in Rome under Jacob Moleschott (1822–1893), his favorite teacher. Moleschott was born and studied medicine in the Netherlands and subsequently worked in several countries. He became a private teacher in Heidelberg, but because his materialistic view ("Ohne Phosphor keine Gedanken" [Without phosphorus no thoughts; phosphorus was thought to be an important substance of the brain as observed in corpses since many years] was one of the propositions from his well-known 1858 book *Kreislauf des Lebens*), problems arose in his relationship with the authorities of the state of Baden.[3]

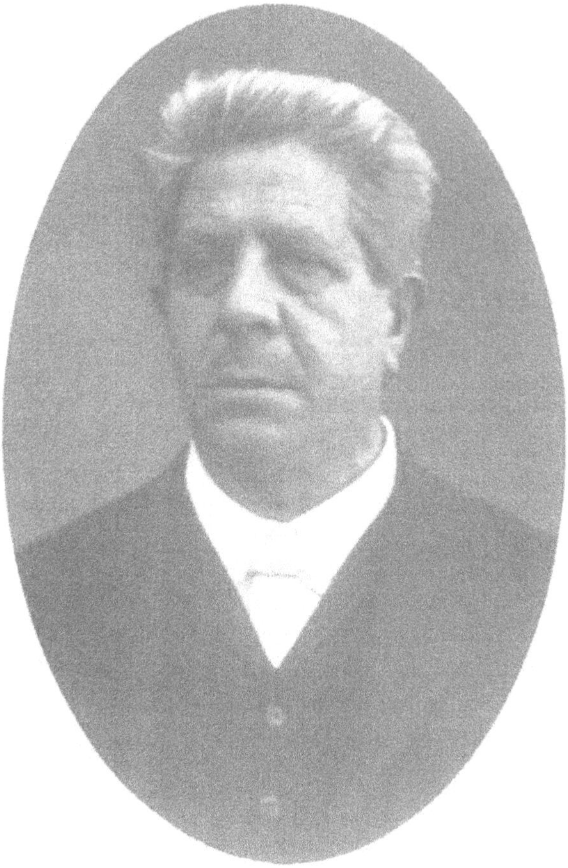

Figure 19–1. Giovanni Mingazzini (1859–1929). Courtesy of Medizinhistorisches Institut, Zurich, Switzerland.

Subsequently, Mingazzini worked under the anatomist Francesco Todaro (1839–1912) and briefly with the psychiatrist and neuroanatomist Bernhard von Gudden (1824–1886) in München, where he performed neuroanatomical work. Mingazzini was appointed professor of psychiatry and neurology at the University of Rome in 1895. He was particularly interested in the nucleus lentiformis and its connections with the inferior frontal gyrus. He postulated a theory on the origin of motor aphasia. The Swedish internist and pathologist Salomon Eberhard Henschen (1847–1930) called the area in front of the left lentiform nucleus, where fibers from Broca's area and the corresponding area in the contralateral hemisphere join, "Mingazzini's field." Mingazzini explained his theory of motor aphasia in *Über die motorische Aphasie* (1907) [On motor aphasia], in which he opposed the view of Pierre Marie (1853–1940), who had criticized the work of Pierre Paul Broca (1824–1880; see Chapter 30). Mingazzini's name is also associated with the acute syndrome of the putamen ("Mingazzini's lenticular hemiplegia").

He was portrayed as a capricious, nervous, and easily unsettled person. Usually he was generous, but in some matters he was strikingly tight-fisted. His assistants knew they could accept the coffee, which he sometimes offered them courteously, but had better refuse the pastry. He also was very absent-minded: he could go to the opera with his wife and return home alone, having forgotten that she had accompanied him.[1] His wife came from Germany and Mingazzini could read German publications without difficulty. He was a good teacher and lectured without notes. His lectures started as early as 7.00 A.M. The walls of his working room were decorated with certificates of honorary memberships and degrees, totalling 43. When Mussolini took power, Mingazzini refused to sign the fascist oath, for which he risked expulsion to the island of Sardinia. He died of a heart attack in 1929.[1,4] He was called "il fondatore della Neurologia Italiana."[5]

Barré described several clinical tests, including clinical signs of lesions of the pyramidal system. Best known is his "Manoeuvre de la jambe" [Leg maneuver], which carried the subtitle "nouveau signe objectif des paralysies ou parésies dues aux perturbations du faisceau pyramidal"[6] [New objective sign of paralysis or paresis caused by disturbance of the pyramidal bundle]. He often said that his teacher Babinski talked about this sign in terms of "qui sera votre signe de l'orteil" ([which will be your toe phenomenon] personal communication, Dr. Michel Bonduelle letter of 27 March 1995). Barré recalled in his article that Babinski had described a number of objective signs for the differentiation between organic and functional paralysis in the period 1896 to 1900. Babinski always applied the term *pithiatique,* as he rejected the term *hystérie* as well as the ideas of Charcot on this subject.

The test served "à aider très notablement le diagnostic dans les cas délicats" (to help considerably in the diagnosis of subtle cases), that is, in latent paresis, notably those caused by pathology of the central motor neuron. The test was carried out with the patient lying prone, the lower legs held up in a 90 degree angle from the bed (Fig. 19–2). In latent paresis, the leg would move downward on the paretic side. If it

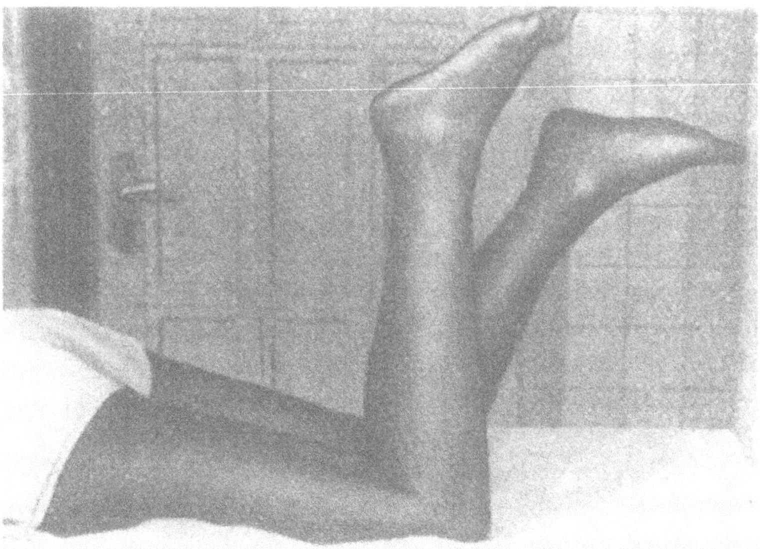

Figure 19–2. Barré's leg maneuver (manoeuvre de la jambe). From Ref. 12.

was not clear enough, the patient could be asked to bend the legs maximally. With this test, one could observe that the leg could be bent less on the paretic side than on the healthy side. Moreover, the patient could be asked once more to hold the legs up in a 90 degrees angle. Due to fatigue from the previous test, the leg on the paretic side would go down more readily. Barré provided ways to reveal latent paresis more clearly, but essentially the test is performed as described. He also observed that pain may complicate the interpretation and, obviously, passive mobility of the joint must be normal. The legs must be held up separately. He wondered whether a patient would be able to simulate a positive test. For this purpose, he advised paying attention to possible contraction of the thigh muscles if the leg on the paretic side goes down. If the leg goes down in a simulating patient, the thigh muscles would contract less than in cases of central motor paresis.

Barré tested the maneuver in more than 500 cases. The test appeared to be negative in peripheral and hysterical paresis. Observations in tabetic patients were variable: flexion as well as extension could be found, while normal strength was observed on testing muscle strength, indicating disturbed proprioception. The test appeared normal in cerebellar disease and was more sensitive than other indirect signs of pyramidal lesions, including Babinski's sign and increased muscle stretch reflexes. Finally, Barré claimed that his test was more sensitive than the test described by Mingazzini: "encore qu'elle soit très intéressante, manquait assez fréquemment quand la manoeuvre de la jambe était très nette[6] [Although it is very interesting, it is frequently absent when the leg maneuver is very clear].

In articles published six years previously, Mingazzini discussed *piccoli segni,* small signs, by which distinction between organic and hysterical hemiparesis could be made.[7–9] Moreover, slight hemiparesis or apparently recovered paresis that had escaped attention at superficial examination could be discovered. He pointed out that "neuropathologists" (as he called neurologists) had searched for similar signs in the preceding years. He admitted that some of these were *indices de luxe,* as they were accompanied by other, more obvious signs.[7] His assistant Romagna-Manoja investigated the technique, validity, and significance of a number of *piccoli segni* that Mingazzini had introduced in the Roman school some years previously. He particularly mentioned the *signe orbiculo-palpébral,* which was found in 55% of 89 hemiplegic or hemiparetic patients. In this test, the examiner tries to open the eyes, while the patient forcefully closes them. One may notice less resistance on the paretic side. Furthermore, he described the *signe orbiculo-labial,* which was positive in 67% of the same group. The test is similar to the previous one, except that in this case the examiner tries to move the lips apart at the corners of the mouth.

To detect slight paresis of the arms, Mingazzini performed the following test: the patient was asked to stretch his arms in front, the hands in the same horizontal plane and the fingers spread. The eyes are closed. Downward movement, oscillation, or sometimes only flexion of the hand after 30 to 60 seconds could indicate organic paresis. He described a similar test for the legs. The patient in supine position raises the legs straight in a 45 degree angle from the bed. "Lo si prega di tenere le gambe divaricate e sollevate in estensione al di sopra del piano del letto, in modo che esse

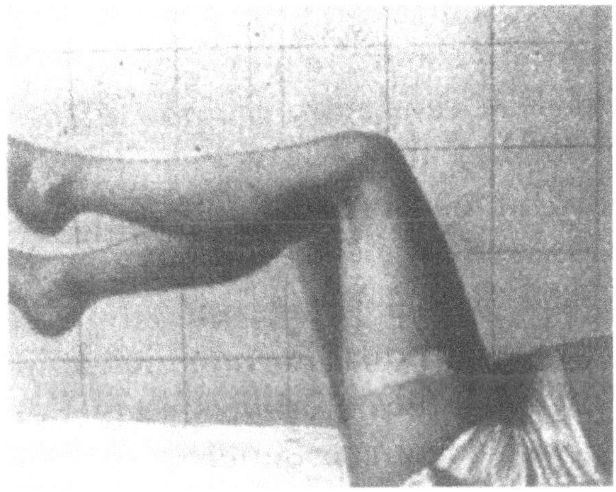

Figure 19–3. Mingazzini's test as carried out by Barré. Mingazzini originally described a variant with extended legs, making a 45 degree angle with the bed. From Ref. 12.

formino con questo un angolo di circa 45°[9] [He is asked to hold the legs spread and elevated in extension above the level of the bed, making a 45 degree angle]. If the leg moves downward too early, an organic paresis could be present. Combinations of several of these four signs and exaggerated muscle stretch reflexes were often observed in lesions of the lentiform nucleus, that is, "Mingazzini's lenticular hemiparesis."

Neither the leg nor the arm sign of Mingazzini is mentioned in many textbooks. Rondot described another way of performing the leg test: the patient's feet rest on the bed, with the knees held in a 90 degree angle.[10] Barré described a second variant in addition to the one mentioned above. The patient is in the supine position and legs are bent 90 degrees at the hip as well as at the knees (Fig. 19–3). Probably the modifications made by Rondot and Barré are more practicable than Mingazzini's test, in particular for elderly patients, but they are less sensitive.

Did Barré really also describe a "Barré" for the arms? Following some research it appears that he indeed presented a short paper at the August 1920 Congrès des aliénistes et neurologistes, entitled "Le signe de l'écartement des doigts" [Finger-spread sign], a test for demonstrating slight paresis of the arms (Fig. 19–4).[11] A healthy person is able to spread the fingers of both hands with the same extent and strength. Barré asked the patient to have his arms stretched in front of him, the palms facing each other, and the fingers spread. Even the slightest central motor lesion would cause decreased ability to perform this test, resulting in a positive *signe de l'écartement.*

Barré discussed the different tests in a review article (1937), indicating that the palms should not touch each other while performing this test.[12] In the same review, he referred to an "arm sign" described by Mingazzini, which has more resemblance to the "Barré sign" as it is carried out today than Barré's original *signe de l'écartement.* Barré indicated that in pyramidal syndromes the arm not only moves downward while performing Mingazzini's arm sign, but it may also demonstrate that it cannot be held completely extended at the different joints (Fig. 19–5). If the arm goes down, one may observe that the fingers, the hand, and the elbow gradually flex and drift. Barré considered his *signe de l'écartement* a refinement of Mingazzini's arm sign.

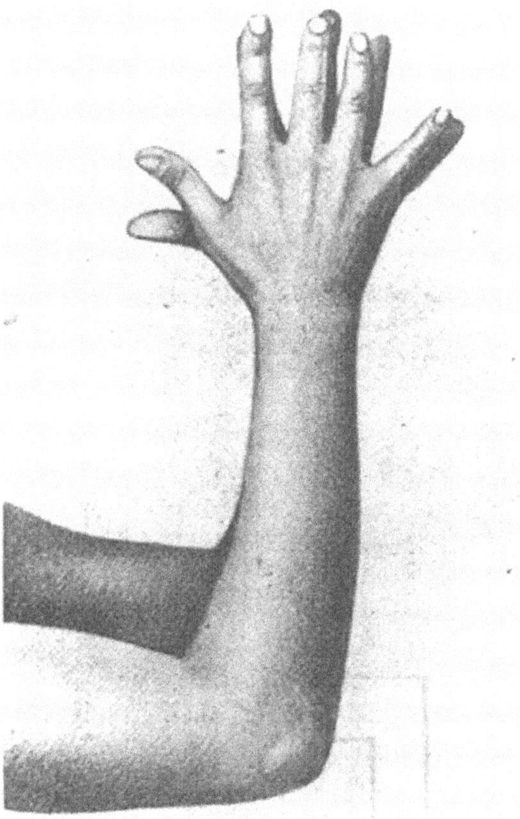

Figure 19–4. Barré's spread finger sign (signe de l'ecartement). From Ref. 12.

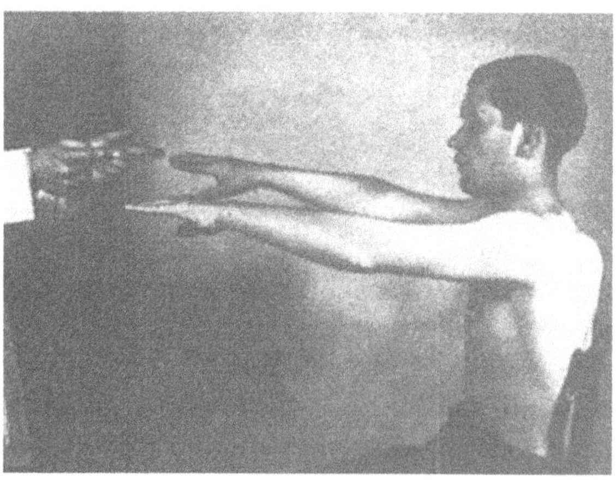

Figure 19–5. Barré's arm test, as often performed nowadays, in fact was first described by Mingazzini. Barré indicated that the arm is not fully stretched in all joints on the paretic side. From Ref. 12.

He argued that paresis in central motor lesions is more pronounced distally in the extremities, which would result in the fact that the *signe de l'écartement* was more sensitive than Mingazzini's arm sign.

Raymond Garcin (1897–1971) payed attention to what he called the *signe de la main creuse* [hollow hand sign] in the 1950s. The sign resembles Barré's finger-spread sign.[13] The arms are stretched forward, with the forearms bent vertically, the wrists and fingers stretched, while the fingers are spread widely. The sign may be positive in chorea, athetosis (among other signs of thalamic syndromes, which may be called pseudo-athetosis), and pyramidal syndromes: the first metacarpal may show adduction and slight flexion. Garcin stated that Barré, describing his *signe de l'écartement,* paid particular attention to the fact that the palm of the hand, in pyramidal syndromes, may be more hollow than at the healthy side. He would not have noticed the adduction–flexion movement of the first metacarpal, which, according to Garcin, was essential. One could conclude that Garcin's sign in fact is the combination of Barré's *signe de l'écartement* and Mingazzini's arm sign.

The relevant literature indicates that Barré especially investigated the leg maneuver, which he had described. It was more sensitive than the sign that had been described six years earlier by Mingazzini. It appears that Barré's arm sign, Barré's test as we still perform it today, was in fact Mingazzini's arm sign (Table 19–1). Barré and Garcin, however, particularly concentrated on phenomena distally in the arms. For this purpose the forearm is pronated and the hand stretched forward.

The test in which the forearm is held supinated in front of the patient while the occurrence of pronation is looked for is called "Barré" by some neurologists. However, "arm pronation test" would be a better name for this test. Several other pronation tests have been described. Babinski reported a similar arm sign in spastic hemiparesis, occurring as a result of predominating pronator tonicity.[14] He mainly used the sign for differentiating organic from hysterical hemiplegia. Adolf Strümpell (1853–1925) wrote that active flexion of the paretic arm is followed by pronation and flexion of the hand, and Samuel Alexander Kinnier Wilson (1878–1937) described combined pronation and internal rotation of the shoulder, occurring when the arms are elevated above the head.[15]

Most of these tests that may distinguish organic from psychogenic paresis are no longer used. The Barré (Fig. 19–5) and the Mingazzini tests (Fig. 19–3), however, may still be valuable.

Table 19–1. History of Barré and Mingazzini Tests

Test	Author	Year of Publication
Arm test*	Mingazzini	1913
	Barré	1920 (finger-spread test)
Leg test†	Mingazzini	1913 (patient lying on the back)
	Barré	1919 (patient lying on the abdomen)

* Now called Barré's test.

† Now called Mingazzini's test.

References

1. Ferraro A. Giovanni Mingazzini (1859–1929). In: Haymaker W, Schiller F, eds. *The Founders of Neurology.* 2nd ed. Springfield, Ill: Charles C Thomas; 1870:348–351.
2. Frank C. Giovanni Mingazzini und seine Schule. *Arch Psychiatr (Berl).* 1930;92:1–7.
3. Moleschott J. *Der Kreislauf des Lebens.* Mainz: Babern; 1852.
4. Nonne M. Giovanni Mingazzini. *Münch Med Wochenschr.* 1930:148–149.
5. Fumarola G. Giovanni Mingazzini. *Policlinico Sezione Pratica.* 1929;36:1900–1902.
6. Barré J A. La manoeuvre de la jambe. *Presse Méd.* 1919;79:793–795.
7. Mingazzini G. Sur quelques "petits signes" des parésies organiques. *Rev Neurol.* 1913;20: 469–473.
8. Mingazzini G. Alcuni "piccoli segni" delle paresi organiche. *Riforma Medica.* 1914;27:78.
9. Scarpino O, Pelliccioni, Magi M, Angeleri F. Originalita del contributo di Giovanni Mingazzini allo sviluppo della neurologia. In: Zanchin G, Premuda L, eds. *Lo sviluppo storico della neurologia Italiana: lo studio dell fonti.* Padova: La Garangola; 1990:233–236.
10. Rondot P. Syndromes of cental motor disorder. In: Vinken P J, Bruyn G W, Garcin R. *Handbook of Clinical Neurology, 1. Disturbances of Nervous Function.* Amsterdam: North-Holland; 1969:169–217.
11. Barré J A. Le signe de l'écartement des doigts. XXIVe Congrès des Aliénistes et Neurologistes, août 1920. *Rev Neurol.* 1920:942. Summary.
12. Barré J A. Le syndrome pyramidale déficitaire. *Rev Neurol.* 1937;67:1–40.
13. Garcin R. Syndrome cérébello-thalamique par lésion localisée du thalamus avec une digression sur le "signe de la main creuse" et son intérêt séméiologique. *Rev Neurol.* 1955;95: 143–149.
14. Babinski J. De la pronation de la main dans l'hémiplegie organique. *Rev Neurol.* 1907; 15:755.
15. De Jong R N, Haerer A F. Case taking and the neurologic examination. In: Joynt R J, ed. *Clinical Neurology.* Philadelphia: Lippincott; 1994;1:1–89.

20

THE REFLEXES OF HOFFMANN, TRÖMNER, AND MAYER

Hendrikus G. J. Krouwer, Paul E. Barkhaus, and Piero G. Antuono

The clinical neurological examination played a key role in the evaluation of the patient in the era preceding high-technology medicine. In contemporary medical practice, laboratory tests and imaging are given greater weight in diagnostic decision making. Therefore the clinical neurological examination has lost ground as the primary tool in clinical localization and in the problem-solving process. The seemingly obsessive and eccentric pursuit of reflexes by early clinicians can be understood through an appreciation of the historical perspective of lack of technology and much greater reliance on bedside skills.

The description of the pathological plantar reflex (see Chapter 18) by Joseph Babinski (1857–1932) in 1896 incited a veritable deluge of "new" reflexes, each, of course, "dignified" by the eponym of its discoverer. Between 1918 and 1935, a total of 76 new pathological reflexes were added to the neurological literature![1] The majority of these were trivial modifications and variations of previously described reflexes, particularly the Babinski response. Robert Wartenberg (1887–1956) eruditely expostulated this fad among early twentieth century neurologists in his 1945 monograph, *The Examination of Reflexes: A Simplification.* Foster Kennedy (1884–1952) referred to the three decades at the beginning of the twentieth century as the "open season for the Hunting of the Reflex."[1]

The lower extremity was the most exploited anatomic region for the majority of the reflex hunters. A few predictably directed their efforts toward the upper extremity in search of a reflex analogous to the Babinski reflex. The latter symbolized the realization of a Holy Grail of the neurological examination as an objective manifestation of central nervous system pathology. As such, it was reasoned that a second Grail in the rostral appendage surely awaited discovery by the keen clinical observer. Of the upper extremity responses subsequently described, the reflexes of Hoffmann, Trömner, and Mayer are the most enduring, with the first two remaining in common clinical use.

Johann Hoffmann (18 March 1857–1 November 1919) was born in Rheinhessen, Germany. Following his education at the Worms Gymnasium, he started his medical studies in Heidelberg. He continued in Strassburg and Berlin, eventually returning to Heidelberg where he obtained his medical degree. He later became an assistant to Wilhelm Erb (1840–1921), who headed the Medizinische Klinik. Hoffmann completed his thesis (1888) on the increased mechanical excitability of sensory nerves in tetany. He was appointed professor in 1891. Ludolf von Krehl (1861–1937), who succeeded Erb after his retirement in 1907, established a separate lectureship for Hoffmann, entitled "Neuropathology and Electrotherapy." Hoffmann lectured extensively on these subjects until his death.[2,3]

His research and publications focused on diseases of the spinal cord, peripheral nerves, and muscles. He described, independently from Guido Werdnig (1844–1919), acute infantile spinal muscular atrophy.[4] In 1900, he reported on female twins with myotonic dystrophy, a disorder that became known as Curschmann–Steinert after the two physicians who published their report nine years later.[5,6]

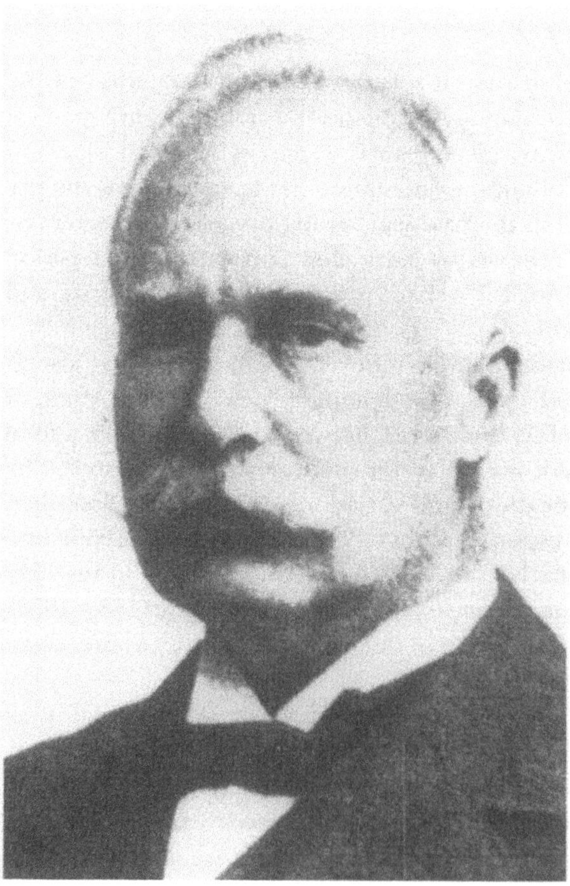

Figure 20–1. Johann Hoffmann (1857–1919). Courtesy of Institut für Geschichte der Medizin, Ruprecht-Karls-Universität Heidelberg.

One may look in vain for a publication by Hoffmann in which he describes "his" reflex. The apparent absence of this original description also frustrated a number of American neurologists who attempted to provide their readers with some background information on this reflex which had attained a somewhat surprising popularity among American neurologists.[7–10] Eventually it was a medical student, Otto Bendheim, from Ann Arbor, Michigan, who extensively researched the medical literature and found that Hoffmann had never written about the reflex attributed to him.[11]

It was Hans Curschmann (1875–1942; see Chapter 44), Hoffmann's resident while doing general medicine training from 1901 to 1904, who cited the reflex in a footnote to an article about neurological abnormalities in a 10-year-old boy with acute nephritis.[12] Biceps and triceps reflexes were diminished bilaterally and "Hoffmann's phenomenon (finger flexion reflex) was negative bilaterally." In this footnote Curschmann further elaborated:

> The phenomenon of J. Hoffmann (not published) entails that the examiner holds the slightly bent fingers of the patient between thumb and index finger and then "snaps" the nail of one of these fingers with his own index finger. A quick flexion of this, or more commonly all of the fingers, will then occur (Fig. 20–2).

Curschmann found this reflex to be frequently present in patients with hyperreflexia secondary to a neurological disease. He did not think it had pathognomonic significance as a "Babinski of the upper extremity," since he had also found the reflex in patients with nonneurological disorders such as hysteria and neurasthenia. He thus anticipated the debate in the ensuing years between proponents of the Hoffmann reflex as a Babinski of the arm[8–10] and opponents who stated that its presence only indicated a state of muscular hypertonia, which may occur in nervous individuals without any organic disorder.[13]

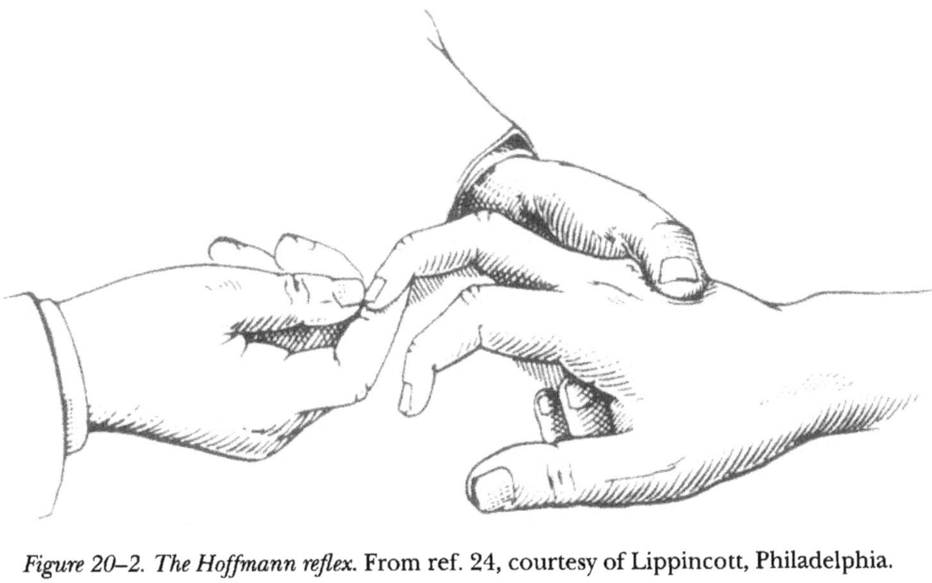

Figure 20–2. The Hoffmann reflex. From ref. 24, courtesy of Lippincott, Philadelphia.

In 1936, Kastein stated in the *Nederlandsch Tijdschrift voor Geneeskunde* that the Hoffmann (and Trömner) reflex is a normal stretch reflex of the finger flexor muscles.[14] Wartenberg emphasized that both reflexes are based on the physiological mechanism of the muscle stretch reflex.[1] The finger flexors contract when they are being stretched rapidly. Hence these reflexes can be elicited in normal subjects. They may, however, be indicative of a pyramidal tract lesion, especially in cases with asymmetric findings and in the presence of other pathological reflexes.

The finger flexion reflex, of which the Hoffmann and Trömner reflexes are merely more complicated variants, can be most easily elicited in the following fashion. The patient sits opposite the examiner, with his hands half-supinated on his knees. The examiner positions his own index finger and middle finger over the slightly flexed distal phalanges of the four fingers of the patient's hand and gently taps his two fingers with his reflex hammer. Flexion of the patient's four fingers and mostly also of the end phalanx of the thumb are seen. The reflex may be modulated by having the patient increase (or decrease) the tension of his four flexed fingers against the examiner's two fingers.

Ernst Trömner (1868–1930) was born in Merano, Saxony. He completed his medical studies in Leipzig in 1893 and eventually started to practice neurology in Hamburg as staff neurologist at the Allgemeines Krankenhaus St. Georg. He actively pursued the discovery of new reflexes. He described a muscle stretch reflex of the

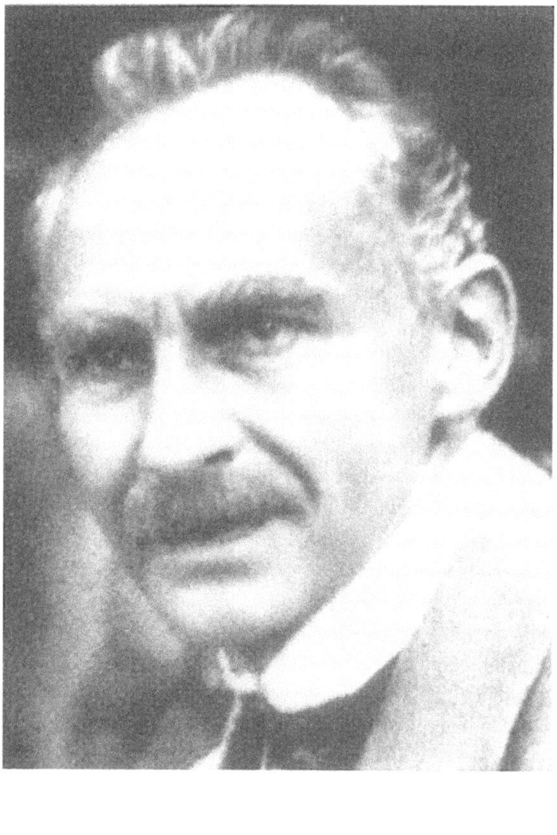

Figure 20–3. Ernst Trömner (1868–1930). Courtesy of Allgemeines Krankenhaus St. Georg, Hamburg.

diaphragm and a variant of the Achilles tendon reflex elicited via the lateral malleolus. In addition, he published a number of review articles about cutaneous and muscle stretch reflexes as well as about the techniques of eliciting reflexes.

His interest in this subject also induced him to design diagnostic equipment such as the muscle plessimeter. This is a broad spatula used to compress a muscle and offer protection against the direct percussion of the reflex hammer. It appears that only the Trömner reflex hammer has endured. At the Mayo Clinic in Rochester, Minnesota, this instrument is given to staff neurologists at the time they begin their appointment.[15]

On 2 January 1912, Trömner introduced his reflex, the *Fingerbeugephänomen* or *Fingerphänomen,* during a meeting of the Hamburg Medical Society. He presented a 29-year-old woman with spastic spinal paralysis secondary to syphilis.[16] He described the reflex as

> a pathognomonic finger reflex . . . a reflex of the arm, analogous to the Babinski, which is as pathognomonic for motor conduction abnormalities above the spinal centers innervating the arm as the Babinski phenomenon for the leg. Thus far, such a phenomenon was missing.

Trömner briefly explained (in this report of no more than 39 lines) the technique of eliciting this reflex. He elaborated on it in more detail in two subsequent publications.[17,18] The patient's hand needs to be placed in a relaxed position, with the fingers slightly bent. The middle finger is held by the examiner at the proximal or middle phalanx (Fig. 20–4). The examiner then flicks the distal phalanx of his own index finger against the volar portion of the distal phalanx of the patient's middle finger. A brief flexor motion of this middle finger as well as the other fingers and

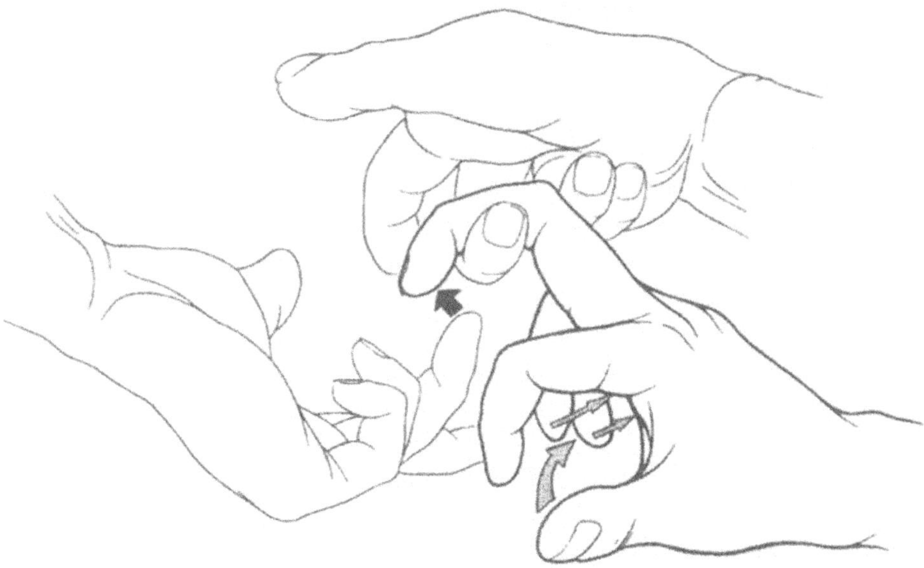

Figure 20–4. The Trömner reflex. From M. Mumenthaler, Neurology. Stuttgart: Georg Thieme Verlag, 1979; permission of Thieme Verlag, Stuttgart, Germany.

frequently the thumb may be seen if, according to Trömner, a lesion of the motor tracts above the level of the fifth cervical nerve has occurred.

Trömner initially thought he had discovered the Babinski of the arm. He continued to do so in an article published in 1913,[17] but he was more cautious in a publication of 1923.[18] In that report he stated that if there was a response of only minor flexion of the fingers, the possibility of "a neuropathic condition" (without further defining or specifying) could be considered. If a more pronounced flexion occurred, then a pyramidal tract lesion was certain to be present, especially if the response was unilateral.[18] Like the Hoffman reflex, the Trömner reflex became the subject of controversy among neurologists with respect to its nature and significance. More than ten neurologists discovered a Babinski of the arm in the years following Trömner's publication. It should—again—be emphasized that all of these reflexes, including the Hoffman and Trömner reflexes, are variants of the finger flexion reflex.[1]

Carl Mayer (9 December 1862–24 April 1936) was born in Vienna, Austria. He completed his premedical school education (Gymnasium) and medical studies in Vienna. He trained at the Psychiatric-Neurologic Clinic headed by Theodor Meynert (1833–1912) and Richard von Krafft-Ebing (1840–1902), remaining on the staff until 1895 when he was appointed professor of neurology and psychiatry in

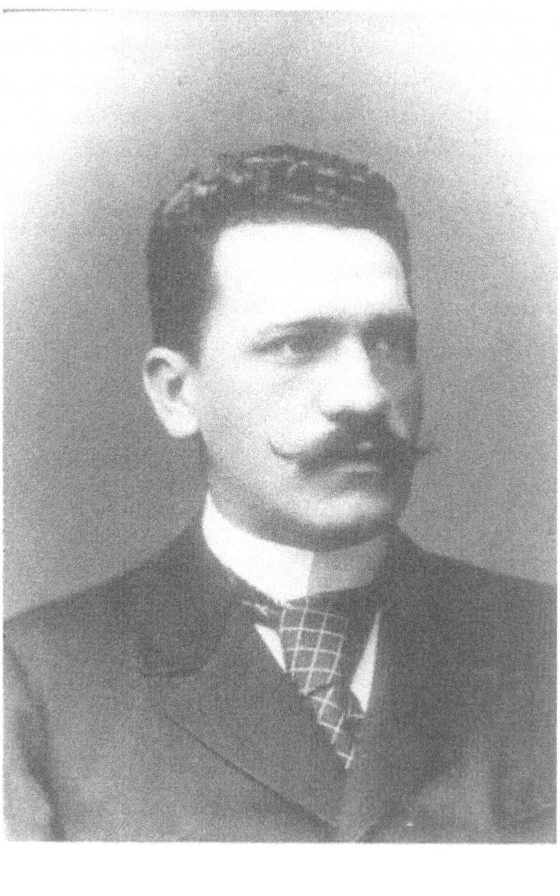

Figure 20–5. Carl Mayer (1862–1936). By courtesy of the Institut für Geschichte der Medizin der Universität Wien.

Innsbruck, Austria. He was an enthusiastic advocate of the inseparable association between these two specialties, and he published in both fields.[19] The topics of his neurological publications include pathologic–anatomical studies on disorders of brain and spinal cord (e.g., tumors, poliomyelitis), the physiology and pathology of yawning, microcephaly, and observations on the encephalitis epidemic as well as on dysphasia and dyslexia.

He devoted a total of 11 publications to his reflex, the finger-thumb reflex, starting in 1915 and 1916.[20,21] In a lecture on war injuries affecting the nervous system held before the Medical Society of Innsbruck on 12 November 1915, Mayer gave a very detailed account of the neurological examination of eight soldiers who developed a "neuritis" of the peripheral nerves of the arm following wound infections. In two of these patients he could elicit a prominent opposition and flexion in the carpometacarpal joint of the thumb, with extension of the distal phalanx, by forceful flexion of the proximal phalanx of especially the third, but also the second and fourth digits.[20] Two weeks later, Mayer commented on these initial observations and stated that these were not an abnormal finding but actually a true reflex which could also be found in most healthy individuals.[21]

He extensively described the examination technique for this reflex: with the patient's hand in supination, the proximal phalanx of one of the three aforementioned fingers needs to be pushed down, slowly but forcefully, by the examiner's thumb (Fig. 20–6); if this downward push is too fast, the reflex cannot be properly evaluated. The examiner is cautioned that if the Mayer reflex is elicited with undue force, it may be painful for the patient and of no clinical value.

Mayer distinguished his reflex from a number of others, including Trömner's, and stated that his reflex could not be compared to any of these.[21] In ten hemiplegic patients the reflex was absent on their paralyzed side but present on their unaffected

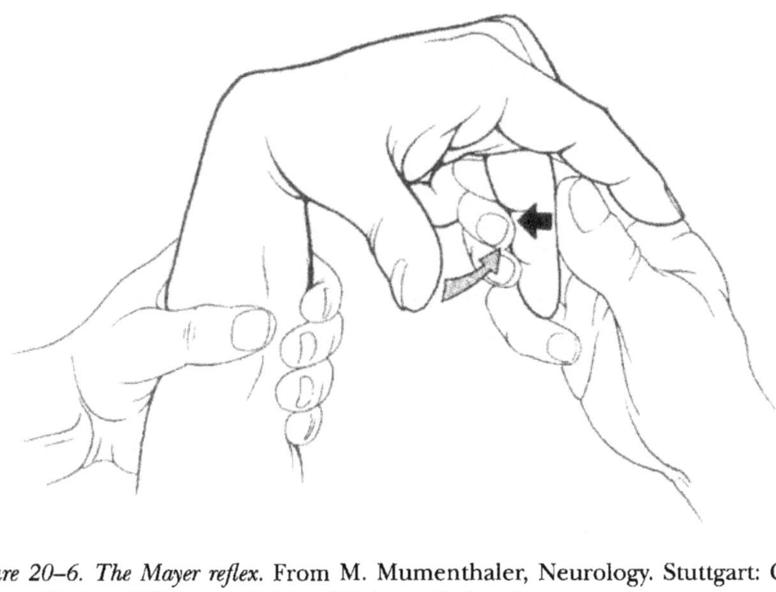

Figure 20–6. The Mayer reflex. From M. Mumenthaler, Neurology. Stuttgart: Georg Thieme Verlag, 1979; permission of Thieme Verlag, Stuttgart, Germany.

(i.e., contralateral) side. Mayer concluded that the absence of the reflex indicated a lesion of the upper motor neuron, analogous to the unilateral absence of abdominal cutaneous reflexes in similar cases.

The pathophysiology of the Mayer reflex has received minimal study. Mayer elaborated in great detail on the physiological mechanisms activated by flexion of the proximal phalanx of the middle finger and the subsequent muscle contractions.[22] He considered it to be a proprioceptive reflex, with the afferent pathway via the C6-T1 nerve roots, and the efferent pathway via the C7-T1 nerve roots. He briefly mentioned the absence of the reflex contralateral to hemispheric lesions, and he raised the possibility of a cortical, subcortical, or even spinal localization of the reflex.[22] Wartenberg pointed out that it is not a muscle stretch reflex but a postural reflex, a component of the so-called negative support reaction.[1] According to Monnier the reflex follows nerve roots C6 through T1, with integration centers in the corresponding spinal segments.[23] Brodman's area 6a or premotor cortex represents its cortical center. The Mayer reflex will disappear as a result of lesions in this area.

The Babinski of the arm, that is, the upper extremity analogue of the plantar extensor response, was not discovered by Hoffman, Trömner, or Mayer. Justified or not, the reflexes of this triumvirate of *fin de siècle* clinical neurologists remain in the neurological examination. Singly or jointly, the reflexes of Hoffmann and Trömner have evolved to form an integral part of the current, standard neurological examination. Both of these reflexes and their significance are discussed extensively in the most recent edition of *DeJong's Neurological Examination.*[24] The Hoffman reflex is particularly popular among American medical students, house officers, and neurologists. The eponyms do, however, obscure the fact that the Hoffmann and Trömner reflexes are variants of the basic finger flexor reflex. When they occur bilaterally and symmetrically, the presence of these muscle stretch reflexes may be entirely within normal limits. When asymmetric or unilaterally present, especially in combination with other pathological reflexes or abnormal findings, they may indicate a lesion of the ipsilateral corticospinal tract. The Mayer reflex may be considered the most sensitive of the three reflexes. Its unilateral absence may be regarded as a subtle sign of an ipsilateral pyramidal tract lesion. It should not be part of the standard repertoire neurological examination and only sought when clinically indicated.

We are grateful to Alfred Kraemer, librarian of the Medical College of Wisconsin, for obtaining some of the historical material and Jayne Rossman for manuscript preparation. Hermann Heuck from the Allgemeines Krankenhaus St. Georg, Hamburg, provided the portrait of Ernst Trömner.

References

1. Wartenberg R. *The Examination of Reflexes: A Simplification.* Chicago: Year Book Publishers; 1945.
2. Schönfeld W. Johann Hoffmann (1857–1919), der Heidelberger Neurologe, Schüler und Freund Wilhelm Erb's. *Ruperto Carola.* 1962;31:184–188.
3. Vogel P. Die Heidelberger Neurologische Schule: Friedreich-Erb-Hoffmann. *Heidelberger Jahrbücher.* 1970;14:73–84.

4. Hoffmann J. Über chronische spinale Muskelatrofie in Kindesalter, auf familiärer Basis. *Dtsch Z Nervenheilk.* 1891;1:95–120.
5. Hoffmann J. Zur Lehre von der Thomsen'schen Krankheit mit besonderer Berücksichtigung des dabei vorkommenden Muskelschwundes. *Dtsch Z Nervenheilk.* 1900;18:198–216.
6. Steinert H. Über das klinische und anatomische Bild des Muskelschwunds der Myotoniker. *Dtsch Z Nervenheilk.* 1909;37:58–104.
7. Keyser T S. Hoffman's [sic] sign or the "digital reflex." *J Nerv Ment Dis.* 1916;44:51–62.
8. Pitfield R L. The Hoffman [sic] reflex: a simple way of reinforcing it and other reflexes. *J Nerv Ment Dis.* 1929;69:252–258.
9. Fay T, Gotten H B. Clinical observations on the value of the Hoffmann sign. *J Nerv Ment Dis.* 1933;77:594–600.
10. Echols D H. The Hoffmann sign: its incidence in university students. *J Nerv Ment Dis.* 1936;84:427–431.
11. Bendheim O L. On the history of Hoffmann's sign. *Bull Hist Med.* 1937;5:684–686.
12. Curschmann H. Ueber die diagnostische Bedeutung des Babinskischen Phänomens im präurämischen Zustand. *Münch Med Wochenschr.* 1911;58:2054–2057.
13. Brain R. *Diseases of the Nervous System.* 2nd ed. London: Oxford University Press; 1940:45.
14. Kastein G W. De aard en het voorkomen van den reflex van het type Troemner, Hoffmann, en Rossolimo, Zukowski. *Ned Tijdschr Geneeskd.* 1936;80:1187–1194.
15. Rooke E D. The Trömner hammer: a historical postscript. *Mayo Clin Proc.* 1960;35:335–336.
16. Trömner E. Fingerbeugephänomen. *Neurol Centralbl.* 1912;31:603–604.
17. Trömner E. Ueber Sehnen- resp. Muskelreflexe und die Merkmale ihrer Schwächung und Steigerung. *Berl Klin Wochenschr.* 1913;50:1712–1715.
18. Trömner E. Zur Technik der Reflexprüfung. *Klin Wochenschr.* 1923;2:1810–1812.
19. Ganner H. Zum Gedenken C. Mayer. *Wien Z Nervenheilk.* 1962;24:177–188.
20. Mayer C. Kriegsneurologische Erfahrungen. *Med Klin.* 1915;37:1017–1022.
21. Mayer C. Zweite Mitteilung über ein Reflexphänomen am Daumen (Finger-Daumenreflex). *Neurol Centralbl.* 1916;35:11–16.
22. Mayer C, Ostheimer S. Ueber reflektorische im Bereich der Extremitäten von den Gelenken her auslösbare Kontraktion von Muskeln. *Arch Psychiatr Nervenkrankh.* 1918;59: 462–483.
23. Monnier M. Defensive functions (flexion reflexes). In: *Functions of the Nervous System.* Amsterdam: Elsevier; 1968:224–249.
24. Haerer APH. *DeJong's The Neurologic Examination.* 5th ed. Philadelphia: Lippincott; 1992: 430–457.

21

THE HOFFMANN–TINEL SIGN

Frank Spaans

Paul Hoffmann was born on 1 July 1884 in Dorpat, Estonia, where his father was a professor of internal medicine.[1] He studied medicine at the universities of Leipzig, Marburg, and Berlin, and in 1911 he was appointed assistant to Max von Frey (1852–1932) at the physiology institute of Würzburg University, where he mostly investigated muscle potentials and reflexes. During World War I he worked in several German field hospitals in France and later at a military hospital in Würzburg, where he wrote the reports about the sign that was later named after him.[2,3] In 1920 he was the first to describe the reflex which can be obtained by electrical stimulation of peripheral nerves, the so-called H (or Hoffmann) reflex. He can be regarded as the founder of modern German neurophysiology.

In 1924, Hoffmann was made director of the institute of physiology of the University of Freiburg-im-Breisgau, an institute which was completely destroyed by an air strike in November 1944. He nevertheless continued his work, initially in a temporary building and later in a newly built institute, until his retirement in 1954. He was given honorary doctorates by the universities of Berlin (Humboldt) and Zürich. Paul Hoffmann died on 9 March 1962.

Jules Tinel was born in Rouen on 12 October 1879, in a family which had produced prominent physicians for five generations.[4] He studied medicine in Paris, where Jules Dejerine (1849–1917) taught him neurology and the pathological anatomy of the nervous system. In 1910, he published his dissertation, *Les Radiculites et le Tabes,* in which he showed, among other things, that any form of meningitis—whether syphilitic or otherwise—involved the nerve roots, particularly the dorsal roots. He then worked for a few years as head of the department at the Salpêtrière in Paris, until World War I broke out and Tinel was assigned to an infantry regiment. In 1915, he founded a regional neurological center at the front, where he devoted himself to the diagnosis and treatment of peripheral nerve

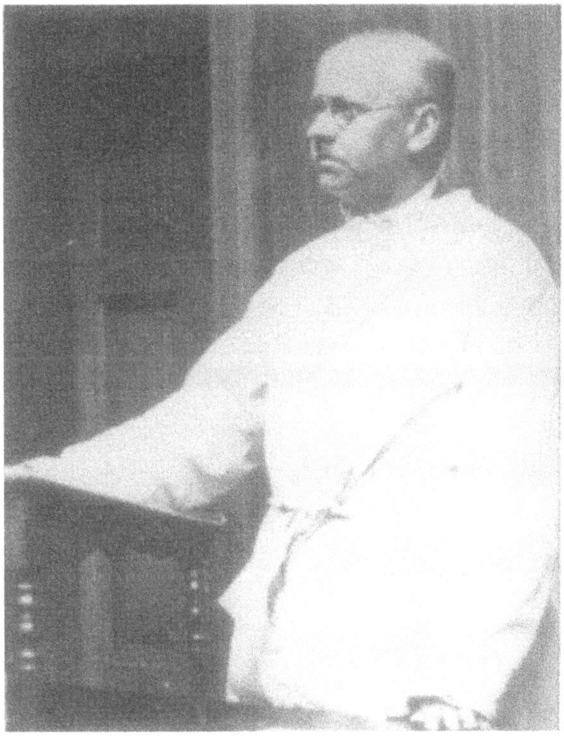

Figure 21–1. Paul Hoffmann (1884–1962). Courtesy of University Archives, Freiburg, Germany.

injuries. The publication that secured him a place in medical history appeared in the same year.[5]

Tinel continued to play an active role in a large number of research areas, though focusing on the autonomic nervous system. In his view, the autonomic nervous system also influenced a person's mental state.

During the German occupation in World War II Tinel concealed Allied pilots. The pilots were helped to cross the Franco-Spanish border by one of Tinel's sons, who later died in a German extermination camp.

After a period in which he suffered various cardiovascular problems, Jules Tinel died in 1952.

In March and August 1915, Hoffmann published two papers in the journal *Medizinische Klinik* about a method that allowed an early assessment of both the success of nerve sutures and the possible spontaneous recovery of nerve injuries.[2,3] In October 1915, Tinel wrote a paper on virtually the same test, based on his experience on the French side of the front.[5] This was at the height of World War I, which meant that peripheral nerve injuries were frequent as a result of bullet wounds; World War II was to provide similar major breakthroughs.

The sign which bears their two names involves radiating tingling sensations in the otherwise anesthetic skin area innervated by an injured nerve, upon light percussion of the area (see Fig. 21–3). The sign was immediately regarded as evidence of the presence of newly formed, extremely sensitive regenerating nerve fibers.

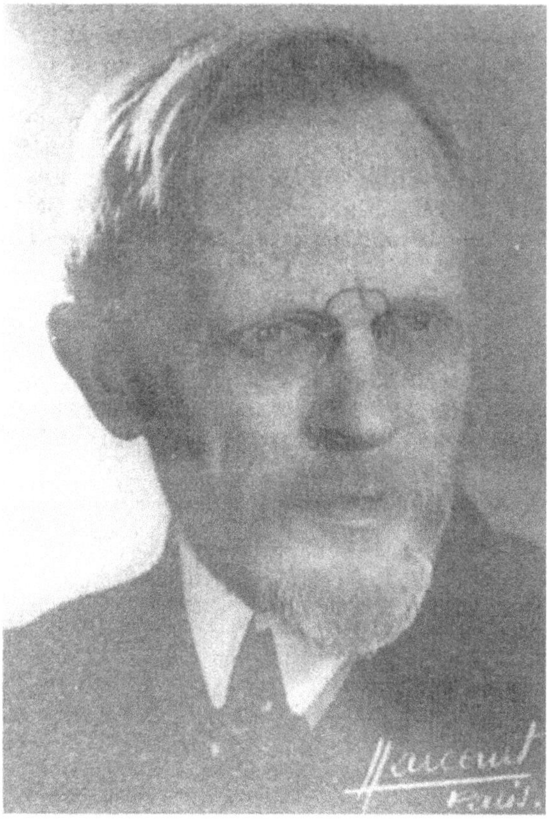

Figure 21–2. Jules Tinel (1879–1952). Permission of La Presse Médicale (1952;979–980), Masson Editeur, Paris.

Originally, Tinel described the occurrence of paresthesias when *pressure* was applied to the injured nerve. In his first publication, Hoffmann did the same, but he already mentioned that slight *percussion* with the extended finger was a better method. In his second publication, he simply referred to the test as *Klopfversuch* (tapping test) and provided a thorough and systematic discussion of the phenomenon (Fig. 21–4). He had found that tapping with the tip of the finger or with the reflex hammer was more effective in eliciting the paresthesias than pressure. Hoffmann emphasized that

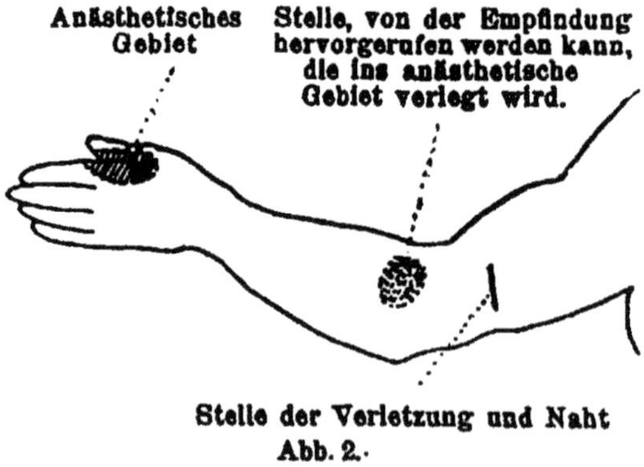

Figure 21–3. Illustration from Paul Hoffmann's first report.[2]

Figure 21–4. Illustration from Paul Hoffmann's second report.[3]

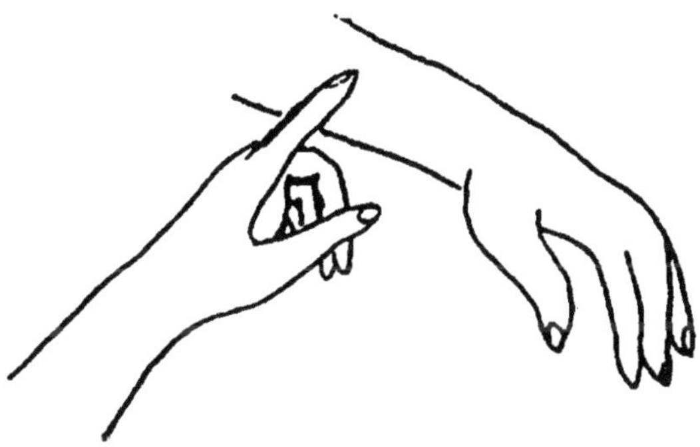

Abb. 1. Handstellung beim Beklopfen des Vorderarms auf der Suche nach auswachsenden Enden des N. radialis.

the percussion had to be light, since paresthesias might otherwise also be found in normal nerves. Often a single tap on a ruptured nerve proved enough to elicit paresthesias in the innervated area, with the paresthesias sometimes persisting for minutes.

Hoffmann also noticed that repetitive stimulation could have a summational effect on the paraesthesias; sometimes this was the only way to elicit them.[3] Both Tinel and Hoffmann pointed out the significance of a positive sign upon mechanical stimulation *at a certain distance distal to the nerve suture or lesion,* since this allowed the conclusion that the nerve axons had proceeded beyond this crucial point. Percussing the nerve along its course allowed the examiner to assess the rate of regeneration. Hoffmann found rates of more than 2 mm a day, a finding which has frequently been confirmed since.

Outside the German-speaking countries this test is usually referred to only as Tinel's sign, probably because the war meant that Tinel's publication received far greater attention than Hoffmann's. In addition, Tinel became a well-known name in English-speaking countries after his book on nerve injuries was translated into English in 1917.[6] In this book he mentions that the sign can be elicited both by *sudden* pressure and by percussion (see the following quotation). At that time Tinel may have been informed about Hoffmann's observations.

> The all important sign is formication. We find that sudden pressure or percussion of the nerve trunk, below the lesion, calls forth a tingling sensation in the cutaneous region of the nerve . . . It appears about the fourth or sixth week . . . Then it gradually becomes more pronounced and it is possible to follow, week by week, in the course of the nerve, the progress of this provoked formication, pari passu with the advance of the axis cylinders. The formication sign is thus of supreme importance since it enables us to see whether the nerve is interrupted, or in the course of regeneration; whether a nerve suture has succeeded or failed, or whether regeneration is rapid and satisfactory.

After a period in which the symptom seemed to have been forgotten, the experience of World War II,[7] and, even more important, the appearance of an English translation of the article in 1972,[8] led to renewed interest in Tinel's publication in the Anglo-American literature. In German-speaking countries, the symptom is often termed

Hoffmann's sign (*das Hoffmannsche Klopfzeichen*) or the Hoffmann–Tinel sign.[9–11] In view of the content of the publications and the order in which they originally appeared, the latter designation would seem to be the correct one. It was also used by Sunderland, an expert on peripheral nerve lesions,[12] although he preferred the noneponymous name *distal tingling on percussion* (DTP).

The original publications by Hoffmann and Tinel show that both were immediately aware of the limitations of their test. For instance, in the early stages of a nerve injury which has not been explored, a negative test result can indicate either a lack of regeneration or a mild lesion, which is not accompanied by axonal degeneration. The Hoffmann–Tinel sign is usually not found until four to six weeks after the nerve injury and can often be elicited for up to one or two years after injury. It is assumed that this is the time it takes for the regenerated axons to rebuild their myelin sheath, making them less sensitive to mechanical stimuli.[10]

Although Hoffmann was acutely aware that the test was suitable for assessing the regeneration of *sensory* axons only, a positive finding upon percussion of the nerve at a certain distance distal to the suture usually augured well for a full recovery. Later experience has shown that the regeneration of motor axons can lag considerably behind that of the sensory axons. In addition, no prognosis can be given about the ultimate extent of reinnervation, let alone about the level of functional recovery to be expected.[7,9,11]

The significance of the sign was initially overrated by many clinicians; it may often have been incorrectly elicited, leading to the sign being dismissed as unreliable. However, a reappraisal occurred during and after World War II, which showed that the sign could indeed have clinical relevance if it is correctly elicited and interpreted.[7,9,11] The nerve should be tapped lightly, going from distal to proximal, until the point is reached where the first tinglings are found. This corresponds to the most distal point to which the regenerating sensory axons—which are depolarized by such stimuli—have progressed. If this point is situated at more than about 8 cm distal to the location of the nerve lesion or suture, this proves that the regenerating nerve fibers have proceeded beyond the site of the lesion. Another important condition is that the patient must be able to locate the paraesthesias precisely in the skin area innervated by the relevant nerve. The Hoffmann–Tinel sign remains the only clinical test to show incipient nerve regeneration.

The further course of regeneration can be monitored by repeating the test at regular intervals. Firm percussion should be avoided, as this may also elicit tingling proximal and distal to the point of regeneration. In the case of injuries to deeper nerves, however, the Hoffmann–Tinel sign can be elicited only by firm percussion. A positive test in this situation means only that sensory axons have indeed formed, but whether these have proceeded beyond the site of the lesion cannot be definitely established. Conversely, the continued absence of the Hoffmann–Tinel sign three months after total axonal disruption indicates that no regeneration or reinnervation is to be expected.[12]

While the Hoffmann–Tinel sign has value in the assessment of regeneration after traumatic nerve injuries, it is also used as a tool in diagnosing compression neuropathies. Neither Hoffmann nor Tinel ever mentioned this application. Although the lack of sensitivity and/or specificity of this sign for the diagnosis of carpal tunnel syndrome (CTS) has been demonstrated in various studies,[13–19] a single publication[20] suggests that there may be subsets of patients in which CTS may be diagnosed by a number of clinical tests including the Hoffmann–Tinel sign. One of the authors' argues for omitting nerve conduction studies because of costs, which varied in their region between $150 and $500. De Krom et al.,[21] however, investigated a large sample from the general population and convincingly demonstrated that the use of any combination of provocative test is inadequate for the diagnosis of CTS and that confirmation of the diagnosis by nerve conduction studies is essential. Novak et al.[22] found the Hoffmann–Tinel test useful in the diagnosis of what they considered to be "cubital tunnel syndrome" (sensitivity 0.70, specificity 0.98); however, maximal elbow flexion combined with pressure on the ulnar nerve just proximal to the cubital tunnel was found to be a more reliable test.

"Tinel-like" percussion paresthesias have been encountered in patients with cervical root lesions[19,23,24] and even in patients with spinal cord injury, where it may be called the "central Tinel sign."[25] In a patient with an ulnar nerve lesion a "motor Tinel sign" has been reported;[26] percussion and palpation of the nerve just proximal to the groove easily provoked shocklike sensations shooting into the little finger with concomitant contractions exclusively in the ulnar innervated hand muscles (recorded by electromyogram).

Using microneurography, Ochoa et al. recorded the electrophysiological correlate of the Hoffmann–Tinel sign in a patient with an amputation neuroma.[27] Yarnitsky and Ochoa paid attention to the fact that paresthesias evoked by tapping over an injured nerve are often painful.[28] They were able to demonstrate in a number of patients that a painful Hoffmann–Tinel sign can be mediated either by myelinated or unmyelinated primary afferents.

References

1. Buck-Gramcko D, Lubahn JD. The Hoffmann-Tinel sign. *J Hand Surg Br* 1993;18:800–805.
2. Hoffmann P. Ueber eine Methode, den Erfolg einer Nervennaht zu beurteilen. *Med Klin.* 1915;11:359–360.
3. Hoffmann P. Weiteres über das Verhalten frisch regenerierter Nerven und über die Methode, den Erfolg einer Nervennaht frühzeitig zu beurteilen. *Med Klin.* 1915;11:856–858.
4. Jules Tinel. *Rev Neurol.* 1952;86:329–330. Obituary.
5. Tinel J. Le signe du "fourmillement" dans les lésions des nerfs périphériques. *Presse Méd.* 1915;47:388–389.
6. Tinel J. *Les Blessures des Nerfs.* Paris: Masson; 1916. English translation: Tinel J. *Nerve Wounds.* London: Ballière, Tindal & Cox; 1917.
7. Napier JR. The significance of Tinel's sign in peripheral nerve injuries. *Brain.* 1949;72: 63–82.
8. Kaplan EB. J. Tinel's "fourmillement" paper. In: Spinner M, ed. *Injuries to the Major Branches of Peripheral Nerves in the Forearm.* Philadelphia: Saunders; 1972:8–13.
9. Jung R. Die allgemeine Symptomatologie der Nervenverletzungen und ihre physiologischen Grundlagen. *Nervenarzt.* 1941;14:493–516.

10. Mumenthaler M, Schliack H. *Läsionen peripherer Nerven.* 6th ed. Stuttgart: Thieme; 1993: 72–73.
11. Ruf H. Über die klinische Verwertbarkeit des Hoffmannschen Klopfzeichens. *Nervenarzt.* 1942;15:377–381.
12. Sunderland S. *Nerves and Nerve Injuries.* 2nd ed. Edinburgh: Churchill Livingstone; 1978:121.
13. Stewart JD, Eisen A. Tinel's sign and the carpal tunnel syndrome. *Br Med J.* 1978;2: 1125–1126.
14. Gellman H, Gelberman RH, Mae Tan A, Botte MJ. Carpal tunnel syndrome: an evaluation of the provocative diagnostic tests. *J Bone Joint Surg* Am. 68:735–737.
15. Gelmers HJ. The significance of Tinel's sign in the diagnosis of carpal tunnel syndrome. *Acta Neurochir.* 1979;39:255–258.
16. Golding DN, Rose DM, Selvarajah K. Clinical tests for carpal tunnel syndrome: an evaluation. *Br J Rheumatol.* 1986;25:388–390.
17. Heller L, Ring H, Costeff H, Solzi P. Evaluation of Tinel's and Phalen's signs in diagnosis of the carpal tunnel syndrome. *Eur Neurol.* 1986;25:40–42.
18. Kuhlman KA, Hennesey WJ. Sensitivity and specificity of carpal tunnel syndrome signs. *Am J Phys Med Rehabil.* 1997;76:451–457.
19. Megele R. Diagnostische Tests beim Karpaltunnelsyndrom. *Nervenarzt.* 1991; 62:354–359.
20. Katz JN, Larson MG, Sabra A, et al. The carpal tunnel syndrome: diagnostic utility of the history and physical examination findings. *Ann Intern Med.* 1990;112:321–327.
21. De Krom MC, Knipschild PG, Kester AD, Spaans F. Efficacy of provocative tests for the diagnosis of carpal tunnel syndrome. *Lancet.* 1990;335:393–395.
22. Novak CB, Gilbert WL, Mackinnon SE, Lay L, Louis S. Provocative testing for cubital tunnel syndrome. *J Hand Surg Am.* 1994;19:817–820.
23. Jabre JF. Can proximal nerve lesions give rise to a "Tinel-like" sign distally? *Muscle Nerve.* 1995;18:1495–1496.
24. Hawley RJ. Can proximal nerve lesions give rise to a "Tinel-like" sign distally? *Muscle Nerve.* 1996;19:1056.
25. Woodward KG, Vulpe M. The proximal tap or "central Tinel" sign in central dysesthetic syndrome after spinal cord injury. *J Am Paraplegic Soc.* 1991;14: 136–138.
26. Montagna P. Motor Tinel sign: a new localizing sign in entrapment neuropathy. *Muscle Nerve.* 1994;17:1493–1494.
27. Ochoa J, Torebjörk HE, Culp WJ, Schady W. Abnormal spontaneous activity in single sensory nerve fibers in humans. *Muscle Nerve.* 1982;5:S74–S77.
28. Yarnitsky D, Ochoa JL. The sign of Tinel can be mediated either by myelinated or unmyelinated primary afferents. *Muscle Nerve.* 1991;379–380.

22

JENDRASSIK'S MANEUVER

Jan Stam

Ernö (Ernst) Jendrassik (1858–1921) was 24 years old when he wrote his first paper on the tendon reflexes.[1] At that time (1883) he worked as a resident in internal medicine in Budapest, as he remained two years later, when he wrote about the maneuver that would immortalize his name in neurology.[2]

Jendrassik was born in 1858 in Cluj in Transylvania, Romania (at that time called Kolozsvár in Hungarian), where his father was professor of theoretical medicine. In 1860, when Ernö was two years old, his father was appointed professor of physiology at the University of Budapest. At age 22, in 1880, Ernö was graduated as a medical doctor. In 1884 and 1885, at the Salpêtrière, directed by Charcot (1825–1893), he worked with Pierre Marie (1852–1940) on cerebral hemiatrophy. Their collaboration resulted in an influential paper[3] and in lifelong friendship. In 1887 Charcot wrote a letter of recommendation for Jendrassik when he tried to obtain a prestigious professorship in Budapest. Charcot's strong tribute ("he possesses the rare, indeed very rare, qualities that are indispensable to study without prejudice, and in a profound manner, the diseased")[4] could not secure Jendrassik's appointment. Six years later, however, in 1893, he was appointed professor of neuropathology at the Medical University of Budapest at the age of 35 years. In 1898 he was elected corresponding member of the Hungarian Academy of Sciences. Ten years later, when he was 50 years old, he became professor of general pathology.

Although Jendrassik specialized in neuropathology, he remained a generalist who believed that neuropathology should be part of general, internal pathology, and he contributed to both fields. His most important activities concerned not the reflexes, but the pathology of neurodegenerative diseases.[5,6] Between 1896 and 1902 he made important contributions to the field of neurogenetic disorders, and he developed his famous doctrine of "heredodegeneration." Remarkably, he developed many of his clear insights into the nature of neurogenetic diseases before the rediscovery of

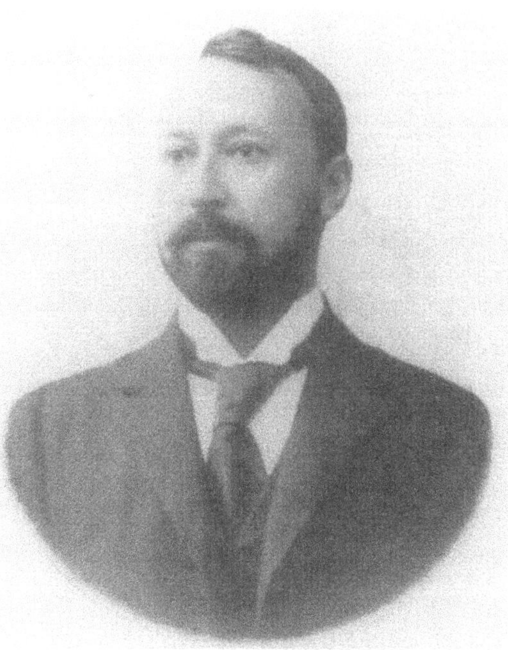

Figure 22–1. Ernö Jendrassik (1858–1921). Courtesy of the Library of the Hungarian Academy of Sciences, Budapest.

Mendel's laws in 1900.[6] In 1903 a reference textbook he wrote on that subject was published in Hungarian. It was translated into German in 1911, as part of the influential handbook edited by Lewandowsky.[7]

Jendrassik's first study of the tendon reflexes was published in 1883, eight years after the discovery of these phenomena by Wilhelm Erb (1840–1921) and Carl Westphal (1833–1890).[1] At that time the nature of the contractions observed after tapping a tendon was far from clear, and their reflex character was hotly debated for many years. Jendrassik chose the side of Erb and others who believed that the contractions were spinal reflexes. He had a clear concept of the reflex arc, and correctly interpreted previous experiments by Tschirjew, concluding

> that for the course of the tendon reflex in the spinal cord . . . it is only necessary that the anterior and posterior roots and the gray matter are intact.[1]

He concluded that the reflexes disappear when the reflex arc is disrupted and observed that

> the pathological increase of the tendon reflexes should in most cases be regarded as the result of the interruption of the inhibiting influence of the brain on the spinal cord.[1]

The maneuver that would bear his name is not mentioned in this first paper, although he rightly pointed out that a voluntary muscle contraction anywhere in the body, such as lifting both arms, causes a physiological increase of the tendon reflexes ("eine physiologische Erhöhung der Sehnenreflexe"). In observing this he revealed a deeper insight than many physicians after him who believed that Jendrassik's maneuver is merely a trick to "divert the patient's attention."

In a second paper, in 1885, Jendrassik examines the relevance of the tendon reflexes for neurologic diagnosis.[2] Previous research had shown that the knee jerk could not be elicited in a number of healthy individuals, which limits its diagnostic value. Jendrassik studied 1000 healthy subjects to examine what we now would call the specificity of the absent knee jerk. First he describes his famous maneuver as follows:

> I put the individual, who has no knee jerk with the normal method, on the edge of a table with the legs as relaxed as possible, and while I tap his patellar tendons I ask him to hook the flexed fingers of the right and left hand in each other, and pull them as hard as possible with the arms extended forward.[2]

In 16 individuals the reflex could not be elicited with the normal technique, but after applying the maneuver, he could easily evoke it in 15 of them. In one patient the knee jerk remained absent, but Jendrassik noticed that this was "a patient suffering from diabetes, in which disease several authors have already missed the knee jerk." He concluded that the significance of the absent knee jerk (in 1.6% of healthy subjects in his study) increased even further by applying his maneuver:

> Since with my method the examination—with the exception of cases where the tendon reflex is lost by a disease—results in 0 per mill, one can obtain a certainty about this symptom, that is hardly possible of any other [symptom].[2]

In his classic monograph (*The Examination of Reflexes: A Simplification*), Robert Wartenberg (1887–1956) mentions Jendrassik's maneuver as one of the many ways to reinforce a tendon reflex and states that any remote muscle contraction has the same effect.[8] He then goes on to give an explanation for the reinforcement: "The explanation for the effectiveness of all these maneuvers is to divert the attention of the patient." This remark, not supported by experimental evidence or by convincing physiological arguments, is probably the source of the erroneous belief that persists today.

Physiological ideas about the Jendrassik effect have been dominated for many years by the theory that the reflex reinforcement was caused by an increased sensitivity of the muscle spindles, by activation via fusimotor gamma efferents. Experiments in the 1940s and 1950s demonstrated that the amplitude of mechanically evoked tendon reflexes increased after Jendrassik maneuvers, whereas the H reflex, which is evoked electrically without stimulation of muscle spindles, did not.[9,10] These observations, however, were contradicted by Landau and Clare, who repeated the experiments and showed in 1967 that the H reflex does increase after muscle contractions elsewhere in the body.[11] After initial confusion, the observations by Landau were finally confirmed by microneurography, which enables direct recording of the nerve volleys in the reflex arc in healthy volunteers. Burke et al. showed that the afferent volleys, evoked by a tendon tap, did not change after a Jendrassik maneuver, although the resulting reflex responses increased normally.[12] This observation excluded modulation of the afferent signal by fusimotor influence. The conclusion from these and other experiments must be that the Jendrassik reinforcement is mediated by a direct effect upon the reflex arc in the spinal cord. This effect may result from a direct neural modulation of the alpha motoneurons or by a change in the strength of the presynaptic inhibition.

Careful recording of the timing of the Jendrassik effect further contributed to clarify the physiological mechanism. Kawamura and Watabene confirmed in 1975 that the H reflex is reinforced by Jendrassik maneuvers.[13] The kind of muscular contraction was not relevant for the reflex reinforcement. Making one or two fists, or merely pressing a button with the thumb, had similar effects upon the reflex amplitude. The time between the conditioning contraction and the reflex was important: the increase in amplitude of the reflex is maximal about 300 ms after the voluntary contraction. Interestingly, about 100 ms *before* a voluntary muscle contraction the reinforcing effect upon the reflexes can already be detected. This phenomenon is part of the physiological changes that occur before any voluntary contraction, the so-called motor preparation, extensively studied by Brunia and his colleagues.[14] Delwaide and Toulouse showed that the Jendrassik effect is propagated in a rostrocaudal direction along the spinal cord.[15]

These physiological studies have proved that the received wisdom that the Jendrassik maneuver is merely a trick to divert the attention of the patient is wrong. This does not imply that mental activity cannot influence the reflexes. Various experiments have shown that mental activity increases the tendon reflexes. When subjects are asked to focus their attention upon one leg the knee jerk in that leg usually becomes more active, even to the extent that some are able to increase the reflexes on one side only.[16] In other words, if one wants to reinforce a reflex, it might be more effective to direct the attention *toward* the examination instead of trying to "divert" it. The simple maneuver discovered by Jendrassik is a bedside manifestation of a complicated neurophysiological process that changes the stimulus–response relation (the "gain") of all muscle spindle reflexes during the preparation and execution of a voluntary movement. One of the many merits of Ernö Jendrassik is not only that he discovered a useful clinical maneuver, but also that he correctly interpreted its physiological significance.

Acknowledgment

I thank Dr. Annemarie de Knecht-van Eekelen (Department of Medical History, Free University, Amsterdam) for her expert help in preparing this paper.

References

1. Jendrassik E. Beitrage zur Lehre von den Sehnenreflexen. *Dtsch Arch Klin Med.* 1883;33: 177–199.
2. Jendrassik E. Zur Untersuchungsmethode des Kniephänomens. *Neurol Zentralbl.* 1885;4: 412–415.
3. Jendrassik E, Marie P. Contribution à l'étude de l'hémiatrophie cérébrale par sclérose lobaire. *Arch Physiol Norm Pathol.* 1885;S3T5:51–105.
4. Antall J, Kapronczay K, Vida T. La correspondance de Jean Martin Charcot, Pierre Marie et Ernö Jendrassik. *Comm Hist Artis Med.* 1978;24:105–135.
5. Van Bogaert L. Hommage to E. Jendrassik. *Ther Hung.* 1958;6:25–26.
6. Czeizel A. A historical evaluation of the doctrine of heredodegeneration. *Comm Hist Artis Med.* 1979;25:159–163.
7. Jendrassik E. Die Hereditären Krankheiten In: Lewandowsky M, ed. *Handbuch der Neurologie.* Berlin: Springer Verlag; 1911.

8. Wartenberg R. *The Examination of Reflexes: A Simplification.* Chicago: Year Book Publishers; 1945:18–19.
9. Sommer J. Periphere Bahnung von Muskeleigenreflexen als Wesen des Jendrassikschen Phänomens. *Dtsch Z Nervenheilk.* 150;1940:249–262.
10. Buller AJ, Dornhorst AC. The reinforcement of tendon reflexes. *Lancet.* 1957;2:1260–1262.
11. Landau WM, Clare MH. Fusimotor function, IV: Reinforcement of the H-reflex in normal subjects. *Arch Neurol.* 1964;10:123–127.
12. Burke D, McKeon B, Skuske NF. The irrelevance of fusimotor activity to the Achilles tendon jerk of relaxed humans. *Ann Neurol.* 1981;10:547–550.
13. Kawamura T, Watabene S. Timing as a prominent factor of the Jendrassik maneuver on the H-reflex. *J Neurol Neurosurg Psychiatry.* 1975;38:508–516.
14. Brunia CHM, Vuister FM. Spinal reflexes as indicator of motor preparation in man. *Physiol Psychol.* 1979;7:377–380.
15. Delwaide PJ, Toulouse P. Facilitation of monosynaptic reflexes by voluntary contraction of muscle in remote parts of the body: mechanisms involved in the Jendrassik maneuver. *Brain.* 1981;104:701–719.
16. Stam J, Speelman HD, van Crevel H. Tendon reflex asymmetry by voluntary mental effort in healthy subjects. *Arch Neurol.* 1989;46:70–73.

23

THE TEST OF LASÈGUE

Hans J.G.H. Oosterhuis

Ernest-Charles Lasègue was born on 5 September 1816 in Paris. His father Antoine, a botanist, served as librarian of the Delessert family. He was soon aware of the extraordinary intelligence and capacities of his son and placed him at the prestigious Lycée Louis-le Grand for the completion of his scientific education. The young Lasègue studied philosophy and retoric, spoke fluent Latin, and was able to translate Greek philosophical texts at first reading.[1]

In 1838, at the age of 22, he was appointed teacher to the school he had just left; there Charles Baudelaire (1821–1867) became one of his pupils. At that time he became a friend of Claude Bernard (1813–1878), whom he assisted in animal experiments and by whom he was persuaded to study medicine. He was definitely converted to this choice in 1839, when he attended the lectures of the famous Armand Trousseau (1801–1867).[1,2]

He became passionately involved in the study of medicine in general and psychiatry in particular. After receiving his doctoral degree in 1846, he soon became fascinated by his work as consultant physician at the Préfecture de Police, where he had to examine many people accused of various crimes. He kept standardized notes of all cases, and when he intended to describe some common pattern of abnormal behavior, he collected all his case notes and wrote an article on it.[3] In 1852 he became Trousseau's *chef de clinique* and in 1853 he became *professeur agrégé* with a thesis on general paralysis of the insane. In the same year he became editor of the *Archives générales de Médicine,* in which he published most of his articles. His knowledge of other languages, unusual in France at that time, was very useful in acquainting him with German and English scientific literature.

In 1862 he was appointed lecturer in mental and nervous diseases, in 1867 he became professor of general pathology, and in 1869 he took the chair of clinical

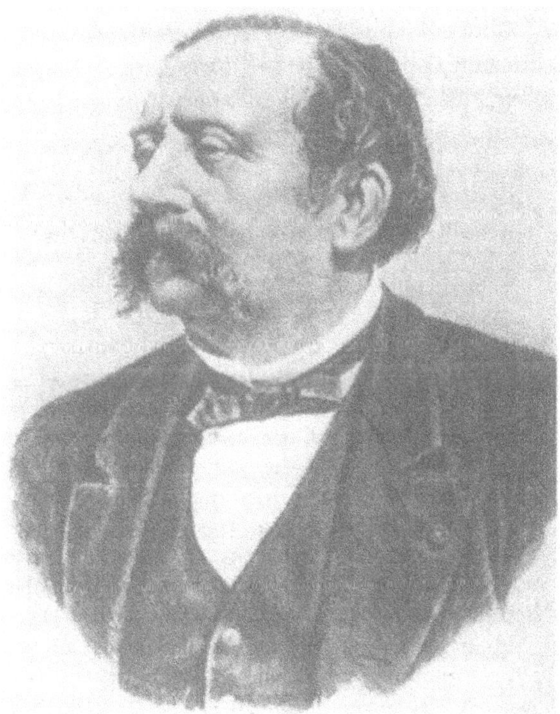

Figure 23–1. Charles Ernest Lasègue (1816–1883). Courtesy of Medizinhistorisches Institut, Zurich, Switzerland.

medicine at La Pitié Hospital, which he occupied until his death, from complications of diabetes, in 1883.[2,3]

Although his 115 scientific papers included many on internal medicine, pediatrics, neurology, and the history of medicine,[4,5] his most original work lies in the field of psychiatry. The main subjects of his psychiatric writings were the "folies à deux," delusion of persecution, exhibitionism, and hysterical anorexia. He was the first to describe the latter condition in detail in 1873 with experience of eight cases, although the English physician William Gull (1816–1890) claimed priority.[3]

It is a strange irony that the test to which his name is attached was in fact not described by him but by one of his pupils. In 1864, in his paper on sciatica, Lasègue distinguished a benign and a grave form with muscle atrophy. The benign sciatica was caused by compression of the muscles and was characterized by paroxysmal bouts of pain that could not be provoked. The more severe form produced a dull continuous pain, radiating into the thigh, provoked by pressure on the nerve and by traction, and was conceived to be related to the hip joint.[6]

This paper is frequently quoted as the first description of the test and the sign of Lasègue, although its description does not occur in this paper.[7] The phenomenon of the start or worsening of pain in the domain of the sciatic nerve by passive elevation of the knee-extended leg was first described by J. J. Forst in his thesis presented on

29 January 1881 at the Medical Faculty of Paris.[8,9] He nevertheless gives full credit to his teacher Lasègue:

> We prefer to confine our description to a clinical sign with great diagnostic value . . . it was our teacher professor Lasègue who drew our attention to this sign. The patient is positioned supine on a bed and the foot of the affected leg is taken by one hand as in [Fig. 23–2, top]. We place our other hand on the knee of the same leg and while stretching the leg in the knee we flex the upper-leg in the hip. The elevation of the leg over a minor distance causes a sharp pain at the place of the tuber ischiadicum, exactly on the place where the nerve comes out. We now lay the leg on the bed again and proceed to another maneuver that is merely intended as a control test. If we flex the leg in the knee, as in [Fig. 23–2, bottom], it is possible to flex the leg in the hip, without pain. To succeed in this maneuver we have to take some precautions. The leg should be flexed slowly in the knee by slipping the heel over the bed, thus avoiding other movements in the hip joint. The explanation of the impaired flexion of the stretched leg in the hip is apparently that the flexors of the hip are balanced by the extensors, which are very powerful. At the elevation of the leg both muscle groups are contracting simultaneously. Therefore the sensation of traction is most probably caused by a compression of the sciatic nerve, by the muscle contraction. By flexion of the leg in the knee we paralyze the extensors of the upper-leg. These are now completely relaxed. The action of the flexors of the upper-leg is now more effective and elevation of the leg is much easier with less compression of the sciatic nerve. Consequently the numbness in the buttock is absent.
>
> We suppose that the sharp pain experienced by the patient can be ascribed to the compression of the nerve by the muscle bulk: this is also the opinion of our teacher professor Lasègue.[8]

Remarkably, Lasègue stated in his paper of 1864[6] that passive flexion or extension of the painful leg is possible without increase of pain. Probably he had not tried the combination of extension in the knee and flexion of the hip.

According to a biographical note, Lasègue conceived the extended-leg test when he had to answer the question of how to discern between patients with real sciatic pain and malingerers.[2] When he saw his son-in-law playing a violin, it occurred to him that the fibers of the sciatic nerve stretched by raising of the leg are extended over the tuber ischii in the same way as the strings are stretched over the bridge of the violin. Forst's explanation that the nerve is compressed by the muscle bulk of the upper leg is apparently not in agreement with the anecdote of the violin.

De Beurmann investigated the shift of the sciatic nerves in corpses in 1884 and found that the sciatic nerve was much more stretched if the knee was extended than flexed; he concluded that stretching of the nerve was the cause of pain in the test of Lasègue.[10] Modern investigators point to an antidromic activation of nociceptors in the peripheral part of the affected root, since the pain can be prevented by a local block of the sciatic nerve.[11]

Independent from Forst, Lasègue, and De Beurmann, the test of the stretched leg was described in 1884 by Lazarevic, a Serbian physician in Belgrade, who also emphasized that the leg should be flexed in the knee, as a control test. He explained the pain as produced by stretching of the nerve. Lazarevic claimed that he had described this test as early as 1880 in a Serbian medical journal, thus preceding the description of Forst.[12]

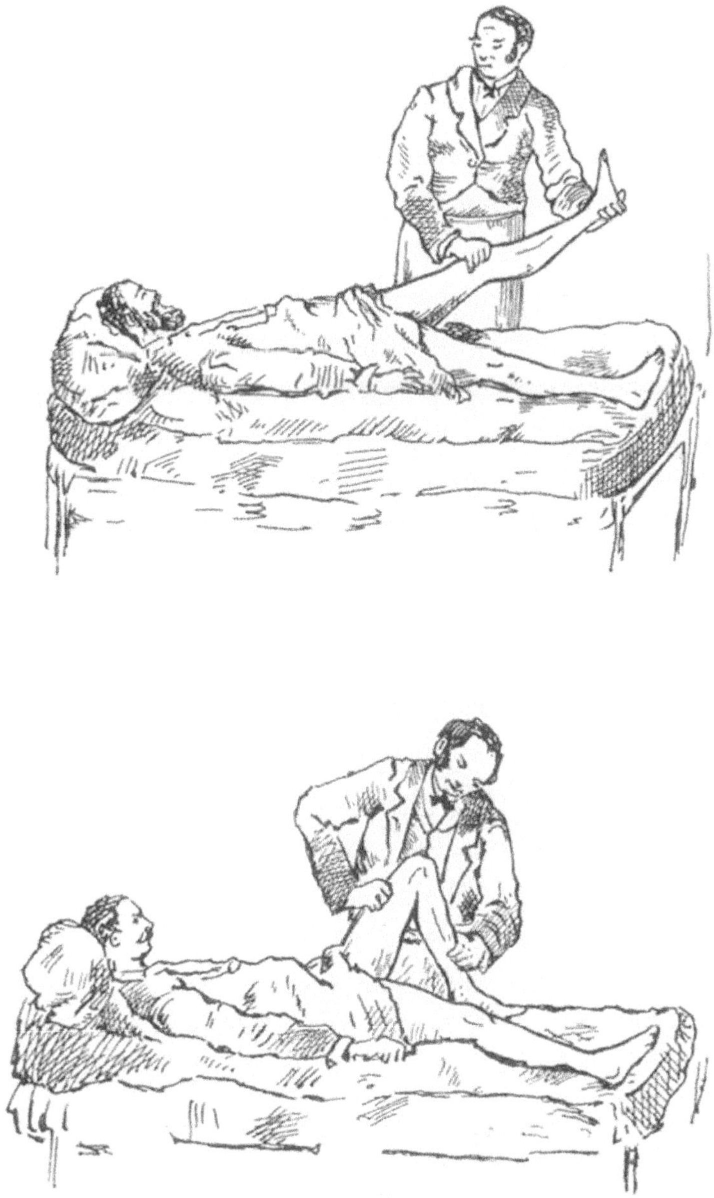

Figure 23–2. The test of Lasègue: first and second maneuver. Original pictures from Forst's thesis.[8] *The text does not explain the raised head and the disappearance of the beard during the second maneuver (!).*

The crossed Lasègue test, radiating pain in the affected leg if the nonaffected leg is raised, was described by the Polish neurologist J. Fajersztajn (1867–1935). He also stated that sciatic pain may be provoked by passive dorsal extension of the foot, if passive raising of the leg to a certain height has not yet caused this pain. This maneuver is usually attributed to Karl Bragard (1890–1973), but it had been described in 1913 as the "Lasègue of the foot" by the Genevan internist Maurice Roch (1878–1967).[9]

The test or sign of Lasègue is mentioned in all textbooks of neurology, although in the recent English and American literature the eponym Lasègue is frequently omitted and the test is referred to as the "straight-leg-raising test." The description is often rather sketchy and many authors do not mention the control test with the flexed knee. Few details can be found about the question of whether the elicited sign consists only of the radiating pain or also of the blockade of further movement by the muscle defense, as is sometimes said. Usually, in order for the sign to be positive, the pain has to radiate beneath the knee and not remain localized only in the back or the thigh, because in these cases the pain is usually of ligamentous origin (pseudo-radicular). Some authors consider 70 degrees as the lowest value of the positive sign; the value of less than 30 degrees is sometimes mentioned as strongly positive.

The sensitivity of the tests of Lasègue for the diagnosis "lumbar disk protrusion" in patients with sciatica varies from 45% to 97% (mean 85%)[14–18] in surgically verified protrusions, and it is highest in the youngest groups.[19] The specificity of the test is less thoroughly investigated in lumbar disk protrusion since patients with sciatica but without a verified disk prolapse are less common, or not considered in the statistics.

In a study of the signs and symptoms of 100 consecutive patients with lumbar disk prolapse or with lateral or central spinal stenosis, respectively, who were all surgically verified, a positive test of Lasègue was found in 88%, 51%, and 35%, respectively; but a test of less than 30 degrees in 43%, 9%, and 4%, respectively; a crossed test of Lasègue was found in this group in 23%, 6%, and 2% respectively.[17] In meta-analysis studies, the crossed Lasègue test had high predictive value for the presence of a herniated disk, which was sequestered in about 50% (sensitivity about 30% specificity 90%–98%).[14]

Reproducibility of any test depends on consistent instructions to and a certain experience of the examiner. When various examiners had to determine the angle of raising, systematic differences of 20 degrees occurred in a quarter to one-third of the cases.[15]

To achieve an optimum reproducibility and accuracy, I would recommend the following procedure for the test of Lasègue:

- The patient lies completely supine.
- The affected leg is extended at the knee with the examiner's hand under the heel and is raised strictly vertically, avoiding rotation of the hip joint.[20]
- Measure with a goniometer at which angle irradiating pain under the knee occurs.

- Perform the same procedure in the nonaffected leg.
- Control that flexion in the hip with flexed knee is not painful.

References

1. Ritti M. Éloge du professeur Ch. Lasègue. *Ann Med-Psychol.* 1885;2(7th ser):88–121.
2. Aird R. Charles Lasègue. In: Haymaker W, Schiller F, eds. *The Founders of Neurology.* 2nd ed. Springfield, Ill: Charles C Thomas; 1970:469–472.
3. Vandereycken W, Van Deth R. Who was the first to describe anorexia nervosa: Gull or Lasègue? *Psychol Med.* 1989;19:837–845.
4. Pozzi L. Charles Lasègue. *Arch Orthop.* 1968;81:227–238.
5. Études médicales du Professeur Ch. Lasègue. 2 vols. Paris: Asselin; 1884. Complete works.
6. Lasègue Ch. Considérations sur la sciatique. *Arch Gén Méd.* 1864;2:558–580.
7. Wartenberg R. Lasègue sign and Kernig sign: historical notes. *Arch Neurol.* 1951;66:58–66.
8. Forst J J. *Contributions à l'étude clinique de la sciatique.* Paris: Faculté de Médicine de Paris; 1881. Thesis.
9. Wilkens R H, Brody I A. Lasègue's sign: neurological classics XXII. *Arch Neurol.* 1969;21: 219–221.
10. Beurmann L De. Note sur un signe peu connu de la sciatique: recherches expérimentales. *Arch Physiol Norm Pathol.* 1884;16:375–380.
11. Xavier A V, McDanal J, Kissin L. Mechanism of pain caused by the nerve root tension test in patients with sciatica. *Neurology.* 1989;39:601–602.
12. Lazarevic L K. Ischias postica contunnii. Ein Beitrag zu deren Differential Diagnose. *Allgem Wien Med Z.* 1884;29:425–426.
13. Karbowski K. Zur Geschichte der Entdeckung des Lasègueschen Phänomens und seiner Varianten. *Schweiz Med Wochenschr.* 1984;114:942–945.
14. Vroomen PCAJ, Krom MCTFM de, Knottnerus J A. Diagnostic value of history and physical examination in patients suspected of sciatica due to disc herniation: a systematic review. *J Neurol.* 1999;246:899–906.
15. Kosteljanetz M, Bang F, Schmidt-Olsen S. The clinical significance of straight-leg raising (Lasègue's sign) in the diagnosis of prolapsed lumbar disc: interobser variation and correlation with surgical finding. *Spine.* 1988;13:393–395.
16. Kortelaïnen P, Puranen J, Koivisto E, Lähde S. Symptoms and signs of sciatica and their relation to the localization of the lumbar disc herniation. *Spine.* 1985;10:88–92.
17. Jönsson B, Strömqvist B. Symptoms and signs in degeneration of the lumbar spine. *J Bone Joint Surg Br.* 1993;75:381–385.
18. Kerr R S, Cadoux-Hudson T A, Adams CBT. The value of accurate clinical assessment in the surgical management of the lumbar disc protrusion. *J Neurol Neurosurg Psychiatry.* 1988;51: 169–173.
19. Spangfort E V. Lumbar disc herniation: a computer aided analysis of 2504 operations. *Acta Orthop Scand.* 1972 (suppl 142):1–93.
20. Breig A, Troup JDG. Biomechanical considerations in the straight-leg-raising test cadaveric and clinical studies of the effects of hip rotation. *Spine.* 1979;4:242–250.

24

KERNIG'S AND BRUDZINSKI'S SIGN

Anton Valkenburg

Vladimir Mikhailovitsch (also known as Woldemar) Kernig was born in St. Petersburg in 1840. Trained by A. Wachsmuth in Dorpat, Estonia, he obtained his medical degree in 1864 with a thesis titled *Experimentelle Beiträge zur Kenntniss der Wärmeregulierung beim Menschen.* He practiced medicine in the Obuchows Women's Clinic in St. Petersburg from 1865 to 1911. From 1873 to 1899, he worked as a practitioner at the St. Petersburg Institution for the Deaf and Mute, and taught internal medicine from 1881 to 1886).[1–3] Kernig died in 1917. Apart from neurological studies, he also published several articles on internal diseases.

Kernig presented his experiences on patients with meningitis at a meeting of the Union of Medical Doctors in St. Petersburg in 1882.[4] His 1884 article, "Ueber ein wenig bemerktes Meningitis-Symptom," included a new sign (neck stiffness in meningitis) that had not been previously described.[5] In the same year, he gave a lecture about this sign at the International Medical Congress in Copenhagen, Denmark. Kernig examined mainly women between 20 and 62 years old and only three children. He published his experiences in a German medical journal:

> If the patients are sat upright, allowing them to sit on the edge of the bed their legs hanging down . . . you will first notice a much more intensive contraction of the neck and back, and second a flexion contraction of the knee joints, occasionally also in the elbow joints, will set in. If one tries to extend the knee of the sitting patient, one succeeds only to an angle of about 135 degrees. In cases in which the phenomenon is very pronounced, the angle will be even more straight . . . the difference between the entire absence of the contraction in the supine position and its presence in the sitting position is so remarkable that it is worthwhile to pay particular attention to this symptom and to look for it in every case.[5] [translated from German]

Kernig examined 15 patients suffering from meningitis (13 cases of epidemic, one of tuberculous, and one of purulent meningitis). He found spontaneous contractions of

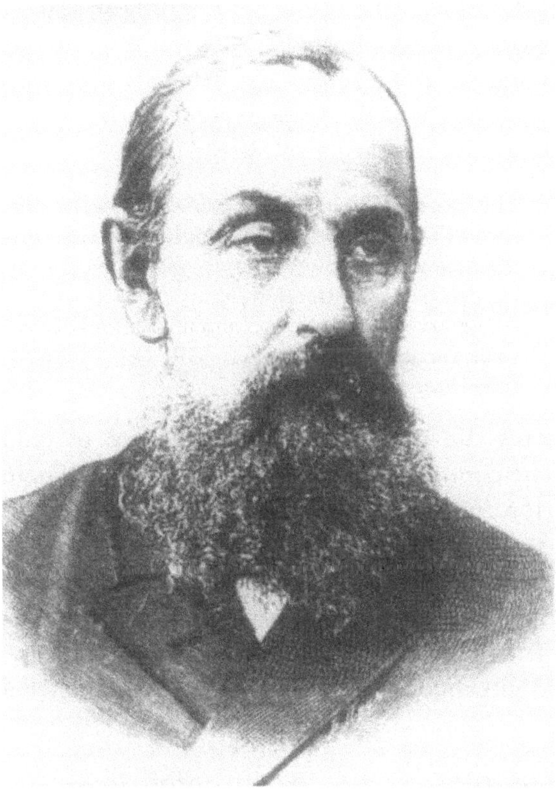

Figure 24–1. Vladimir Mikhailovitsch Kernig (1840–1917). From *Vsemiznaya illustratziya* (1894), vol. 51, p. 394.

the limbs in the supine position in three. In eight patients spontaneous contractions were not present in the supine position, but did occur in a sitting position. However, the contractions of the legs disappeared in the standing position. Subsequently, Kernig examined the patients again in the supine position. If he tried to extend the leg to a right angle with the trunk, he noticed a contraction at a certain degree of flexion of the thigh on the trunk. He concluded that in the supine as well as in the sitting position, a contraction might occur at the knee joint if the upper leg is at a certain angle to the trunk. He ended his article with an extensive description of six cases with a positive "Kernig's sign." In these cases, meningitis was suspected but could not be proved. Following autopsy, a definitive diagnosis of meningitis was made. These observations soon fell into oblivion. The sign was not even mentioned in textbooks.[6]

Arnold Netter (1855–1936), discoverer of antibodies in human convalescent serum of patients suffering from poliomyelitis (1910), studied Kernig's sign during an epidemic of cerebrospinal meningitis in Paris in 1898.[7] He proved that the sign is almost constantly present in but not specific for meningitis, as had been stated by Kernig. It may also be present in other diseases including sciatica, typhoid fever, intracerebral hemorrhages, cerebral tumors, and tabes dorsalis.

Kernig's sign has been described many times since, and it indicates an irritation of the cerebrospinal membranes. Nowadays, Kernig's sign is tested while the patient is in the supine position. Authors who refer to Kernig's original article mention the examination of the sitting patient only and suggest that the sign tested in the supine position was described later, but this is a mistake. Kernig described both methods in his original article, although he emphasized the examination in the sitting patient.

Throughout the years, several modifications of testing appeared. William Osler (1849–1919), for example, wrote in 1899:

> The patient should be propped up in bed in the sitting position, then, on attempting to extend the leg on the thigh there is contraction of the flexors which prevents the full straightening of the leg. On the other hand, in the recumbent posture the leg can be fully extended. Many patients with meningitis are not in a condition to sit up, and the test can be equally well made by flexing the thigh on the abdomen, when on attempting to extend the leg, if meningitis be present, the limb cannot be fully extended.[8]

Kernig did not mention the presence of pain while performing the maneuver. Some clinicians interpret the occurrence of pain, rather than a contraction, as a criterion for a positive Kernig's sign. Thus this sign conforms with the Lasègue sign (see Chapter 23).

Jozef Polikarp Brudzinski was born in Bolew, Poland, on 26 January 1874.[1,9,10] Like Kernig, he studied in Dorpat at first. He completed his studies in Moscow in 1897, after which he specialized in pediatrics. He was initially trained under Jakubowski in Krakau, and subsequently he worked with Theodor Escherich (1857–1911) in Graz, where he

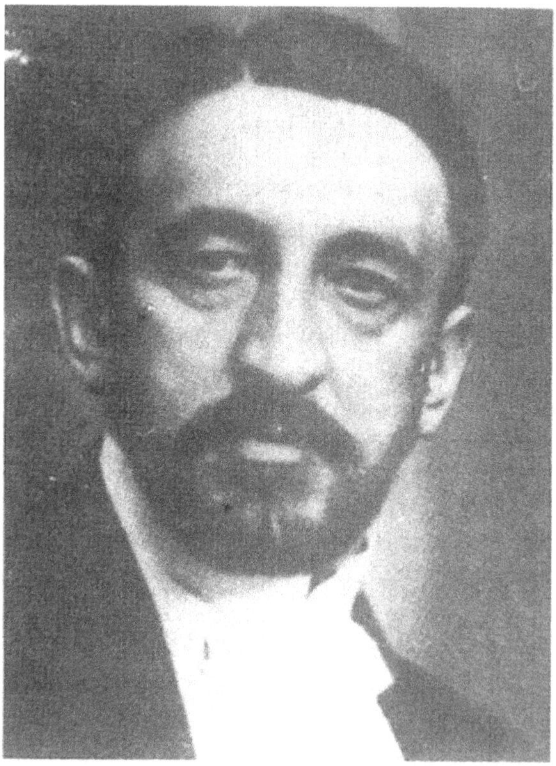

Figure 24–2. Jozef Polikarp Brudzinski (1874–1917). Courtesy of the Biblioteka Glówna, Akademia Medycna, Lodz, Poland.

studied the bacterial flora of the gastrointestinal tract of infants. Later he worked under Jacques Joseph Grancher, Jean Bernard, and Antoine Marfan in Paris, and with Anders in Warsaw. He was associated with the Anne-Marie Pediatric Hospital in Lodz, Poland, after 1903. In 1908, he set up the first Polish journal of pediatrics: *Przeglad Pedyatryczny.* Two years later, he moved to Warsaw and set up the "Karl and Maria-Child Hospital," where he became chief physician. Following the German occupation of Poland, he was involved with the reestablishment of the Polish University in Warsaw, which he opened as rector in 1915. Brudzinski was a devoted teacher and spent much time with his students. Suffering from nephritis, he died at the age of 43, in Warsaw, on 18 December 1917. Next to his neurological studies, his work on the bacterial flora of the bowels (the cause of dysentery, streptococcus enteritis, and proteus vulgaris in the stools of infants) and prevention of infectious diseases was also notable.

Brudzinski's name has been associated with several signs of meningism. He described the first sign in 1908: "Ueber die kontralateralen Reflexe an den unteren Extremitäten bei Kindern."[11] In this article he first discussed several theories about associated movements of extremities, mainly in children. Subsequently, he gave an extensive description of a number of children suffering from hemiplegia, developmental disorders, and meningitis. In many of these children he found an "identical contralateral reflex." This reflex could be elicited in the supine position when the examiner passively bends the hip and knee on one side, resulting in flexion of the contralateral leg. Sometimes a "reciprocal contralateral reflex" may appear. This occurs if the leg that is flexed in response to passive flexion of the other leg extends spontaneously. In six out of eight cases of tuberculous meningitis, Brudzinski found the identical contralateral and in one the reciprocal contralateral reflex. In one patient he found neither. He found only identical contralateral reflexes in two cases of epidemic meningitis. Apart from the signs already known, including neck stiffness and Kernig's sign, these reflexes may contribute to the diagnosis.

Following extensive study of this reflex, Brudzinski noticed a new sign in patients suffering from meningitis. He described it minutely in a French medical journal in 1909; "Un signe nouveau sur les membres inférieurs dans les méningites chez les enfants".[12] While testing for neck stiffness, flexion of the legs in knee and hip joints occurred. Brudzinski called it "le signe de la nuque" (neck symptom):

> Passive forward flexion of the neck causes flexion of the lower extremities in the knee and hip joints, and the limbs sometimes execute a very extensive flexion on the pelvis . . . The technique of testing for the sign of the neck is very easy; one takes the head of the child that is lying supine, in the left hand, and bends the head and the neck while pushing the right hand on the child's chest to prevent it from raising . . . only, sometimes, in very young children, one does not easily succeed in holding the legs extended because of the child's anxiety; in this case, one gently retains them at the region of the knee joint. To prevent errors, it is important to do repeated examinations.[12] [translated from French]

Brudzinski studied the frequency of several signs and reflexes in 42 patients (21 with tuberculous and 21 with nontuberculous meningitis).[12] Kernig's sign, Babinski's sign, the contralateral reflex, and Brudzinski's neck symptom appeared in 57%, 50%, 66%, and 97% of the patients, respectively. By this time, Kernig's sign was well known and widely used. Brudzinski finished his 1909 article by concluding that the neck-symptom was positive in nearly all cases of meningitis and that the contralateral reflex has the same value as the other signs already known in meningitis.

Brudzinski described two other symptoms in 1916, which, however, did not become well known clinically; the "cheek sign" and the "symphysis sign." The cheek sign consisted of a rapid reflex elevation of the arms and simultaneous flexion of the elbow joints elicited by pressure on both cheeks just below the zygomatic bone. Brudzinski observed the symptom in 98% of patients with tuberculous meningitis (42 cases). In cases of nontuberculous meningitis the cheek sign was positive less often. In 85 cases of children with symptoms of meningitis this sign was positive in 81% of cases. The symphysis sign consisted of flexion contracture of both legs elicited by pressure with the thumb and index finger over the symphysis pubis. Brudzinski found this symptom in all children with tuberculous meningitis. In his article, he advised these tests in all children suspected of tuberculous meningitis.[13]

Of all the tests of Brudzinski described, the neck symptom (Brudzinski 1) is best known and most tested, followed by the contralateral reflex (Brudzinski 2).

Several pathophysiological explanations for the occurrence of Kernig's sign were proposed at the beginning of the twentieth century:[6] (1) irritative lesions of the pyramidal tract, diminishing its functional activity;[14] (2) exaggeration of a normal reflex in a cerebral lesion;[15] (3) slight predominance of antagonists in hypertonic muscles resulting from a disturbed equilibrium between active hypertonic flexors and, less, hypertonic extensor muscles;[16] (4) irritation of the spinal cord and cauda equina in meningitis inducing hypertonia of the flexor muscles;[17] and (5) contraction of the flexor muscles of the knee as a defensive mechanism against painful stretching of the inflamed sciatic nerve in meningitis, when the leg is bent at the hip joint.[18]

Brudzinski did not have a clear explanation for the symptoms he described. He suggested muscular hypertonia of the legs and physiological predominance of the extensor muscles of the neck as well as the back, over the flexor muscles of the lower limbs.[12]

Later, the signs of Kernig and Brudzinski were explained as tonic neck reflexes; however, an underlying lesion of the brainstem was not considered likely.[19] Using autopsy data, O'Connell in 1946 extensively described the possible pathophysiological mechanisms, speculating that an inflammation of the meninges causes hypersensitivity of the nerve roots. If the roots are stretched by certain movements of the head, neck, and legs, reflex muscular hypertonia will develop to protect the spinal nerve roots from painful stimuli:[20]

> It is a justifiable assumption that the spinal nerve-roots as they traverse the inflamed meninges (indeed, as has been shown, roots which are themselves inflamed) will be hypersensitive to mechanical stimulation by compressing or stretching.

This remains the most satisfactory theory today.[21]

References

1. Hall G W. Neurologic signs and their discoverers. *JAMA*. 1930;9–5:703–707.
2. Pagel J. *Biographisches Lexikon der hervorragender Ärzte des neunzehnten Jahrhunderts*. Berlin: Urban & Schwarzenberg: 1901: 851.
3. Pearce JMS. The signs of Kernig and Brudzinski. *J Neurol Neurosurg Psychiatry*. 1992;55:1141.
4. Kernig W. Ein Krankheitssymptom der acuten Meningitis. *St Petersb Med Wochenschr.* 1882; 7:398.
5. Kernig W. Ueber ein wenig bemerktes Meningitis-Symptom. *Berl klin Wochenschr.* 1884; 21:829–832.
6. Hassin G B. Kernig's sign and its pathogenesis. *Med Rec.* 1905; 68:413–415.
7. Netter A. Diagnostic de la Méningite cérébro-spinale (Signe de Kernig, Ponction lombaire). *Sem Méd.* 1898;281–284.
8. Osler W. The Cavendish lecture on the etiology and diagnosis of cerebro-spinal fever. *Br Med J.* 1899;2:1517–1528.
9. Fischer I. *Biographisches Lexikon der hervorragender Ärzte der letzten fünfzig Jahre.* München: Urban & Schwarzenberg; 1962:181–182.
10. Kyle R A, Shampo A. Jozef Brudzinski. *JAMA*. 1979;241:1620.
11. Brudzinski J. Ueber die kontralateralen Reflexe an den unteren Extremitäten bei Kindern. *Wien Klin Wochenschr.* 1908;21:255–261.
12. Brudzinski J. Un signe nouveau sur les membres inférieurs dans les méningites chez les enfants. *Arch Méd Enf.* 1909;12:745–752.
13. Brudzinski J. Ueber neue Symptome von Gehirnhautentzündung und Reizung bei Kindern, insbesondere bei tüberkulösen. a) Ueber das Wangenphänomen; b) Ueber das Symphysisphänomen. *Berl Klin Wochenschr.* 1916;25:686–690.
14. Sailer J. The unilateral occurrence of Kernig's sign as a symptom of focal brain disease. *Am J Med Sci.* 1902:772.
15. Bull E. Ueber die Kernig'sche Flexionscontractur der Kniegelenke bei Gehirnkrankheiten. *Berl Klin Wochenschr.* 1885;22:772–774.
16. Chauffard A. Du signe de Kernig dans les méningites cérébrospinales. *Phys pathol Presse Méd.* 1901:153.
17. Roglet P. *Contribution à l'étude du signe de Kernig dans les Méningites. Sa valeur diagnostique et séméiologique, sa pathogénie.* Paris: Faculté de Médicine de Paris; 1900. Thesis.
18. Piéry. Signe de Kernig et signe de Lasègue: Pathogénie du signe de Kernig. *Lyon Méd.* April 1904.
19. Wartenberg R. The signs of Brudzinski and of Kernig. *J Pediatr.* 1950;37:679–684.
20. O'Connell JEA. The clinical signs of meningeal irritation. *Brain.* 1946;69:9–21.
21. Simpson J F. Meningeal signs and symptoms. In: Vinken P J, Bruyn G W, eds. *Handbook of Clinical Neurology.* Amsterdam: North Holland Publishing Company; 1969;1:536–549.

25

MORO'S REFLEX

Rianne J. Wennekes

Ernst Moro was born the youngest of eight children, in Leibach (Austrio-Hungarian Empire) on 8 December 1874.[1–3] He planned to study botany but changed his mind and started his medical studies at the University of Graz. Following graduation in medicine, he became assistant to Theodor Escherich (1857–1911), professor of pediatrics. In 1899 he took his doctoral degree and in 1902 he followed Escherich to Vienna. In June 1904 he married Margarete Mathilde Honigswald, and they had one daughter. He returned to Graz in the same year, and became a pediatrician in 1906.

From 1906 to 1911 Moro worked in the university's pediatric clinic *(U-Kinderklinik)* in Munich (1907) under Escherich's successor Meinhard von Pfaundler (1872–1947). Finally, Moro succeeded Emil Feer (1864–1955) as head of pediatrics at Heidelberg, Germany's oldest university, in 1911; the Kinderklinik was situated in a convalescent home, the Louisenheilanstalt. He remained head of pediatrics for 25 years, doing much fundamental work in such fields as vitamin and calcium metabolism, allergy and skin disease, and the pathogenesis of infantile diarrhea. By the end of his scientific career he had published a pioneering monograph on seborrheic dermatitis and atopic eczema. In 1936, at the age of 62, he resigned because of ill health as well as scientific-political activities against him (not unusual at that time in German pediatric-academic circles). He spent his remaining years in Heidelberg, together with his wife and daughter. He died on 17 April 1951.

Moro was basically a morphologist, preferring to see and not to imagine things. He wrote about 186 papers in the field of pediatrics based on his clinical experience and eminent observational capacities. His lectures were outstanding, given in the tradition of classical clinical lectures of the German or French school. In addition, he displayed many artistic qualities, and practiced calligraphy as well as painting, especially copying the old masters.

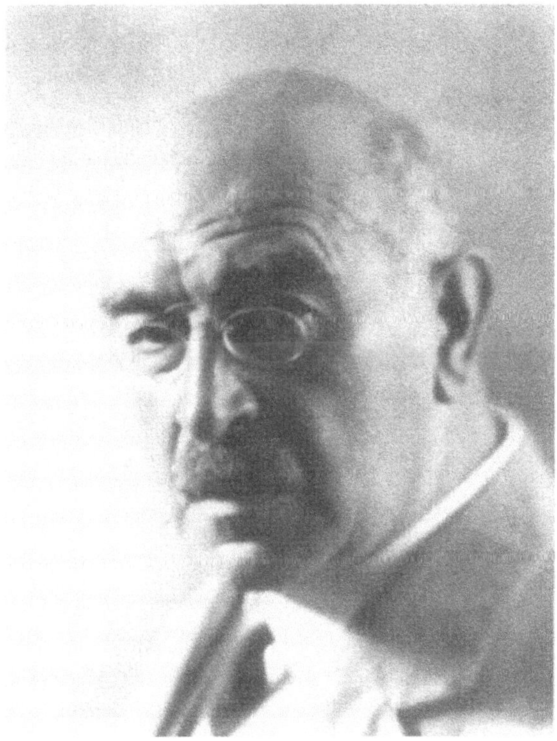

Figure 25–1. Ernst Moro (1874–1951). Courtesy of Universitätsarchiv Heidelberg.

On 7 May 1918, Ernst Moro presented a lecture entitled "Das erste Trimenon" [The first trimester] at a meeting of the Society of Natural History and Medicine in Heidelberg. In this lecture he discussed some features he observed during the first three months of an infant's life. At the end he described a behavioral observation, that is, the reflex that later came to bear his name:[4]

> Zum Schlusse möchte ich Ihnen noch über eine kleine Beobachtung berichten . . . Legt man einen jungen Säugling auf den Wickeltisch und schlägt man zu beiden Seiten mit den Handen auf das Kissen, so erfolgt ein eigenartiger Bewegungsreflex, der ungefähr folgendermassen verläuft: Beide Arme fahren symmetrisch auseinander um sich hierauf unter leicht tonischen Bewegungen im Bogen wieder annähernd zu schliessen. Ein ähnliches motorische Verhalten zeigen gleichzeitig beide Beine. [Fig. 25–2]

[Finally I would like to mention a minor observation . . . If a young infant is laid down on the dressing table and one beats the pillow on both sides with the hands, a particular reflex movement is elicited, proceeding as follows: both arms move apart symmetrically and subsequently converge archlike with slightly tonic movements. The legs show a similar motor behavior at the same time.]

The *Umklammerungsreflex* (clasping reflex) described by Moro is most easily obtained in the first weeks of life and gradually becomes less clear and less frequent until it is difficult to obtain by the end of the third month. He specified the reflex

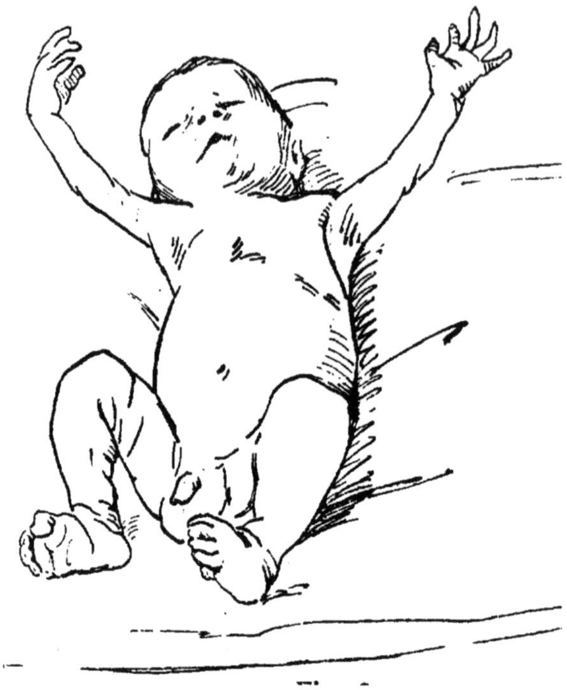

Figure 25–2. The Moro reflex. From Ref. 4.

may be elicited for a longer period in premature infants. Moro had observed the clasping reflex several years earlier:

> Dieser Bewegungsreflex ist mir schon vor vielen Jahren aufgefallen. Zu einer befriedigenden Deutung seines Wesens bin ich aber erst kürzlich gelegentlich der Lektüre von F. Dofleins Tierbiologie geführt worden.

[I have noticed this motor reflex for many years. Only recently was I led to the satisfactory interpretation of its nature after reading F. Doflein's *Animal Biology*.] After attending the lecture by Doflein he recognized the analogy with the behavior of newborn animals. Doflein divided the newborn animals into four groups; *Beutelsäuglinge* (marsupial infants), *Lagersäuglinge* (hole infants), *Brustsäuglinge* (breast infants), and *Laufsäuglinge* (walking infants). The Brustsäuglinge, humans included, are not able to walk immediately after delivery, and have to be carried by their mother. That is why they have special clasping abilities (instincts). Newborn apes, for instance, have a strong clasping reflex, and they are able to hold the skin of their mothers tightly. Figure 25–3 pictures a mother orangutan holding her baby, illustrating the "clasping" movement. Moro speculated that the clasping reflex, as observed in newborn infants, was an effort by the baby to grasp its mother. He called it "Umklammerungsreflex" because he assumed it to be an anxiety response. He recognized its possible diagnostic significance. In a later paper, he described the persistence of the reflex in children with delayed mental development.[5]

The Moro reflex has probably been the primitive reflex most commonly used to evaluate the neurological status of the newborn infant, despite the continued absence of consensus concerning the proper stimulus for eliciting the reflex

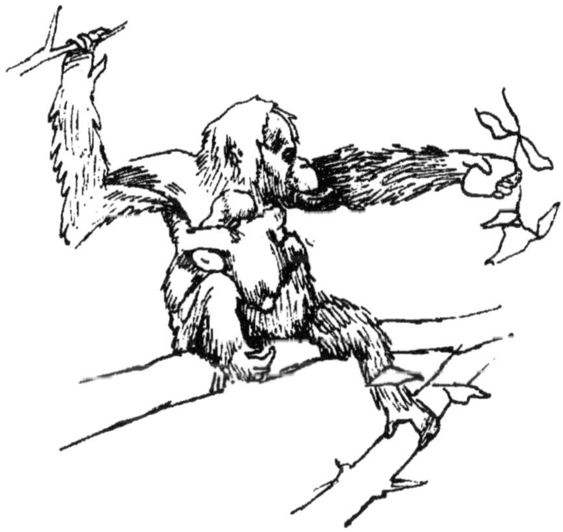

Figure 25–3. The Umklammerungss-reflex, *or clasping reflexes.* From Ref. 4.

response and the absence of general agreement on the response to be expected (qualification of the reflex).[6]

In Moro's original description, the striking, with both hands, of the pillow on which an infant was lying elicited the (Moro) reflex. Moro also observed that manipulation of the baby in other ways than beating the pillow would give rise to the reflex response. Magnus and de Kleyn suggested that these movements in infants were of labyrinthine origin.[7] Later, Schaltenbrand, Pieper, Isbert, and Prechtl agreed with him.[8] Thomas and Hanon, applying the same stimulus as Magnus, that is, holding the baby in a semiseated position and letting the head fall back suddenly by 30 degrees, concluded that the Moro reflex is a response not to vestibular stimulation but rather to proprioceptive stimulation originating in the neck.[9] Prechtl and Beintema described the head drop as well as dropping the whole body as a stimulus to elicit the reflex.[10] They advised though to use the head drop maneuver; the examiner lifts the infant's head and gently allows it to fall back into his hand, eliciting abduction and extension of the arms, followed by adduction and flexion.

Touwen also used the slapping of the examining table near the baby's head as a stimulus.[11] In applying this original stimulus, it is important to keep the head of the infant in the middle position, as the response can be asymmetric otherwise. The normal timetable for the appearance and disappearance of the Moro reflex depends on the stimulus chosen to elicit the reflex. The head drop maneuver fades quickly (in 78% of the infants the response disappeared at the age of 20 weeks) while the whole body drop maneuver elicits a Moro response that persists for a longer period (a slight response was still visible at the age of 36 weeks).

In 1921, Freudenberg already observed that the secondary adduction of the arms, as well as extension of the legs, was not always present.[12] Goldstein, Landis, Hunt, and Clarke (1938)[13] emphasized the abduction and extension of the arms to be the main and primary component of the Moro reflex. They considered the adduction to be a secondary phenomenon. Parmelee described the sequence of appearance. The abduction movement is dominant in the first weeks after birth, while the adduction movement is recognized in the older infant.[14] In 1984, Capute and associates graded the primitive reflexes for strength and completeness of response. They described their evaluation in a longitudinal study of full-term infants, and later also in premature infants, from birth through infancy.[15] The primitive reflexes and their developmental course have been useful components of neurologic examination in infancy ever since. They help to assess the integrity of the central nervous system, or, more specifically the brainstem maturation.[16]

Gordon and Sandford noticed that persistence of a Moro reflex into the second year of life referred to pathology of the central nervous system.[17,18] An asymmetrical response should raise suspicion of peripheral neurological (brachial plexus problems) or nonneurological (fractured clavicle) disorders of the arm. In children with neurological pathology (i. e., cerebral palsy), the persistence of some primitive reflexes until the age of two (i.e., Moro, asymmetric tonic neck reflex, tonic labyrinthine reflex) seemed to be a good predictor of motor development (future ambulation).[19–21]

For a number of years, the newborn infant's behavior was believed to consist of a repertoire of primitive reflexes reflecting the dominance of subcortical neural centers. As neural maturation occurs, these primitive reflexes diminish, disappear, or are integrated into more complex functional movements. Because several limitations of this hierarchical model of motor control have been pointed out and because the distinction between reflex and voluntary movement is blurred, it is no longer accepted that development just proceeds from reflex-driven to voluntary behavior. The nervous system probably produces variable emergent motor strategies to meet the task at hand ("dynamic systems theory"). Within this framework, primitive reflexes are mostly termed infantile reactions.

Many neurological assessment scales have been developed to evaluate the neurological development of preterm and full-term newborn infants.[22] Observation of spontaneous motor behavior and of head and body positions is considered more important than investigations requiring active manipulations of the infant including the evaluation of primitive reflexes or infantile reactions. However, the Moro reflex remains one of the neonatal primitive reflexes applied most often.[23]

References

1. Opitz H. Kinderaertzliche Praxis. *Gesellsch Pediat D D R.* 1930;19:350–351.
2. Kleinschmidt H. Ernst Moro. *Monatsschr Kinderheilk.* 1951;99:311–312.
3. Hoefnagel D, Lüders D. Ernst Moro (1874–1951). *Pediatrics.* 1962;29:643.
4. Moro E. Originalien aus der Heidelberger Kinderklinik das erste Trimenon. *Münch Med Wochenschr.* 1918;65:1147–1150.

5. Moro E. Zur Persistenz des Umklammerungsreflexes bei Kindern mit zerebralen Entwicklungshemmungen. *Münch Med Wochenschr.* 1920;67:360.
6. Parmelee A M. A critical evaluation of the Moro reflex. *Pediatrics.* 1964;31:773–788.
7. Magnus R, Kleyn A de. Die Abhängigkeit des Tonus der Extremitätenmuskeln von der Kopfstellung. *Pflügers Arch Ges Psychol.* 1912;145:455.
8. Prechtl HFR. Neurological diagnosis of cerebral injury in the newborn. In: *Proceedings of the Symposion Prenatal Care.* Groningen: Noordhoff; 1959.
9. Thomas A, Hanon F. Les premiers automatismes. *Rev Neurol.* 1947;79:641.
10. Prechtl HFR, Beintema D. The neurological examination of the full term newborn infant. *Little Club Clinics in Developmental Medicine* no 12. 1964:45–47.
11. Touwen BCL. *De neurologische ontwikkeling van de zuigeling.* Utrecht: Bohn, Scheltema & Holkema; 1984:112–121.
12. Freudenberg E. Der Morosche Umklammerungs-reflex und das Brudzinskische Nachenzeichen als Reflexe des Säuglingsalters. *Münch Med Wochenschr.* 1921;68:1646.
13. Goldstein K, Landis C, Hunt WA, et al. Moro-reflex and startle pattern. *Arch Neurol Psychiatry.* 1938;40:322.
14. Parmelee A H. A critical evaluation of the Moro reflex. *Pediatrics.* 1964;33:773.
15. Capute A J, Palmer F B, Shapiro B K, Wachtel R C, Ross A, Accardo P J. Primitive reflex profile: a quantification of primitive reflexes in infancy. *Dev Med Child Neurol.* 1984;26:375–383.
16. Allen M C, Capute A J. The evolution of primitive reflexes in extremely premature infants. *Pediat Res.* 1986;20:1284–1289.
17. Gordon M G. The Moro embrace reflex in infancy; its incidence and significance. *Am J Dis Child.* 1929;38:26.
18. Sandford H M. The Moro reflex in the newborn. *Am J Dis Child.* 1933;46:337.
19. Blasco PA. Primitive reflexes: their contribution to the early detection of cerebral palsy. *Clin Pediatr Phila.* 1994;33:388–397.
20. Trahan J, Marcoux S. Factors associated with the inability of children with cerebral palsy to walk at six years: a retrospective study. *Dev Med Child Neurol.* 1994;36:787–795.
21. Watt J M, Robertson CMT, Grace MGA. Early prognosis for ambulation of neonatal intensive care survivors with cerebral palsy. *Dev Med Child Neurol.* 1989;31:766–773.
22. Mandich M, Simons CJR, Ritchie S, Schmidt D, Mullet M. Motor development, infantile reactions, and postural responses of preterm at risk infants. *Dev Med Child Neurol.* 1994; 36:397–405.
23. Dubowitz L, Mercuri E, Dubowitz V. An optimality score for the neurologic examination of the term newborn. *J Pediatr.* 1998;133:406–416.

26

ROMBERG'S SIGN

Jan M. Keppel-Hesselink and Peter J. Koehler

One might assume that neurology started as an independent specialty when a chair was founded for Jean-Martin Charcot in 1882. Some 40 years earlier, Moritz Heinrich Romberg (1795–1873) formulated the first blueprint of systematic neurology by publishing a two-volume neurological reference book.[1] He formulated the eponymous test in the second edition of that book.

Moritz Romberg was born in Meiningen (Thüringen) on 11 November 1795.[2,3] After his father's death he moved to Berlin with his mother. He went to high school and subsequently studied medicine. He graduated in 1817 with a thesis on congenital rickets, providing a classical description of achondroplasia.[4] He decided to devote his further studies to nervous diseases. Three years later, he visited the Viennese physician Johann Peter Frank (1745–1821), who was particularly interested in the study of the spinal cord but became better known for his endeavors to improve public health. His most famous publication in this respect was *System einer vollständigen medicinischen Polizei* [System of a comprehensive medical police], which was published in nine volumes between 1777 and 1817. In it he ascribed an important role to the state in improving public health. Frank had an important influence on Romberg.

Romberg became physician to the poor in Berlin in 1820, a position he held for 25 years. He dealt with more than 200 neurological patients a year in the ancient Charité hospital. During this period, he translated several English textbooks into the German language, the most important of which was Charles Bell's *The Nervous System of the Human Body*.[5,6] Romberg was an admirer of this English physician, who probably inspired him to write his textbook. He was among the persons who incorrectly attributed the discovery of the function of the ventral and dorsal roots to Charles Bell; François Magendie (1783–1855) in fact had provided the first correct description (see Chapter 29).

Figure 26–1. Moritz Romberg (1795–1873). Courtesy of Medizinhistorisches Institut, Zurich, Switzerland.

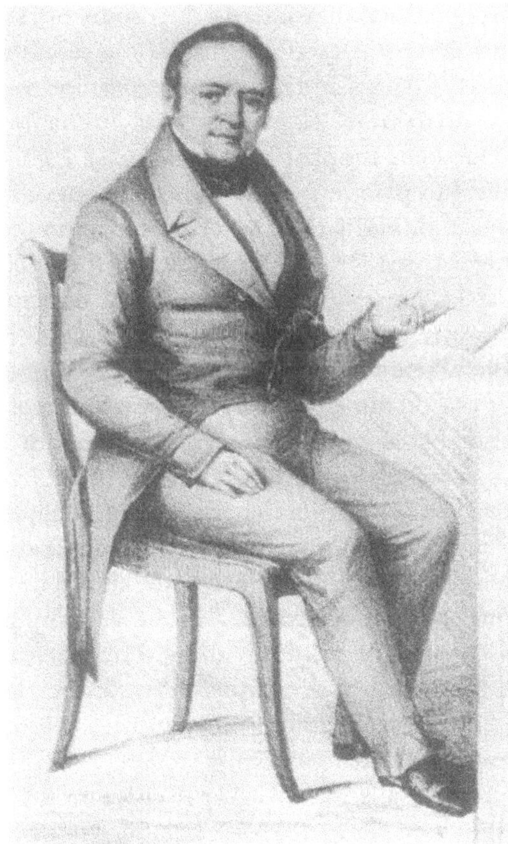

Not until 1830 did Romberg start an academic career, when he was appointed *Privat-Dozent* (associate professor) of special pathology and therapy at the University of Berlin. In 1831 and in 1837 he directed the cholera hospital. He was appointed extraordinary professor of pathology in 1838 and director of the university hospital in 1840.

Romberg's most important book, *Lehrbuch der Nervenkrankheiten des Menschen,* was published between 1840 and 1846. Three editions followed by 1857. The book is considered the first systematic neurological textbook and was translated into English in 1853. The structure of the book was similar to other textbooks on medicine that were published in that period, classifying disease in a way Linnaeus had done for plants. William Cullen (1710–1790), who had coined the term *neurosis* and applied it to nervous diseases, classified diseases into (1) fevers, (2) neuroses, (3) cachexias, and (4) locales. Cullen's classification influenced Philip Pinel (1745–1826), who recognized neuroses of the senses, cerebral function, locomotion and voice, nutrition, and sexual function. The class of neuroses may be regarded a mixture of modern neurology and psychiatry, although other diseases were still classified within this category.[7] In this tradition, Romberg, in his textbook, called the first class of nervous diseases "neuroses of sensibility," subdivided in subcategories (e.g., hyperesthesia and anesthesia). Similarly, "neuroses of motility" was subdivided into hyperkinesia and akinesia. Describing the various diseases, Romberg emphasized the parts that fit into the system and did not pay attention to symptomatology, course, and prevalence.

Apart from "Romberg's test," his name became also associated with progressive facial hemiatrophy: the *syndrome of Parry–Romberg* and *Romberg–Howship symptom* refers to pain in the thigh, in the area of the obturator nerve, due to incarcerated obturator herniation. Romberg was appointed full professor of special pathology and therapy in 1845. In the middle of the 1860s, compelled by age and frequent gout attacks, he resigned his position of director of the outpatient clinic and his chair. However, he remained active at the faculty. He had suffered from a heart disorder for several years when he died at the age of 77 on 16 June 1873.

We do not encounter the description of Romberg's sign in the first edition of his textbook. Not until the second edition, in 1853,[8] did Romberg describe it as a sign typical of tabes dorsalis. This term (from Latin: "wasting" of the dorsal columns) was used for a syndrome characterized by lightning pains, ataxia, and urinary incontinence, as well as some other symptoms and signs. It was observed in the tertiary stage of neurosyphilis, but this was not known until the end of the nineteenth century; the spirochete was discovered in the beginning of the twentieth century. However, the disease had been known under terms such as *consumption of the backbone* as referred to in the Hippocratic corpus. It was associated with sexual excesses—not with venereal disease—through the centuries.[9] Romberg was not the first to describe tabes dorsalis. His teacher Ernst Horn (1774–1848) had inspired his students to work on tabes dorsalis, resulting in five doctoral theses between 1817 and 1827, and published a paper in 1813.[9,10] Romberg referred to his colleague (at the Berlin Charité hospital) Robert Froriep (1804–1861), who drew attention to atrophy of the lower posterior spinal column and nerves in a case of tabes dorsalis. In the English translation of the second edition of Romberg's textbook we read:

> I was not a little surprised to find the atrophy so confined . . . If he is ordered to close his eyes while in the erect posture, he at once commences to totter and swing from side to side . . . It is now ten years since I pointed out this pathognomic sign, and it is a symptom which I have not observed in other paralyses.[11,12]

Romberg indeed classified the disease as a "neurosis of motility." However, he was aware that anesthesia of the muscles alone without loss of power invariably accompanies tabes dorsalis.[11,12] Knowledge of position sense or sense of muscular action was already present in the first part of the nineteenth century. In his *Nervous System of the Human Body* (1830; translated by Romberg, see above) Charles Bell referred to

> returning muscular nerves [that] are associated with the nerves of sensibility to the skin, but they are probably very distinct in their endowments, since there is a great difference between conveying the sense of external impressions and that of muscular action.

Six years later, however, Bell wrote about "consciousness of muscular exertion," which he called a sixth sense, referring to an army captain who "could feel the touch of a lady's petticoat on the calf of his legs" without being able to "tell the position of his feet without looking at them."[12] The next important paper on tabes dorsalis was written by Duchenne, who applied the term *ataxie locomotrice.*[13,14]

One of the early signs of tabes dorsalis is the decrease of sense of touch and proprioception, whereas the sense of temperature and pain remain intact. The feet are numb when the patient is standing, walking, or supine, and the skin may feel like it is covered with fur. The sensation of standing and walking is also abnormal. The sensation is described as if the soles of the feet are in contact with wool, soft sand, or a balloon filled with water. The gait becomes insecure and the patient tries to improve it by consciously taking bigger steps. From the beginning of the disease, the patient keeps his eyes directed at his own feet. If he is asked to close his eyes while standing upright, he immediately starts to sway. The unsteady gait is worse in the dark.

Romberg effectively used this observation: on eliminating optic control—by closing the eyes or in the dark—insecure gait is displayed. We now know that this is caused by the absence of feedback by the dorsal columns. Romberg did not yet associate his observation with the dorsal column lesion. This association was made a few decades later by William Gowers (1845–1915). Nor did Romberg associate the phenomenon with what is now called ataxia.

During the century after Romberg's first description, the test gradually gained recognition. William Hammond (1828–1900), who was the first to describe athetosis, described the symptom in 1876, not mentioning Romberg.[15] A patient consulted Hammond because of symptoms indicating locomotor ataxia. The first sign of the disease that the patient had noticed was the inability to remain standing while he was washing himself in the morning with his eyes closed. On examination, the patient indeed could not stand with his eyes closed.

A few years later, in 1880, a presentation on locomotor ataxia by Gowers was published in the *Lancet.*[16] He described five persons suffering from Friedreich's ataxia in a family with nine children.[17] The least affected 22-year-old son had no symptoms but displayed an abnormal Romberg's test, absent knee tendon reflexes and sensory disturbances of the legs. Furthermore, he noted that this hereditary type of ataxia, first described by Nikolaus Friedreich (1825–1882) in 1863,[18] was very rare, and that there usually was a medical history of syphilis.

How difficult it was in those days to separate and distinguish between neurological syndromes based on principles of localization. This is apparent from the book by the Tübingen professor Carl Liebermeister (1833–1901), who discussed Romberg's sign, *das Romberg'sche Symptom,* in lesions of peripheral nerves.[19]

The fact that the feet need to be placed together while carrying out Romberg's test is an addition found over and over again in twentieth-century papers on the subject. In the third part of his textbook (1898),[20] Adolf Strümpell (1853–1925) described Romberg's sign as loss of balance when closing the eyes, similar to Romberg's description.

On studying the medical literature, Romberg's name is found in eponyms including "Romberg's sign," "Romberg's symptom," "Romberg's phenomenon," and "Romberg's test." In all instances, however, the same phenomenon is referred to. The sign was identified early in the history of neurology, at a time when neurological examination did not yet exist, a few decades before the description of the knee tendon reflex and 40 years before the description of Babinski's sign. In Romberg's day, neurological patients were only observed. The fact that he made his observations indicates great acuity, as the sign cannot be found just by watching: the physician must provide some particular instructions. Although this seems to be a detail, it in fact is not, as the physician has to enter into a dialogue with the patient, providing specific instructions. One step further on the way to formal and systematic neurological examination was to approach the patient, that is, sensing the muscle tone and testing the muscle stretch reflexes. This phase was not reached until the 1870s. The observation that Romberg's sign was described relatively early in the history of neurology is probably due to the fact that the sign was directly associated with a symptom, uncertainty of gait in the dark.

The initial association of Romberg's sign with tabes dorsalis gradually decreased in the course of the nineteenth century. The presence of an abnormal test gradually evolved from tabes to other afflictions accompanied by sensory ataxia. We have to realize that the understanding of the structure and function of the pathways of the spinal cord was limited in the days of Romberg. This is the reason why the test was not associated with disordered function of the dorsal columns until the end of the nineteenth century. Only then was it possible to distinguish between cerebellar and tabetic ataxia. This is one of the reasons why the test was no longer used solely in the context of tabes dorsalis at the end of the nineteenth century.

References

1. Romberg M H. *Lehrbuch der Nervenkrankheiten des Menschen.* 2 vols. Berlin: Duncker; 1840–1846.
2. Viets H. Moritz Heinrich Romberg (1795–1873). In: Haymaker W, Schiller F, eds. *The Founders of Neurology.* 2nd ed. Springfield, Ill: Charles C Thomas; 1970:506–509.
3. Waldenburg L. Moritz Heinrich Romberg. *Berl Klin Wochenschr.* 1873;10:289–290.
4. Romberg M H. *De rachitide congenita.* Berlin: Platen; 1817.
5. Bell C. *The nervous system of the human body.* London: Longman; 1830.
6. Romberg M H. *Bell's physiologische und pathologische Untersuchungen des Nervensystems.* Berlin: Stuhr; 1832.
7. Reynolds E H. Structure and function in neurology and psychiatry. In: Reynolds EH, Trimble M R, eds. *The Bridge between Neurology and Psychiatry.* Edinburgh: Churchill Livingstone; 1989:38–55.
8. Romberg M H. *Lehrbuch der Nervenkrankheiten des Menschen.* 2nd ed. Berlin: Duncker; 1851;1:185.
9. Schiller F. Venery, the spinal cord and tabes dorsalis before Romberg: the contribution of Ernst Horn. *J Nerv Ment Dis.* 1976;163:1–9.
10. Horn E. Bemerkungen über die wichtigsten Erkrankungen. *Horns Arch Med Erfahrung.* 1813;236:8.
11. Romberg M H; Sieveking E H, trans. *Manual of the nervous system of man.* London: Sydenham Society; 1853;2:396.
12. Schiller F. Staggering gait in medical history. *Ann Neurol.* 1995;37:127–135.
13. Duchenne de Boulogne GBA. De l'ataxie locomotrice progressive; recherches sur une maladie caracterisée spécialement par les troubles généraux de la coordination des mouvements. *Arch Gén Méd.* 1858;12:641–652.

14. Pryse-Phillips W. *Companion to Clinical Neurology.* Boston: Little, Brown and Company, 1995.
15. Hammond W. *A Treatise on the Diseases of the Nervous System.* New York: Appleton; 1976: 589–590.
16. Gowers W R. Ataxy in several members of a family. *Lancet.* 1880;ii:618.
17. Keppel Hesselink J M. Een discussie uit de vorige eeuw: multipele sclerose of tabes of de ziekte van Friedreich. [Romberg's test; a century of discord over its implementation] *Ned Tijdschr Geneeskd.* 1986;131:2353–2356.
18. Friedreich N. Ueber degenerative Atrophie der spinalen Hinterstränge. *Arch Pathol Anat Berl.* 1863;26:391–419.
19. Liebermeister C. *Vorlesungen über die Krankheiten des Nervensystems.* Leipzig: Vogel; 1886:38.
20. Strümpell A. *Lehrbuch der Speciellen Pathologie und Therapie der inneren Krankheiten.* Leipzig: Vogel; 1895:3:241.

27

THE NO-REBOUND PHENOMENON OF STEWART–HOLMES

Nicolaas J. M. Arts and George W. Bruyn

The (no-)rebound phenomenon is a valuable diagnostic tool that, in our opinion, is regrettably underused in neurological examinations. This is probably largely due to a misunderstanding about (or lack of comprehension of) the essential point of this sign, despite its lucid description by Stewart and Holmes.[1–3]

Thomas Grainger Stewart, the third son of the well-known Sir Thomas (Grainger Stewart) and his wife Jessy Dingwall Fordyce, daughter of the parson Dr. R. Macdonald, was born in Edinburgh on 2 December 1877. The shy, rather introverted youth was of above-average intellectual endowment. He took the bachelors in medicine and surgery in 1900, became a member of the Royal College of Physicians (RCP), Edinburgh, in 1902 and of the RCP, London, in 1904. Between a stint as house physician at the Edinburgh Royal Infirmary and his moving to London he studied in Munich. He was awarded the gold medal for his M.D. thesis in 1912 and elected Fellow of the RCP, London, a year later.

At the National Hospital, Queen Square, he was house physician, resident medical officer, assistant pathologist, assistant physician, and became honorary (consultant) physician in neurology, discharging his duties as such for nearly 40 years (1908–1948). His retirement was due in 1942, but because of staff absences in the war, he continued attending outpatient clinics. He also was neurologist to the West London Hospital (1909–1939), the Central London Ophthalmological Hospital (1929–1938), the Metropolitan Hospital, St. Vincent's Cripple Home, St. James' Hospital, and the Charing Cross Hospital (1909–1937). In addition, he built up his private practice in Queen Anne Street, where he also lived in a small flat on a floor above. He left for a large mansion in Ennismore Gardens in 1922 and married the wealthy Lady Frances Sophia Harvey, the widow of Sir Patrick Playfair.

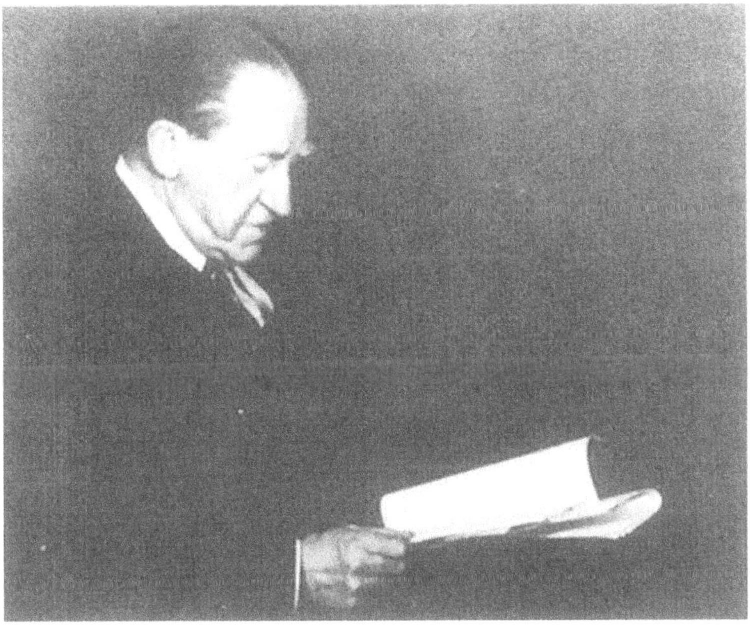

Figure 27–1. Thomas Grainger Stewart (1877–1957). Courtesy of the Institute of Neurology, National Hospital, Queen Square, London.

In addition to the two authoritative papers that founded the eponym,[1,4] Stewart, together with another Presbyterian Scot, Aldren Turner (son of the distinguished anatomist Sir William Turner), wrote a neurological textbook of great detail and merit,[5] that must have taken a long gestation period because Stewart disliked teaching and writing, and Turner, a stickler for meticulous precision, was even more unhurried in manner than Stewart was. His paper in the *Lancet* on frontals tumor–induced tremors (1906) is nearly forgotten. He was associated with Gordon Holmes, another staff-member at the National Hospital, (see below) in another eponym, "Holmes–Stewart syndrome," which essentially is the same as the "Jacksonian cerebellar fits,"[6] that is, decerebration attacks. His last paper was written with Greenfield in 1927 on Schilder's diffuse sclerosis.[7]

The initial bond of friendship between Holmes and Stewart gradually cooled; indeed, it deteriorated to the point of a fistfight, coats off, in the laboratory of the hospital, an event preserved by Steiner et al.[8] After that, they scarcely spoke to each other. Now, Stewart was certainly not the only one with whom Holmes had bitter quarrels bordering on violence. Holmes was (erroneously) said to have had but few friends: Francis Walshe, Charles Symonds, Greenfield, and William Adie, whose exquisite personalities probably rendered them more tolerant than others. But Stewart, though kind and hospitable to staff and friends, could at times be disagreeable: gruff, reserved, conservative, high-principled, laconic, apparently devoid of emotion, and noted for his sparse, overcautious, oligosyllabic speech. The difference of background may have been crucial. Holmes came from a humble Irish home and had to fight for his position. Stewart came from an academic, cultured, Protestant "milieu."

Stewart, of ruddy hair, fair complexion, and sturdy build, had the natural manners of an aristocrat; he knew and courteously addressed by name colleagues, nurses, technical and administrative staff, for whom he displayed amiable attention, and was always cheerful and considerate. He detested teaching, persuading young Macdonald Critchley to take over his paid teaching duties at the West London Hospital. But after a few months, he forgot to remunerate Critchley for his troubles, which may have been a matter of mere amnesia but, on the other hand, admirably fits the picture of the proverbially tightfisted Scotsman.

Stewart's lack of haste during ward rounds or physical examination was as legendary as irritating; he seemed to be bereft of any sense of time. He was a sound clinician, inspiring at the bedside, as his Norwegian pupil Georg Monrad-Krohn used to point out.

Having been a golfer and angler, Stewart soon discovered the all-absorbing passion of his life: deer hunting, which he had learned in Glen Etive, Argyll, while still a boy. Every late autumn he returned to Scotland for two months, to stalk deer, indefatigably. The Stewarts rented the Rothiemurchus property in the Cairngorms every year for this purpose. To this day, a certain deer track across a steep scree in the wooded Braeriach is still called "the Doctor's Walk." Often, when early sunset forced the hunt to close, he took the evening train to London to see patients and return by night train to Aviemore for the full day's stalking. The story goes that the gamekeeper or one or two "guns" from his hunting party had to grab him by ankles and feet to stop him hanging over a precipitous escarpment to obtain a better shot.

Stewart was Dr. Marcia Wilkinson's first cousin once removed by marriage, and she remembers him and his wife "Bo" when they came to stay with her parents between the late 1920s and 1930s. He was a gruff man who seemed to like less and less the age in which he lived and at any rate insisted on his predinner single malt (personal communication, letter, April 1994).

In the mid-twenties he developed an undefined disease, after recovery from which he was changed, lacking in vigor and joie de vivre, rarely smiling, introverted, slow, and suffering from progressive deafness. He withdrew unobtrusively from professional activities between the end of the war and the early 1950s and died, without issue, at Farnborough, on 18 March 1957.

Gordon Morgan Holmes was born in a Yorkshire Protestant family on 22 February 1876 in Castlebellingham, Ireland.[9–14] He was a shy and solitary child. The early death of his mother and problems with his stepmother reinforced these character traits. He studied medicine at Trinity College in Dublin and qualified in 1899. As a clinical assistant at the Richmond Asylum in Dublin he did so well that he was awarded the Stewart scholarship, which enabled him to go to Frankfurt for two and a half years, to study comparative and human anatomy with Karl Weigert (1845–1904) and Ludwig Edinger (1855–1918). In 1902, he was appointed house physician to John Hughlings Jackson (1835–1911) at the National Hospital, and in 1909 he became a member of the honorary staff. Later, he also became consulting physician at Charing Cross Hospital and Moorfields Royal Ophthalmic Hospital.

At the outbreak of World War I, Holmes immediately volunteered for military service but was rejected on account of myopia. Determined to serve in France, he joined the staff of a Red Cross hospital just behind the front line.[15] His skills and his enormous capacity for work attracted the attention of the War Office; his disqualification was revoked and Holmes was appointed consultant neurologist to the British armies in France. The subject of myopia was never raised again.

The war offered excellent opportunities for Holmes to continue his studies of the cerebellum and start research on the visual cortex,[15,16] because the British helmet, which resembled a bedpan, rested high on the head leaving the occiput exposed to bullets and shrapnel. The numerous young soldiers whose occipita were hit were perfect subjects for examination.

At the front, Holmes belonged to a staff of 10 doctors who had to treat 900 acute military cases. Convoys of up to 300 wounded men might arrive daily. Holmes coped with all his military duties, performed all the neurological postmortems, and, in addition, was simultaneously engaged in three major research projects. Between 1914 and 1918 he published 18 papers, half of them exceeding 30 pages. Most had been written at the front, at night, in the most difficult conditions.

In France, at the Red Cross hospital, Holmes met Dr. Rosaly Jobson, a Scottish captain in the British army, and a top-class athlete. They married in 1918 and had three daughters. After the war, Holmes became a very active member of the neurological community. In 1933 he was elected Fellow of the Royal Society; in 1951 he was knighted. Holmes retired in 1941. After enduring the London blitz, during which the houses on either side of their house were damaged, Gordon and Rosaly moved to a country house in Farnham, Surrey. There, Holmes's main interest was in his large garden. He also spent much time reading and playing golf. He died in his sleep, early in the morning of 29 December 1965, aged 89.

Holmes was a dark, tall, and powerful man, described by his pupils in terms like volcanic, tornadolike, brusque, demanding, almost bullying. He was tireless, but prone to migraine and duodenal ulcer. In the *Lives of the Fellows of the Royal College of Physicians of London,*[17] we find the following characterization:

> With his tall, powerful frame and his hawk-like eyes under beetling brows and spectacles, he intimidated candidates for the College Membership [examination] until they found that direct answers to direct questions brought out the kindliness for which he was known to his intimate friends.

Holmes had strong likes and dislikes and no great gift for wit, diplomacy, or compromise. He was an irascible martinet devoted to detailed observation and collection of data. At the front, he came into collision with Harvey Cushing (1869–1939) about the treatment of war casualties,[15] and his frienship with Stewart ended with the previously mentioned fistfight. However, his interminable feud with Samuel Alexander Kinnier Wilson (1878–1937) was one-sided, according to Holmes's house physician Macdonald Critchley:

> Wilson was a vain and touchy man, jealous of Holmes, and he would ostracise anyone who stayed in the other camp. Holmes for his part could not care less, and simply ignored his colleague.[13]

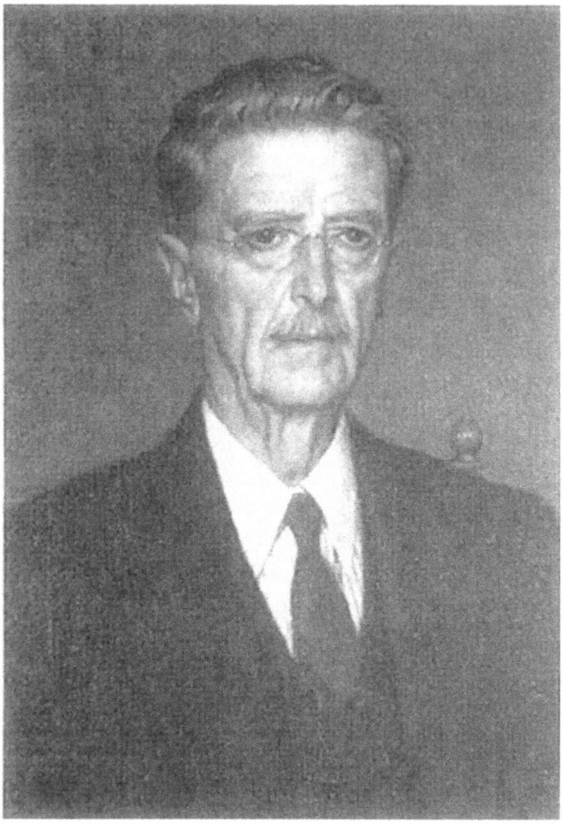

Figure 27–2. Gordon Morgan Holmes (1876–1965). Courtesy of the Institute of Neurology, National Hospital, Queen Square, London.

The story goes that whenever Holmes and Wilson made their respective rounds in Queen Square, each with his own retinue of doctors of all ranks, and they met in the passageways, neither of them would budge to make way for the other party. Lengthy blockages ensued, which could only be dispersed when the head nurse intervened.[18]

Holmes made many contributions to neurology, especially to our knowledge of the cerebellum and the visual cortex.[19,20] He was the first to challenge the universally accepted theory about of the unitary function of the cerebellum. In cerebellar disturbances he discerned the components: asthenia, ataxia, absence of rebound, and adiadochokinesis. This work was the basis for his Croonian Lectures to the Royal College of Physicians (1922).[21] He also developed the modern standard clinical neurological examination, with its subdivision in higher cortical functions, cranial nerves, locomotion and coordination, sensibility, and reflexes.[22] His collaboration with Henry Head on the visual pathways and the optic thalamus remains a classical model of neurological research.[23,24]

He edited *Brain* from 1922 until 1937. Here also his work was exemplary: "He exercised critical control over neurological literature in England," wrote an anonymous author in an obituary in the *British Medical Journal*.[25]

The original description of the "rebound phenomenon" figures in Stewart and Holmes's 1904 paper,[1] though Holmes first applied this designation in 1917:[2]

> There is one phenomenon which we have repeatedly observed associated with, and apparently due to, hypotonia. When a person attempts to execute a movement against resistance with a normal limb, and the resistance is suddenly removed, the limb rapidly moves a short distance in the desired direction till abruptly checked, or it may recoil. In a spastic limb the amount of recoil is excessive; in functional cases there may be neither primary movement nor recoil. In homolateral cerebellar disease the range of movement is excessive, generally continued till it is no longer mechanically possible, and there is little or no recoil. This absence of recoil must be attributed to the inability of the antagonistic muscles to react in tone to the sudden strain to which they are exposed (reflex muscle tone).
>
> The simplest way to test this phenomenon is to request the patient to flex the forearm as strongly as he can, the elbow being firmly supported and the movement effectually resisted by the observer grasping the wrist. The resistance is suddenly relaxed by releasing the wrist.[1]

Normally, this movement is almost immediately stopped by the myotatic antagonistic reflex contraction of the patient's triceps muscle; indeed, it will revert in a brisk, short-lasting recoil of the patient's forearm toward the examiner. This rebound movement is the essential point: in cerebellar lesions the recoil is absent and the patient's forearm and fist may well continue their trajectory, causing the patient to autoinflict a black eye or swollen nose (the careful examiner will prevent this happening by holding his other hand in front of the patient's face). In spastic pyramidal disorders the recoil (=rebound) will be potentiated and the examiner runs the risk just specified.

The misapprehension of the essential component in this sign—the "*no*-rebound" in cerebellar pathology (or, alternatively, the "enforced" rebound in upper pyramidal lesions)—has gained firm foothold in quite a few textbooks and papers[26–28] and, moreover, the eponym has even been truncated to the name of Holmes.[29]

The value of the Stewart–Holmes test (because it is a test rather than a sign or phenomenon) lies in the fact that it requires crude strength of proximal muscles, whereas all other cerebellar or coordination tests (diadochokinesis, finger–finger, finger–nose, heel–knee tests, etc.) call on the execution of tasks by fine motoricity of distal muscles. The test is independent of the patient's handedness, a factor which the prudent examiner keeps in mind on interpretation.

A cogent pathophysiological explanation of the cerebellar role in the reactive antagonistic muscle contraction still pertains, as does the discriminative diagnostic value of the test in centromedian versus lateral cerebellar hemisphere lesions. Holmes entertained the idea that muscular hypotonia—as is usual in cerebellar lesions—underlies the phenomenon; others ascribe it to delayed relaxation of the agonist or delayed reciprocal activation of the antagonist muscles.[30]

References

1. Stewart T G, Holmes G M. Symptomatology of cerebellar tumours. *Brain.* 1904;27:522–592.
2. Holmes G M. The symptoms of acute cerebellar injuries due to gunshot. *Brain.* 1917; 40:461–535.

3. Holmes G M. Clinical symptoms of cerebellar disease and their interpretation. *Lancet.* 1922;I:1177–1182, 1231–1237; II:59–65, 111–115.
4. Holmes G M, Stewart T G. On the connection of the inferior olives with the cerebellum in man. *Brain.* 1908;31:125–137.
5. Stewart T G, Turner JWA. *A Textbook of Nervous Diseases.* London: Churchill; 1910.
6. Jackson J H. Case of tumor of the middle lobe of the cerebellum. *Brain.* 1906;29:425–440.
7. Stewart T G, Greenfield J G. Encephalitis periaxialis diffusa. *Brain.* 1927;50:1–29.
8. Steiner T J, Capildeo R, Rose F C. The neurological tradition of the Charing Cross Hospital, In: Rose F C, Bynum W F, eds. *Historical Aspects of the Neurosciences.* New York: Raven Press; 1982:347.
9. Walshe FMR. Gordon Morgan Holmes 1876–1965. In: *Biographical Memoirs of Fellows of the Royal Society, 12.* London: Royal Society, 1966.
10. Penfield W. Sir Gordon Morgan Holmes (1876–1965). Obituary. *J Neurol Sci.* 1967; 5:185–190.
11. Breathnach CS. Sir Gordon Holmes. *Med Hist.* 1975;19:194–200.
12. Lyons JB. Sir Gordon Holmes: a centenary tribute. *Irish Med J.* 1974;69:300–302.
13. Critchley M. Gordon Holmes, the man and the neurologist. In: Critchley M. *The Divine Banquet of the Brain.* New York: Raven Press; 1979.
14. Parsons-Smith B G. Sir Gordon Holmes. In: Rose F C, Bynum W F, eds. *Historical Aspects of the Neurosciences.* New York: Raven Press; 1982.
15. Lepore F E. Harvey Cushing, Gordon Holmes, and the neurological lessons of World War I. *Arch Neurol.* 1994;51:711–722.
16. Fishman R S. Gordon Holmes, the cortical retina, and the wounds of war. *Doc. Ophthalmol.* 1997;93:9–28.
17. Trail R R. *Lives of the Fellows of the Royal College of Physicians, 5.* London: Royal College of Physicians, 1968.
18. Bruyn G W. Personal communication. The story was related to him by Holmes's sister, W. Penfield and D. Denny Brown in May 1975.
19. Holmes G M; Walshe FMR, ed. *Selected Papers.* London: Macmillan; 1956.
20. Holmes G M; Phillips C G, ed. *Selected Papers.* Oxford: Oxford University Press; 1979. This is a more extensive collection than the Walshe edition, with a near-complete bibligraphy.
21. Holmes G M. The Croonian Lectures: On the clinical symptoms of cerebellar disease. *Lancet* 1922;I:1177–1182, 1231–1237;II:59–65, 111–115. Reprinted in: Refs. 19 and 20.
22. Holmes G M. *Introduction to Clinical Neurology.* Edinburgh: Livingstone; 1946.
23. Head H, Holmes G M. Sensory disturbances from cerebral lesions. *Brain.* 1911;34: 102–254. Reprinted in: Head H. *Studies in Neurology, I.* London, Oxford University Press; 1920.
24. Head H, Holmes G M. A case of lesion of the optic thalamus with autopsy. *Brain.* 1911;34:255–271. Reprinted in: Head H. *Studies in Neurology, I.* London: Oxford University Press; 1920.
25. Sir Gordon Holmes, C.M.G., C.B.E., M.D., F.R.C.P., F.R.S. *Br Med J.* 1966;1:111–112. Obituary.
26. Baker A B. *Clinical Neurology.* 2nd ed. New York: Hoeber-Harper; 1962.
27. Grinker R R, Bucy PC. *Neurology.* 5th ed. Springfield, Ill: Charles C Thomas; 1949.
28. Scheid W. *Lehrbuch der Neurologie.* 4th ed. Stuttgart: Thieme; 1980.
29. Angel R W. The rebound phenomenon of Gordon Holmes. *Arch Neurol.* 1977;34:250.
30. Chain F, Lhermitte F, Scherrer J. Exploration de l'activité motrice chez l'homme normal et le cérébelleux. *Rev Neurol (Paris).* 1961;105:330–345.

IV

Syndromes

28

ADIE'S SYNDROME

George W. Bruyn and William Gooddy

William John Adie was born in Geelong, Australia, on 31 October 1886. His education at the Flinders School there was cut short at the early age of 13 years, because of his father's death in 1899. He had to help in the dire situation of the family, soon finding a job as errand boy in an office. His employer was quite satisfied by William's efficient work and, struck by the young boy's quick intelligence, paid for evening courses of further education, and young Adie passed the final exam of the secondary "school" in 1905. Soon he found employment as practice assistant with the local general practitioner, Dr. Arthur South. The work inspired him to become a physician. Goddess Fortuna smiled upon him a second time: his uncle, a brother of his late father, in Boston, gave him £19 for a one-way trip from Melbourne to England, promising financial help in the first years of study. (This proved to be unnecessary, as the university and governmental authorities allowed him an annual stipend because of his excellent study results.) The uncle tried in vain to persuade him to emigrate to the United States but William much preferred Edinburgh.

Adie began the study of medicine at Edinburgh University and graduated in 1911 so brilliantly that he won a postgraduate traveling scholarship. This allowed him to spend two years of further training at various hospitals in Berlin, Munich, Vienna, and Paris, the good old *Wanderjahr* or *peregrinatio academica* that used to be customary but, alas, is neither rule nor practice any more. During this study-tour, Adie, at the same time, acquired a thorough knowledge of foreign languages. On his return, he obtained the position of resident medical assistant to James Collier at the National Hospital, Queen Square, London.

World War I saw him, as volunteer, join the colors; he was posted as medical officer with the 1st Northamptonshire Regiment. Were it not for a severe measles infection that kept him bedridden, he would have been involved (and possibly perished) in the retreat near Mons during which his regiment was decimated. Soon

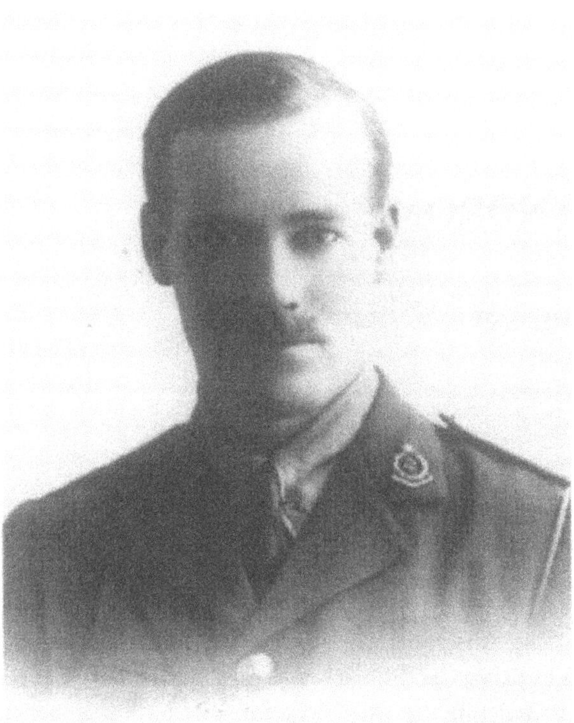

Figure 28–1. William John Adie (1886–1935). Courtesy of Mrs. Critchley.

after, he was posted with the 1st Leicestershire Regiment and earned repeated citations of merit by Sir Douglas Haig, because he saved the lives of many soldiers by improvising a protective mask made from pieces of torn-off clothing, soaked in urine, during the first mustard gas attacks. Toward the end of the war he served as neurological specialist in the 7th General Hospital of the 2nd Army Center, treating cranial gunshot wounds.

After demobilization Adie received appointments at the Charing Cross, Royal Northern, and National hospitals, as well as at the Royal London Ophthalmic (Moorfields). He became a member of the Royal College of Physicians (RCP) in 1919, won the gold medal for his M.D. thesis (1920), and was elected Fellow of the RCP in 1926, after which he joined the honorary consultant staff of the National Hospital. There, his natural talents blossomed in the professional contacts with the nucleus of men who made Queen Square the Mecca of neurology: Collier, Greenfield, Critchley, Symonds, Wilson, Holmes. With the first, he wrote the section "neurology" in the then-authoritative *Textbook of the Practice of Medicine* by Price, with the second a lucid essay on myotonic dystrophy[1] and with the third on forced grasping and groping.[2] Other papers were on subarachnoid hemorrhage in migraine (he was a migraineur himself), on multiple sclerosis, familial paroxysmal paralysis, Tay–Sachs disease, and congenital myotonia.

William J. Adie was a godsend for students: he had a knack for reducing the most complicated clinical problems to the essential elements, by discarding irrelevant trivia and joining what is left in a well-structured diagnosis. This he accomplished by rational argument with the students whose remarks he took as "au serieux" as those of his equals. He kept the patient the center of attention, emphasizing points of history and physical examination and calling on auxiliary laboratory methods only as a means of confirmation. His was the method of rational discourse and discriminating observation, like that of a Sherlock Holmes in a white coat. The story went that he identified the profession of a patient to be examined at one of his teaching sessions from the way in which the man walked into the room: the patient confirmed that he was indeed a waiter. Possessing tolerance, humane warmth, unselfishness, invariable accessibility, and being devoid of the haughtiness that unfortunately seems to be an ingredient of persons of lower caliber risen beyond their intrinsic potential, Adie was the "compleat" neurologist, a noble physician.

In his leisure time, which offered him the opportunity to restore the balance from professional pressures, he proved to be an untiring tennis player, skater, ski fan, and ornithologist, glued for hours on end to binoculars at his country house on the Sussex Downs.

Adie married Lorrain Bonar from Edinburgh in 1916. Their union was blessed with the births of a son and a daughter. The last three years of his life were an ordeal. During a holiday in Mallorca he developed coronary thrombosis, followed by a series of cardiac infarctions in 1933 and 1934. An ultimate infarction terminated his life on 17 March 1935. None of the obituaries that appeared in the medical press had a more catching title than the long one published in the daily newspaper *Geelong Advertizer:* "Geelong boy who made good in London."

The relatively rare combination of myotonic pupils and nonelicitable tendon reflexes may lead the less neurologically versed physician astray because of its resemblance to neurosyphilis.

The syndrome was set out in detail by Adie in a series of publications based on his observations in 15 patients and 12 cases reported previously by others.[3] Though his review of previous reports was incomplete, he showed that many earlier authors either failed to notice or mention the areflexia or they failed to grasp fully the significance of the combination. Those who did not were Ware,[4] Piltz,[5] Morgan and Symonds (who diagnosed their cases as *forme fruste* of encephalitis lethargica),[6] Reitsch,[7] Strassburger,[8] Saenger (who diagnosed Thomson's congenital myotonia),[9] Nonne,[10] Axenfeld,[11] and Moore.[12] Those who did were Markus,[13] and Weill and Reys,[14] who clearly preceded Adie's description and, accordingly, were entitled to be eponymously eternalized. Indeed, Markus's patient was reexamined nearly 30 years later by Weber,[15] who used the term "Markus syndrome." Indeed again, in an extensive critical review, the eponymic monstrosity "syndrome of Markus–Weill and Reys–Holmes–Adie" was created to do justice to chronological priority.[16] Legendary and fervent antieponymic Robert Wartenberg, while (incorrectly) in favor of "Weill–Reys syndrome," suggested the worse term "pseudotabetic pupillotonia."[17]

The neurohistorian hits upon something peculiar in this matter: Morgan,[18] Symonds (the later Sir Charles),[19] and Holmes (the later Sir Gordon, eminent neurologist and meritorious neuro-ophthalmologist)[20] published more or less synchronously with Adie on the pupillotonia–areflexia association, all four of them in different journals without referring to each other, although they knew each other very well and were in frequent professional contact. Each one of them must have known what the other three were brewing. This is no mere coincidence but an inexplicable constellation, which one cannot discard by invoking terms such as vanity or strife. Morgan and Symonds never were granted eponymous rewards. The term "Holmes– Adie syndrome" was later used by some authors,[21,22] perhaps out of veneration for Sir Gordon rather than justifiable veracity, because Adie clearly had worked for many years, at Moorfields, to collect the personal series of cases. Holmes, it is true, presented a larger case series, but he stressed the ocular symptoms to the detriment of the significance of the areflexia he observed.

Clearly, the term "Adie syndrome" won eventually because of Adie's paper in the journal *Brain.* Even the proverbially chauvinistic French, who obstinately hang on to such terms as "Claude Bernard syndrome" (instead of Horner's) or "crises Bravais–Jacksoniennes" (instead of Jacksonian fits) yielded to "syndrome d'Adie" where one would expect them to use "syndrome de Weill–Reys." One might ascribe this to the fact that it was a French professor of neurology, Jean-Alexandre Barré (of the "Guillain–Barré syndrome"), who coined the eponym "Adie's syndrome" in 1934; running true to French style, he soon changed his mind and proposed "Weill–Reys syndrome" as the eponym to be preferred. In the earlier French literature one may encounter the eponym "Maladie d'Adie," honoring his exemplary treatises on idiopathic narcolepsy, both in his gold medal–awarded M.D. thesis and in a subsequent paper.[23] It could not honor his originality or priority, because elsewhere on the continent this disease had been referred to as "morbus Gélineau-Redlich" despite Alexander Westphal's first observations. The Adie eponym spread rapidly to such an extent that the names of later authors were attached to it occasionally, for example, in the blatantly false eponym "Kehrer–Adie syndrome" in German literature.[24]

The eponym denotes the following set of symptoms:

1. A larger, sometimes oval-shaped pupil which reacts scarcely or not at all with constriction upon incident light, neither directly nor consensually, but reacts retardedly (and often excessively) to accommodation so that the abnormal and initially larger pupil becomes smaller than its fellow. During the patient's sojourn in a darkened room, the abnormal pupil dilates and, on subsequent exposure to light, contracts very slowly. This unilateral abnormality may occur bilaterally (exceptionally).
2. The myotonic pupil is associated with one or more unelicitable muscle stretch reflexes of one or both legs (knee jerk and/or Achilles jerk).
3. This association is noticed two to three times more frequently in young women than in men.
4. The underlying segmental paresis of the sphincter iridis is progressive over the years[25] and is occasionally associated with segmental hypohydrosis[21,26] (in which case it is known as "Ross syndrome") or cardiac dysfunction.[27] Adie's

syndrome may be hereditary. Walsh disclosed that the dog of A. Earl Walker's wife had Adie's syndrome; so had the dog's parents and grandparents.[28]

The pathophysiology of Adie's syndrome has been largely clarified. As the marked constriction of the abnormal (without response of the normal) pupil to instillation of one drop of 2.5% solution of methacholyl indicates, there is (segmental) denervation hypersensitivity of the pupilloconstrictor. This is confirmed by the excessive reaction to instillation of 0.125% pilocarpine and by the normal response to mydriatics. Adie already suspected the presence of a postganglionic parasympathetic fiber lesion. Subsequent research indicated the ciliary ganglion and its short nerves as the site of the lesion,[29] as did the occurrence of hippus in the abnormal pupil.[30]

Neuropathological workup revealed quasi-absence of ganglion cells and of axons in the ciliary ganglion, only small nonmyelinated axons "de passage" being present. With respect to the muscle stretch areflexia, its neuropathological basis consists of spinal dorsal root ganglia degeneration.[31,32] Because the tonic vibration reflex, mediated by polysynaptic input from Ia afferents, remains normal, as does the magnetic stimulation test, whereas there are increased afferent central conduction times and impairment of T and H reflexes, the cause must be sought in presynaptic dysfunction of Ia monoafferents.[33]

References

1. Adie W J, Greenfield J G. Myotonic dystrophy. *Brain.* 1923;46:73–127.
2. Adie W J, Critchley M. Forced grasping and groping. *Brain.* 1927;50:142–170.
3. Adie W J. Pseudo-Argyll Robertson pupils with absent tendon reflexes: a benign disorder simulating tabes dorsalis. *Br Med J.* 1931; 1:928–930; Argyll Robertson pupils, true and false, *Br Med J.* 1931;2:136–138; Tonic pupils and absent tendon reflexes: a benign disorder sui generis; its complete and incomplete forms, *Brain.* 1932;55: 98–113; Tonic pupils and absent tendon reflexes, *Br J Ophthalmol.* 1932;16:449–461.
4. Ware J; Ware M, ed. *Observations on the Treatment of the Epiphora or Watery Eye.* London: T & G Underwood: 1818.
5. Piltz J. Über neue Pupillenphänomene. *Neurol Zentralbl.* 1899;18:248–254.
6. Morgan O G, Symonds C P. A series of cases with rapid onset of unequal pupils and failure of accommodation. *Guy's Hosp Rep.* 1927;77:13–15.
7. Reitsch W. Beitrag zur Pupillotomie mit Akkommodationstonie. *Klin Monatsschr Augenheilkd* 1925;74:159–164.
8. Strasburger J. Pupillenträgheit bei Accommodation und Convergenz oder myotonische Pupillenbeweging. *Neurol Zentralbl.* 1902;21:738–740, 1052–1054.
9. Saenger A. Über myotonische Pupillenbewegung. *Neurol Zentralbl.* 1902; 21:837–839, 1137–1139.
10. Nonne M. Über die sogenannte myotonische Convergenzträgheit lichtstarrer Pupillen. *Neurol Zentralbl.* 1902;21:1000–1004.
11. Axenfeld Th. Tonische Akkomodation. *Klin Monattbl Augenheilk.* 1919;62:59–68.
12. Moore R F. The non-luetic Argyll Robertson pupil. *Trans Ophthalmol Soc UK.* 1931;51: 203–209.
13. Markus Ch. Notes on a peculiar pupil-phenomenon in cases of partial iridoplegia. *Trans Ophthalmol Soc UK.* 1906;26: 50–58.
14. Weill G, Reys L. Réaction tonique d'une pupille à la convergence et parésie de l'accomodation avec aréflexie à la lumière chez un sujet atteint de crises tétanoides et d'aréflexie

des membres inférieurs. *Rev d'OtoNeuroOcul.* 1926;4:422–441; *Arch Ophthalmol.* 1926;43: 441–455.
15. Weber F P. The original case of Markus-syndrome shown 27½ years later. *Proc R Soc Med.* 1933;26:530–531.
16. Loewenstein O, Loewenfeld I E. Pupillotonic pseudotabes (syndrome of Markus-Weill and Reys-Holmes-Adie). *Survey Ophthalmol.* 1965;10:129–185.
17. Wartenberg R. Adie's syndrome. *JAMA.* 1951;45:1152.
18. Morgan O G. Internal ophthalmoplegia with absent tendon jerks. *Proc R Soc Med.* 1931;24:867–868.
19. Symonds C P. Internal ophthalmoplegia with absent tendon jerks. *Proc R Soc Med.* 1931, 24:868–869.
20. Holmes G. Partial iridoplegia with symptoms of other diseases of the nervous system. *Trans Ophthalmol Soc UK.* 1931;51:209–228.
21. Hardin Jr W B, Gay A J. The phenomenon of benign areflexia: review of the Holmes-Adie syndrome. *Neurology.* 1965;15:613–621.
22. Lucy Jr D D, van Allen M W, Thompson H S. Holmes-Adie syndrome with segmental hypohydrosis. *Neurology.* 1967;17:763–778.
23. Adie W J. Idiopathic narcolepsy. *Brain.* 1926;49:257–306.
24. Kehrer F A. *Die Kuppelung von Pupillenstörung mit Aufhebung der Sehnenreflexe.* Leipzig: Thieme; 1937; Zur Pathologie der Pupillen. *Z Neurol Psychiat.* 1923;81:345–358.
25. Thompson H S. Segmental palsy of the iris sphincter in Adie's syndrome. *Arch Ophthalmol.* 1978;96:1615–1620.
26. Petajan J H, Danforth R C, d'Alessio D. Progressive sudomotor denervation and Adie's syndrome. *Neurology.* 1965;15:172.
27. Berkowits J S, Zweifach P H. Cardic autonomic dysfunction in patients with tonic pupils. *Neurology.* 1970;20:1096–1102.
28. Walsh F B, Hoyt W F. *Clinical Neuroophthalmology.* 3rd ed. Baltimore: Williams & Wilkins; 1969;1:496–501.
29. Schwarz G A. Dysautonomic syndromes in adults. In: Vinken P J, Bruyn G W, eds. *Handbook of Clinical Neurology.* Amsterdam: North Holland Publishing Company; 1975;22: 259–260.
30. Thompson H S, Corbett J J. Spasms of the iris sphincter. *Ann Neurol.* 1980;8:547–549.
31. Harrimon DGF, Garland H. The pathology of Adie's syndrome. *Brain.* 1968;91: 401–418.
32. Selhorst J B, Madge G, Ghatak N R. The neuropathology of the Holmes-Adie syndrome. *Ann Neurol.* 1984;16:138.
33. Paresi G, Macaluso G M, Medici D. On the cause of tendon areflexia in the Holmes-Adie syndrome. *Electromyogr Clin Neurophysiol.* 1994;34:111–115.

29

BELL'S PALSY

Antoine Keyser and John M. S. Pearce

Charles Bell was born in the neighborhood of Edinburgh in 1774.[1] His father died in 1779, leaving his mother solely responsible for the burden of raising four sons. Charles, the youngest son, was devoted to his mother. He went to Edinburgh High School, where he became friends with David Allan, a painter, known as the "Hogarth of Scotland," who encouraged Charles's draftsmanship.[2] He received his basic medical education in Edinburgh. Like his elder brother, John Bell (1763–1820), he devoted himself to surgery. In those days, as in ours, this required a thorough knowledge of human anatomy. During his medical training, he had already published a two-volume book on anatomical dissection. Later he contributed a chapter on the anatomy of the nervous system to a book edited by his brother under the title *Anatomy of the Human Body*,[3] where the family's artistic gifts are shown in many of John's engravings of bones, joints, and wounds. His brother George Joseph Bell (1770–1843) was a professor of Scots Law, his preferment in Edinburgh being backed by the family friend Sir Walter Scott.

Charles studied medicine in his home town under Joseph Black (1728–1799), Alexander Monro (1733–1817), and John Gregory (1725–1773), being elected a member of the Edinburgh College of Surgeons in 1799. His brother John was in dispute with Dr. Gregory, and both John and Charles were excluded from promotion.

While writing on the anatomy of the nervous system Charles became aware of the fact that the anatomical study of the cranial nerves was seriously neglected and that much of what was considered as "knowledge" was uncritically transmitted from generation to generation without any empirical verification.

In 1799, he finished his studies. Subsequently he was appointed to the staff at the Royal Infirmary. A longstanding conflict between John Bell and members of the Edinburgh Medical Faculty eventually caused Charles Bell to move to London in

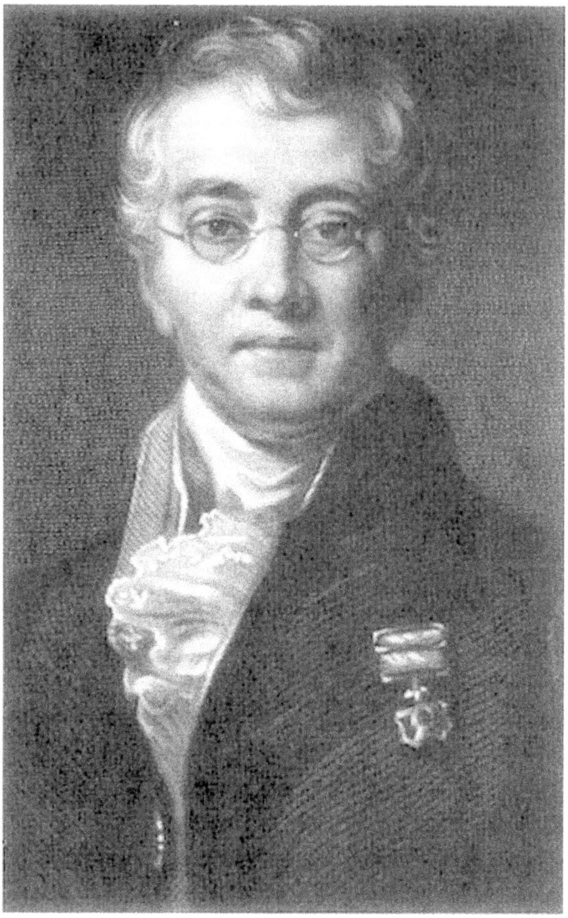

Figure 29–1. Charles Bell (1774–1842). *Courtesy Medizinhistorisches Institut, Zurich, Switzerland.*

November 1804. His coach stopped for the weekend at Huntingdon and he walked the remaining journey down the Great North Road.

His fame as an artist was wide spread, and within a few days of arrival he had been received by Astley Cooper, Sir Joseph Banks, and Matthew Baillie, but despite these contacts he secured no permanent position. He took a dilapidated house in Leicester Street, Leicester Square, with his brother George; his basic diet of barley was funded by payments for lectures to students of anatomy and art.

There had been little interest in neurology at this time. Charles was frustrated by the prevailing doctrine that nervous fluid was derived from the brain and transmitted by nervous tubes. He established a surgical practice and became one of the founders of the Middlesex Hospital and the Middlesex Medical School, with which he was affiliated in later years. This hospital played a major role in the care of the wounded from the various battles fought at the beginning of the nineteenth century (Corunna, Waterloo).

This busy profession of surgeon did not supplant Bell's prolific scientific activities, as can be deduced from the series of publications on the anatomy of the peripheral and cranial nerves. He also maintained his interest in the arts. In 1806 he published *Essays on the Anatomy of Expression in Painting,* intended mainly for artists.[4]

It was well received, and he was flattered that the Queen read a copy. But Bell remained impoverished despite the praises and attentions of many famous and titled doctors and artists. His many lectures and patients eventually brought financial rewards, and he continued to prosect on the anatomy of the brain. His publications were numerous: *The Anatomy of the Brain* (1802)[5] explained in a series of engravings, including 12 beautiful plates, some in color; *A Series of Engravings explaining the Course of the Nerves* (1803) included nine fine quarto plates; and *A System of Operative Surgery founded on the basis of Anatomy* (1807), dedicated to his friend William Lynn.

He married Marion Shaw on 3 June 1811 and moved to 34 Soho Square. With the help of his wife's dowry he bought a share in the Great Windmill Street School of Medicine, owned by the surgeon James Wilson. William Hunter (1718–1783) had founded the school as an institution that taught anatomy, philosophy, and surgery. It contained a museum where Bell worked and to which he added his own specimens and drawings.

In 1813 he was appointed to the Middlesex Hospital and studied gunshot wounds at Haslar Hospital after the battle of Corunna in 1809. A sensitive man, he was greatly distressed:

> I have stooped over hundreds of wretches in the most striking variety of woe and misery . . . Each day as I awake, still I see the long line of sick and lame slowly moving from the beach: it seems to have no end.[6]

Waterloo summoned on 22 June 1815. Without a passport, eight days later he hastened to Brussels, operating from morning till night, but always painting and sketching. Returning to London he was appointed professor of anatomy and surgery at the Royal College of Surgeons in 1824.

In 1828 he was appointed professor of physiology and surgery at the recently founded London University and King's College, but he abandoned this position in 1830, dissatisfied by the bureaucratic rules he had to comply with. He received public recognition, as is apparent from the fact that he was knighted in 1833 by King William IV. In 1834 he received the gold medal of the Royal Society. In 1835, aged 61, he left London after accepting the Chair in Surgery at Edinburgh University. He visited Italy in 1840, but on return, his health failed, probably due to angina.

Visiting a friend near Worcester, he died suddenly on 29 April 1842 and was buried in the neighboring Hallow churchyard, adjacent to the old yew tree that sheltered some sheep near the river, which he had sketched the previous day. The *Letters of Sir Charles Bell* were published in 1870. A long biographical article appeared in the *Edinburgh Review* of April 1872, saying of him: "Never passed away a gentler, truer, or finer spirit" (p. 429).

In a variety of fields, Charles Bell has contributed to our knowledge of the nervous system. He demonstrated the relationship between the special sense organs and those circumscribed brain areas where the nerve tracts from the sense organs ended. Another contribution of considerable weight was the demonstration of the motor and sensory functions of the anterior and posterior spinal nerve roots.

As happens so often in important discoveries, a number of contemporary scientists developed similar ideas during approximately the same period. Georg Prochaska

(1749–1820) had suggested this type of organization some years before. In France, François Magendie (1783–1855) conducted experimental studies on animals and in fact was the first to prove the function of the anterior and posterior spinal roots.[7,8] In the literature this became known as the "law of Bell–Magendie." Charles Bell had found in anesthetized animals that posterior root transection did not abolish motor function, and that anterior root stimulation could elicit muscle contraction. He did not, however, at this stage establish the sensory function of the dorsal roots. His results were published in a pamphlet privately circulated among friends, and only after the publication by Magendie did he come forward to claim his priority.[8,9]

Bell's name is perpetuated in various eponyms, for instance, the long thoracic nerve (Bell's nerve). He was extraordinarily talented in painting and drawing; a number of his publications are illustrated by his own art, for example, *The Anatomy of the Brain.*[5] He made important contributions concerning the intracerebral course of the trigeminal and facial nerves and about their many functions.

Nowadays the name of Sir Charles Bell in clinics worldwide remains connected to Bell's palsy. This attribution stems from his first description of the clinical signs after loss of function of the facial nerve motor component.[10] He communicated his observations on the facial nerve in a lecture for the Royal Society in 1826. He gave a more detailed description in the same journal in 1829.[11] (Fig. 29–2) In his text on the nervous system he recognized several causes, mentioning

> a man shot with a pistol ball, which entered the ear and tore across the portio dura at its root . . . The next instance was in a man wounded by the horn of an ox. The point of the horn entered under the angle of the jaw and came out before the ear, tearing across the portio dura . . . The forehead of the corresponding side is without motion, the eyelids remaining open, the nostril has no motion in breathing, and the mouth is drawn to the opposite side. The muscles of the face by long disuse are degenerated, and the integuments of the wounded side of the face are become like a membrane stretched over the skull . . . In this man the sensibility of the face is perfect. The same nerve (portio dura) has been divided in the extirpation of a tumour before the ear, and the immediate effect has been horrible distortion of the face by the prevalence of the muscles of the opposite side, but without loss of sensibility; and that distortion is unhappily increased when a pleasurable emotion should be reflected in the countenance.[11]

The so-called Bell's phenomenon was clearly described for the first time in a case history incorporated in his 1830 monograph *The Nervous System of the Human Body.*[12] Moritz Romberg translated this influential volume into German a few years later. In it, Bell described "a very remarkable turning up of the cornea in an attempt to close the eyelids," and further on,

> the patient is not at all aware of the eye being turned up; although he can turn it up by a voluntary act, and be conscious of it at the same time . . . the cornea is still safe although the eye lid does not descend, yet the eye ascends to the eye lid; and it is wiped, cleaned and moistened by the partial performance of the act of winking.

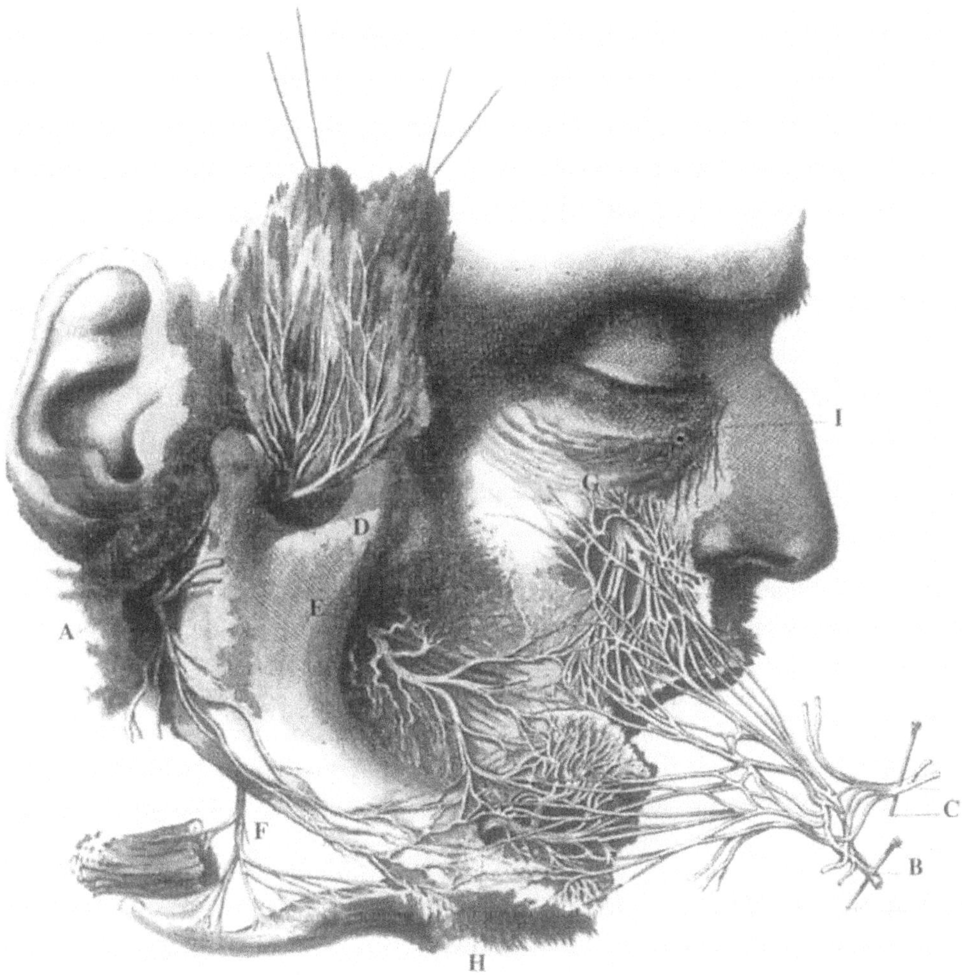

Figure 29–2. Facial and trigeminal nerves drawn by Charles Bell.[11]
In this figure the superficial nerves of the face are turned off, and the distribution of the third division of the fifth to the muscles of the jaws and cheek exposed.

A. The portio dura of the seventh or respiratory nerve of the face coming from the stylomastoid foramen; the principal branches are cut and folded forwards.

B. The trunk of the portio dura of the seventh, dissected off the face and pinned out, while it is left at its connections with the branches of the fifth on the cheek and lips.

C. The branch of the third division of the fifth nerve, which joins the plexus of the portio dura before the ear . . .

D. In this figure the masseter muscle is dissected from the jaw-bone and lifted up to show D, the branch of the fifth pair of nerves going into the muscle.

E. The Ramus Buccinalis-labialis, that branch of the fifth nerve which goes to the buccinator, triangularis, levator labiorum, and orbicularis muscles.

F. That branch of the fifth nerve which separating from the mandibulo-labialis goes to the muscles which depress the lower jaw.

G. The suborbitary nerve, a branch of the fifth nerve.

H. The mandibulo-labalis, a branch of the fifth nerve coming out from the bone to the muscles and integuments of the lip and chin.

I. A branch of the fifth nerve descending from the orbit. D, E, F, are muscular branches of the fifth nerve, and are motor nerves. C, G, H, I, are sensitive branches of the same nerve which join the branches of the portio dura in its universal distribution.

These phrases by Bell for the first time in medical history gave an exact description of what now is called "Bell's phenomenon."[13] The facial nerve he called "the respiratory nerve of the face." It ministered "*to the motions of the face which are connected with respiration*":

> In all the exhilarating emotions, the eyebrows, eyelids, the nostrils and the angles of the mouth are raised. In the depressing passions it is the reverse.[11]

Bell subsequently corrected an earlier ambiguous remark, that the fifth and seventh cranial nerves innervated the muscles of the face:

> The sensibility of the head and face depend upon the fifth pair of nerves . . . the portio dura of the seventh nerve is the principal muscular nerve of the face.[10]

Bell's original 1829 paper to the Royal Society provided a brief but unmistakable description of facial paralysis of lower motor neuron type. He clearly separated it from facial weakness of upper motor neuron lesions, though this terminology was not then in use. His account of the upturning of the globe was graphic and important, and it received more attention from Gowers, and later Kinnier Wilson, than his account of facial palsy. Avicenna had much earlier described spastic, atonic, and convulsive types of facial palsy.[14] Bell generously cited the French neurologist Roux, who had described his own facial nerve paralysis in a letter to Professor Descot. He did not mention a sketchy account of Douglas (1704, cited by Bird)[15] or Nikolaus Anton Friedreich (1761–1836), who comprehensively described three cases of peripheral facial paralysis in 1798 (an English translation appeared in the *Annals of Medicine* in 1800).[16] He was the grandfather of Nikolaus Friedreich of Heidelberg, who elucidated the hereditary ataxia (see Chapter 48).

But the nature of the condition was first exposed and taught by Bell, who merits full credit for this important clinical description. The variable involvement of the nerve to the stapedius, causing transient hyperacusis, and to the chorda tympani, producing impairment of taste, were elaborated at a later date, but well described, inter alia, by Todd, Gowers, and Wilson. The limited diagnostic and prognostic roles of electrophysiological studies were developed in the 1950s.

References

1. Pearce JMS. Sir Charles Bell (1774–1842). *J R Soc Med.* 1993;86:353–354.
2. Gordon-Taylor G, Walls E W. *Sir Charles Bell: His Life and Times.* Edinburgh: Livingstone, 1958.
3. Bell J, Bell C. *Anatomy of the Human Body.* (4 vol.) Edinburgh: Cadell & Davies; 1797–1804.
4. Bell C. *Essays on the Anatomy of Expression in Painting.* London: Longman; 1806.
5. Bell C. *The Anatomy of the Brain.* London: Longman; 1802.
6. Bettany G T. *Eminent Doctors: Their Lives and Their Work.* 2nd ed. London: John Hogg; 1885;1:248.
7. Magendie F. Expériences sur les fonctions des racines des nerfs rachidiens. *J Physiol Exp Pathol.* 1822;2:276–279.
8. Cranefield P F. *The Way In and the Way Out: François Magendie, Charles Bell and the Roots of the Spinal Nerves.* Mount Kisco, NY: Futura; 1974.

9. Bell C. *Idea of a New Anatomy of the Brain.* London: Straham & Preston; 1811. Reprint in: *Med Classics.* 1936;1:105–120.
10. Bell C. On the nerves; giving an account of some experiments on their structure and functions, which lead to a new arrangement of the system. *Phil Trans.* 1821;111:398–424.
11. Bell C. On nerves of the face, being a second paper on the subject. *Phil Trans.* 1829;119:317–330. Reprinted in: *Med Classics.* 1936;1:152–169.
12. Bell C. *The Nervous System of the Human Body.* 2nd ed. London: Longman; 1830. 3rd ed. London: Spottiswode; 1844.
13. Zulch, K J. "Idiopathic" facial paresis. In: Vinken P J, Bruyn G W, eds. *Handbook of Clinical Neurology.* Amsterdam: North-Holland Publishing Company; 1970;7:241–296.
14. Gruner O C. *A Treatise on the Canon of Medicine of Avicenna Incorporating a Translation of the First Book.* London: Luzac & Co; 1930.
15. Bird T D. Nicolaus A. Friedreich's description of peripheral facial nerve paralysis in 1798. *J Neurol Neurosurg Psychiatry.* 1979;42:56–58.
16. Friedreich N A. De paralysis musculorum faciei rheumatica. *J Erfindungen Gotha.* 1798; 8:no. 25, quoted in: *Ann Med Edinb.* 1800;5:214–222.

30

BROCA'S APHASIA

David Moffie and Francis Schiller

Pierre Paul Broca (1824–1880) was born on 28 June 1824 in Sainte-Foy-la-Grande, a small town in the Dordogne, east of Bordeaux, in a Calvinist family.[1] His father, who had served as a surgeon in Napoleon's army, was a general practitioner. Paul attended the local primary and high schools. He wanted to study at the École Polytechnique to become an engineer, but he changed his mind and studied medicine instead. This was probably owing to his father's insistence on his taking over his practice.

As a 17 year old, Paul traveled to Paris by stagecoach to study medicine. He earned some extra money as an assistant-teacher at the Collège Sainte-Barbe, where in fact he was a jack of all trades. After six months he had his own accommodations with financial support from his parents. After passing his non-resident assistant (*externe*) examination, he did anatomical and surgical work to prepare himself for the resident examination. At the end of December 1844 he went to work at the Hôpital de Bicêtre, a psychiatric institute where Philippe Pinel (1745–1826) once worked. In December 1846 he became a resident in surgery at the Hôtel-Dieu and, at the same time, demonstrator of anatomy. In the years that followed he studied problems of cancer, aneurysms, and also muscle diseases. He described muscular dystrophy in 1851,[2] before Duchenne (see Chapter 46), and published on rickets. Many years later (1878) he defined the comparative neuroanatomy of the *grand lobe limbique* and the olfactory system.[3]

In 1857 he married Adèle Lugol (1835–1914), whose father, Jean Lugol (1786–1851), was known for Lugol's solution (*L'emploie de l'iode dans les maladies scrofuleuses;* "the use of iodine in scrofulous diseases"). They had three children. The oldest, Auguste (1859–1924), became a pediatric and early years neurosurgeon. In 1860, together with some friends, Broca founded the Société d'Anthropologie, which was to play an important role in the discussion of aphasia.

Figure 30–1. Paul Broca (1824–1880).
From A. Dayot, *Le second Empire.*
Paris, Ernest Flammarion, n.d.

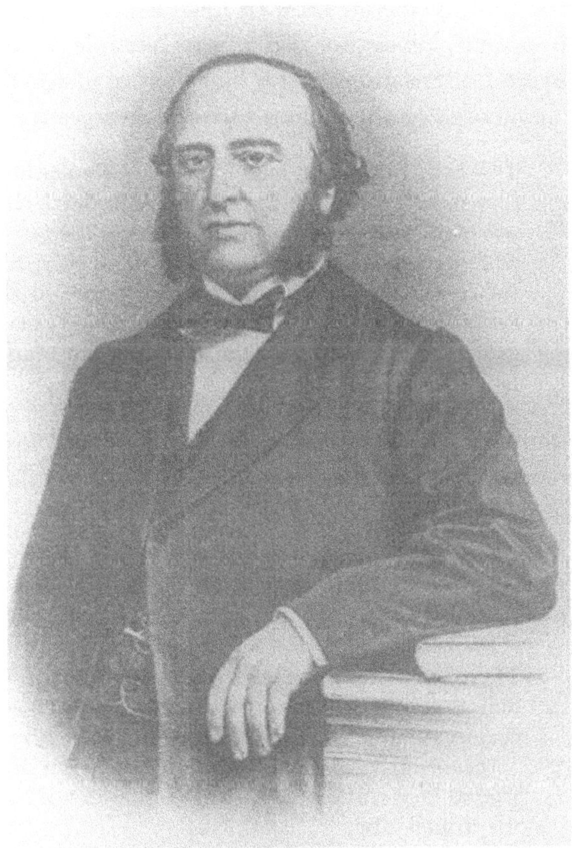

His interest in speech disturbances intensified during the 1860s, in relation to his neuroanatomical and anthropological work, which earned him his fame in clinical neurology. Politically, Broca was a man of the left, a staunch supporter of the 1848 revolution in Paris and a lifelong republican. During the riots and the Commune in 1871, after the Franco-Prussian War, he stayed in Paris and helped to run the Assistance Publique. Less known is his bold act in saving the money of this institute during the Commune. He was a courageous man, and loyal to his friends. He supported Brown-Séquard's career (see Chapter 31). In 1880 Broca was honored by his appointment as a lifetime senator of the French republic, an honor given to prominent scholars and physicians. On 8 July of the same year he died, probably as the result of coronary artery occlusion.

According to Franz Joseph Gall (1758–1828), each one of our human capacities has its own location within the brain, which are expressed in the externally visible features of the skull and face. This theory, epitomized as phrenology and craniology, had numerous adherents for many years, but was discredited by clinical facts.[4]

Jean-Baptiste Bouillaud (1796–1881) concluded from clinical observations that speech disturbances could be caused by abnormalities in the frontal lobes.[5] Exact localization remained a point of dispute. As a result of a discussion at the Société d'Anthropologie on 18 April 1861, Broca presented the brain of a 51-year old epileptic patient, Leborgne, also a right hemiplegic with complete loss of speech but preserved understanding, who had died of gangrene of his paralyzed right leg.[6] Broca commented on the patient's speech disturbance:

> This loss of speech in individuals who are neither paralyzed nor idiots constitutes a very specific symptom for which I consider it useful to invent a special name. So I will name it aphemia . . . for it is only the faculty of articulating words that these patients lack. They hear and understand everything that is said to them; they are in full possession of their senses; they produce vocal sounds without difficulty; they execute with their tongue and lips movements that are far more elaborate and energetic than is required for the articulation of sounds.[7, 8]

Broca wondered whether the disturbance was due to a kind of "locomotor ataxia, limited to the articulate speech." or to the "loss of a special kind of memory, the memory of the procedure which one has to follow in order to articulate words." He favored the latter view.[1(p178)]

On inspection of the brain, the left third frontal convolution and the insula proved to show pathological changes. The posterior part of the left third frontal gyrus was most affected. Broca summarized:

> These were the organs destroyed: the small inferior marginal convolution of the temporal lobe (superior temporal); the small convolutions of the insula, and the corpus striatum; finally, in the frontal lobe, the inferior portion of the transverse (precentral) convolution and the posterior half . . . of the second and third frontal convolutions . . . Three quarters of the cavity at least was carved out of the frontal lobe.[1(p185),7]

As the lesion had been a progressive one and aphemia had been the main sign for many years, Broca reasoned the third frontal convolution, which was in the center of the defect, should be the center for speech. He assumed the paresis was due to the lesion of the corpus striatum, no motor as the cerebral convolutions were still assumed to be on motor organs.[1(p186)] Broca discussed the subject of cerebral localization. "Although I believe in the principle of localization, I have been and still am asking myself, within what limits does this principle apply?"[1(p179)]

In November 1861, a second relevant autopsy was performed on the brain of a patient (called Lelong) with *aphémie.* Again, serious abnormalities were found of the third and the second frontal convolutions on the left side, especially in their posterior part:

> I will not deny my surprise bordering on stupefaction when I found that in my second patient the lesion was rigorously occupying the same site as in my first; not only were the same convolutions affected but they were so at the same point, i.e., immediately behind that middle third, opposite the insula, and precisely on the same side (left).[1(p187)9]

Broca published on left cerebral dominance in 1865.[10]

Armand Trousseau (1801–1867), the famous internist at the Hôtel-Dieu changed the term *aphémie* to *aphasie.*[11] The term *motor aphasia* for this speech abnormality was introduced by Carl Wernicke (1848–1904) in 1874, to distinguish it from the *sensory aphasia* localized in the temporal lobe, as well as from *conduction aphasia.* (See Chapter 38).

In the meantime a question of priority had arisen about the discovery of the localization of *aphémie,* caused by lesions of the left hemisphere, which was claimed by Gustave Dax (1815–1874) in Montpellier. His father, Marc Dax (1770–1837), had observed, written about, but not published several dozen cases with loss of speech and left hemisphere lesions. The famous "Broca–Dax controversy" was born.[12]

On 24 March 1863, two years after presenting the brain of Leborgne, and in response to some criticism, especially regarding an aphasic patient of Charcot showing no frontal lesion but an extensive lesion at the upper border of the left Sylvian fissure, Broca said:

> Instead of being exclusively localized in the posterior portion of the third frontal convolution, might the seat of articulate speech not extend to the inferior parietal convolution which is directly continuous with it? Several anatomists are known to consider the two convolutions as one, calling them the convolutions around the Sylvian fissure (circonvolution d'enceinte—Foville).[1(p190)]

Broca's conclusions were attacked in 1906 by Pierre Marie (1853–1940), in a paper with the provocative title "La troisième circonvolution frontale gauche ne joue aucun rôle spécial dans la fonction du langage" [The left third frontal convolution plays no special role whatever in the function of speech].[13] Marie critically reviewed the location problems after studying the brains of Broca's patients, which were preserved intact in the Musée Dupuytren. (Figs. 30–2 and 30–3) Marie discovered that the destruction was more extensive, with additional pathology in the parietotemporal region, than was previously reported. This was confirmed by computed tomography, performed on these intact brains many years later.[14]

After Marie's criticism of the different localizations of the various forms of aphasia, other authors such as Kurt Goldstein (1898–1965) and Henry Head (1861–1940) came to the fore with holistic views, rejecting a distinct localization.[15] For decades these holistic ideas dominated the discussions on aphasia but after

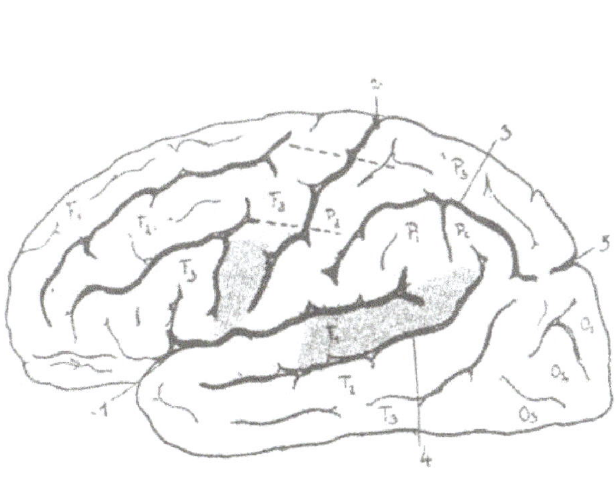

Figure 30–2. Left hemisphere of a brain of an aphasia patient. According to Broca, this lesion supports his theory about localization in the third frontal convolution. However, the lesion in Wernicke's center is much more severe than in the center of Broca.[22]

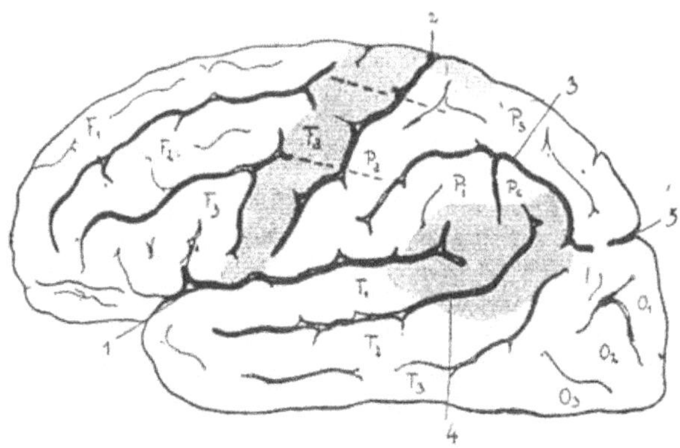

Figure 30–3. Left hemisphere of the brain of patient Foucault. In this case, too, Broca thought that the aphasia was localized in the third frontal convolution. However, the lesion in Wernicke's center is much larger than that of the third frontal convolution.[22]

1945, the pendulum once again swung to those who insist on the localization of cortical functions.

Anatomical investigations of Broca's area seem to support a special role of the left hemisphere in speech,[16] confirming the old ideas of Broca. Thus the term Broca's aphasia is still in use and rightly so. In right-handers it has a well-defined location in the left hemisphere. In mild cases of Broca's aphasia, which are differentiated from pure motor aphasia by some authors, this lesion lies in the Broca area, the third frontal gyrus on the left side. Usually there is a gradual recovery, but an agrammatical and stammering speech pattern remains. In severe cases of Broca's aphasia, in which dysarthric or anarthric problems play a role, the lesion is more extensive and reaches into the striatum. These forms are often combined with hemiplegia.[17–20]

The severity of the different components of motor aphasia and the extent of the lesions of the subcortical and deep periventricular white matter areas are correlated.[21]

References

1. Schiller F. *Paul Broca: Founder of French Anthropology, Explorer of the brain.* 2nd ed. New York: Oxford University Press; 1992.
2. Broca P P. Nouvelles observations sur l'altération graisseuse des muscles et sur leur prétendue transformation fibreuse. *Bull Soc Anat.* 1851;26:379–390.
3. Broca P P. Le grand lobe limbique et la scissure limbique dans le séries des mammifères. *Rev Anthropol.* 1878; 1(2nd ser):385–498.
4. Finger S. *Origins of Neuroscience.* New York: Oxford University Press; 1994:371–385.
5. Bouillaud J B. Recherches cliniques propres à démontrer que la perte de la parole correspond à la lésion des lobules antérieurs du cerveau, et à conformer l'opinion de M. GALL, sur le siège de l'origine du langage articulé. *Arch Gén Méd (Paris).* 1825;8(1st ser):25–45.
6. Broca P P. Perte de la parole; ramollisement chronique et destruction partielle du lobe antérieur gauche du cerveau. *Bull Soc Anthrop Paris.* 1861;2:235–238.
7. Broca P P. Remarques sur le siège de la faculté du langage articulé, suivie d'une observation d'aphémie (perte de la parole). *Bull Soc Anat.* 1861;6:330–336.
8. Eling P. Paul Broca. In: Eling P, ed. *Reader in the History of Aphasia.* Amsterdam: Benjamins; 1994:29–58.
9. Broca P P. Nouvelle observation d'aphémie produite par une lésion de la moitié postérieure des deuxième et troisième circonvolutions frontales gauches. *Bull Soc Anat.* 1861;36:398–407.

10. Broca P P. Du siège de la faculté du langage articulé dans l'hémisphere gauche du cerveau. *Bull Soc Anthrop.* 1865;6:377–393.
11. Trousseau A. De l'aphasie. In: Trousseau A, ed. *Clinique Médicale de l'Hôtel-Dieu de Paris.* 2nd ed. Paris: Baillière; 1865;2:571–626.
12. Critchley M. The Broca–Dax controversy. In: *The Divine Banquet of the Brain.* New York: Raven Press; 1979:72–82.
13. Marie P. La troisième circonvolution frontale gauche ne joue aucun rôle spécial dans la fonction de langage. *Sem Méd.* 1906;26:241–247.
14. Castaigne P, Lhermitte F, Signoret J L, Abelanet R. Description et étude scannographique du cerveau de Leborgne. La découverte de Broca. *Rev Neurol.* 1980;136:563–583.
15. Brain R. *Speech Disorders.* London: Butterworths, 1961.
16. Galaburda A M. La Région de Broca. *Rev Neurol.* 1980;136:609–616.
17. Geschwind N. *Selected Papers on Language and the Brain.* Boston: Reidel; 1974.
18. Benson D F. Syndromes of aphasia. In: Heilman KM, Valenstein E, eds. *Clinical Neuropsychology.* 3rd ed. New York: Oxford University Press; 1993: 23–25.
19. Leischner A. *Aphasieen und Sprachentwicklungstörungen.* Stuttgart: Thieme; 1979.
20. Kertesz A. Aphasia. In: Vinken P J, Bruyn G W, Klawans H L, Frederiks JAM, eds. *Handbook of Clinical Neurology, 45: Clinical Neuropsychology* (rev ser 1). Amsterdam: Elsevier Science; 1985:287–331.
21. Alexander M P, Naesa M A, Palumbo C L. Correlations of subcortical CT lesions sites and aphasia profiles. *Brain.* 1987;110:961–991.
22. Marie P. *Travaux et Mémoires, I.* Paris: Masson; 1926.

31

THE BROWN-SÉQUARD SYNDROME

Peter J. Koehler and Michael J. Aminoff

The Brown-Séquard syndrome occurs following unilateral lesion of the spinal cord. Paralysis and disturbed proprioception are found ipsilateral to the lesion, whereas diminished pain and temperature appreciation, starting one or two segments below the level of the lesion, are found contralaterally. The syndrome may have many different causes.[1]

Charles-Edouard Brown-Séquard was born on the isle of Mauritius in 1817. He was the son of a French mother (Séquard) and an American father (Brown).[2,3] As the island had come under British rule in 1814, he was born a British subject. His father, a merchant sea captain from Philadelphia, died before his birth during a voyage to India. Charles-Edouard set off for Paris with his mother in 1838 to pursue a literary career, but he was discouraged by the author Charles Nodier (1780–1844). Thus it was that he came to the study of medicine. During his studies, he worked at the private laboratory of the "free professor" and physiologist Martin-Magron (1810–1872), whose pupils included Pierre Paul Broca (1824–1880). In 1842, Brown-Séquard became a non-resident assistant (*externe*) under the well-known internist Armand Trousseau (1801–1867). Following the death of his mother in 1842, lonely and depressed, he interrupted his studies to visit Mauritius, but he returned to Paris and resumed his studies in 1843. He published a thesis for his doctorate in 1846, under the surname of Brown.[4] As he wrote later, he added the name "Séquard" to honor his mother, but also to distinguish himself from other "Browns."

Starting in 1848, Brown-Séquard worked under Pierre Rayer (1793–1867) at the Charité hospital. He became secretary of the recently founded Société de Biologie in the same year. He left for Philadelphia in 1852, according to letters of introduction, because of his republican ideas. The coup d'état by Louis Napoleon (1808–1873) had taken place in December 1851, followed seven months later by the establishment of the second empire. Presumably the fact that he had no fixed appointment also played a role. Moreover, it was expected that Claude Bernard (1813–1878), rather than Brown-Séquard, would succeed François Magendie (1783–1855) as professor of medicine at the Collège de France. Brown-Séquard lectured in many cities in the United States and crossed the ocean many times until 1878, the year in which he succeeded Bernard at the Collège de France.

Brown-Séquard was professor at the newly founded Medical College of Virginia in Richmond for a brief period in 1854 but then returned to France. He accepted an appointment at the newly founded National Hospital for the Paralysed and Epileptic in London in 1859. Despite the fact that he had established a prosperous practice and was considered a leading specialist in the field of epilepsy, he left London within three and a half years. John Hughlings Jackson (1835–1911; see Chapter 15) worked as his assistant for some time during this period, and Brown-Séquard probably had an important influence on him.[5] From 1864 to 1866, he was professor at Harvard University. In 1868, Charles-Edouard returned to Paris with his 12-year-old son, Edouard. His wife had died in the previous year. Although the *Journal de la Physiologie,* which he started in 1858, had been discontinued within seven years, he founded a new journal, *Archives de Physiologie normale et pathologique,* with Jean-Martin Charcot (1825–1893; see Chapter 41) and Edmé-Felix-Alfred Vulpian (1826–1887) as coeditors. Brown-Séquard was appointed *charge du cours* of experimental and comparative pathology at the Paris faculty of medicine in 1869. Because of his British nationality, he was not eligible to occupy the vacant chair of Rayer, who had died in 1867, but some have questioned his abilities to occupy the chair. He resigned in 1872

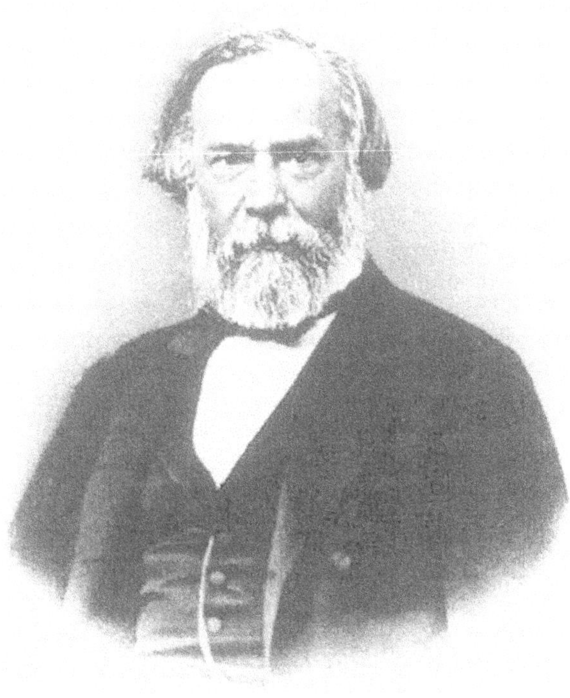

Figure 31–1. Charles-Edouard Brown-Séquard (1817–1894). Courtesy Archives de l'Académie des Sciences, Paris.

and left for the United States, where he married Maria Carlisle, who died after the birth of their daughter Charlotte. He lectured at several places in the United States and England during the years that followed. He married Elisabeth Emma Dakin in 1877 and in the following year settled permanently in Paris. He received accolades for his work in the field of neurophysiology during the first half of the 1880s. During the second half of this decade he became preoccupied with the effect of organ extracts and injected himself with testicular extracts derived from animals, which he believed to improve his physical condition. He died of a stroke on 1 April 1894, shortly after the death of his wife.

Brown-Séquard was a hard worker. Ambition probably was the most important reason to travel from one country to another until he achieved his aim: a professorship in Paris and the opportunity to perform experimental investigations. The following citations provide impressions of his character and physique. Brown-Séquard wrote about himself in a case story:

> The first patient . . . thirty-four years old, of strong constitution, but reduced from several causes to a lamentable state of health. For eight years he had been working very hard, taking no exercise, and living almost all the time in a vitiated atmosphere. He slept very little, and usually passed 18 or 19 hours a day writing, reading or experimenting. His diet was miserable, and, with the object of avoiding the need of much food, he took a great deal of coffee.[6]

Another characterization is given by a newspaper article of 1854, when he stayed on his native island, Mauritius:

> [Il] était un petit homme sec, à la chevelure noire, ondée et qui commençait à s'argenter. La vivacitéde son parler, l'agitation dans la marche et cette mobilité nerveuse dans les yeux faisent de lui une personnalité étrange . . . il entrait comme un coup de vent, ne s'asseyait jamais; il était toujours agité et, à peine arrivé pressé de s'en aller.[2(p193)]

[He was a small, unfeeling man with wavy black hair, starting to become gray. The liveliness of his speech, his agitated gait, and that nervous movement of his eyes made him a strange personality . . . he entered like a blast of wind, never sat down; he was always restless, and hardly arrived before he was in haste to leave.] The Parisian professor of chemistry Marcelin Berthelot (1827–1907) portrayed him in 1855:

> J'ai encore devant les yeux cette figure originale fine et bienveillante, brunie par le climat de son ile natale; ces yeux vifs et doux, toujours en mouvement et toujours inquiets, animeés à la fois par un sentiment affectueux pour les amis de la science, par une curiosité sans cesse en éveil qui le poussait à en pénétrer les secrets, et aussi je ne sais quelle timidité qu'entretenait sans doute son impuissance à dominer la vie pratique.[2(p194)]

[I still see before me that original delicate and kind face, burnished by the climate of his native island; those alert and gentle eyes, always moving and always anxious, at the same time animated by a warm feeling for the friends of science, by a ceaselessly watchful inquisitiveness that insisted on penetrating its secrets, and also I do not know what timidity that apparently governed his inability to control a practical life.]

Brown-Séquard performed research in several fields. He studied rigor mortis and the action of vasomotor nerves. On the latter subject his ideas were in conflict with those of Claude Bernard. His concept of artificially induced hereditary epilepsy received much criticism, although the resulting concept of "Brown-Séquard's spinal epilepsy" was applied by Charcot, Wilhelm Erb (1840–1921), and Friedrich Leopold Goltz (1834–1902) and was used until the twentieth century. Charles Darwin (1809–1882) applied the hereditary aspects for the foundations of his theories.[7] His theories on cerebral localization conflicted with the prevailing views at that time that cerebral functions could be localized in defined centers; instead, he formulated a network theory that shows similarities with present views.[8]

His experiments on the function of the adrenal glands met much criticism but established that these glands are essential to life; thus he has come to be recognized as a founding father of experimental endocrinology. Toward the end of his career, he payed attention especially to the production and testing of testicular and other organ extracts, but this was largely misunderstood by the lay public and scientific community. Nevertheless, he is considered one of the pioneers of modern hormone replacement therapy.

The beginning of the description of the syndrome published a few years later can be found in his 1846 thesis.[4] It comprises a report of experimental research on the pathways that conduct sensory impressions in the spinal cord using laboratory animals. He demonstrated that sensibility below the level of the lesion following section of one or both posterior columns remained intact. This finding, of course, was contrary to the generally accepted view. Charles Bell (1774–1842) and François-Achille Longet (1811–1871), for example, had demonstrated that sensory pathways after entering the spinal cord follow an uncrossed ipsilateral course, by way of the posterior columns. In fact, the Dutch scientist Isaäc van Deen (1805–1869), highly respected by Brown-Séquard, performing research with frogs in his medical practice, had already established that "the animal did not experience real loss of sensibility in the hindleg ipsilateral to the side of hemisection of the spinal cord."[2,9–11] However, Van Deen did not find that sensitivity in the contralateral hindleg was lost.[12]

Particularly during the period from 1846 to 1855, Brown-Séquard performed research that enabled him to demonstrate that sensory pathways, after entering the spinal cord and ascending in the posterior columns over a short distance, cross to the contralateral side before ascending to the brain. (Fig. 31–2) In 1849 he wrote:

> Aussitôt après avoir coupé une moitié latérale de la moelle sur un mammifère, à la région dorsale, la sensibilité paraît très diminuée, dans le membre postérieur du côté de la section. La sensibilité manque complètement dans l'autre membre postérieur. Quelquesfois j'ai trouvé la sensibilité intacte ou à peu près dans le membre postérieur correspondant au côté de la section.[13]

[Immediately after cutting one lateral half of the spinal cord of a mammal, at the thoracic level, sensation in the hind limb on the side of the section seems very decreased. Sensation was absent in the other hind limb. Sometimes I have found the sensibility intact or almost so, in the hind limb on the side of the section.]

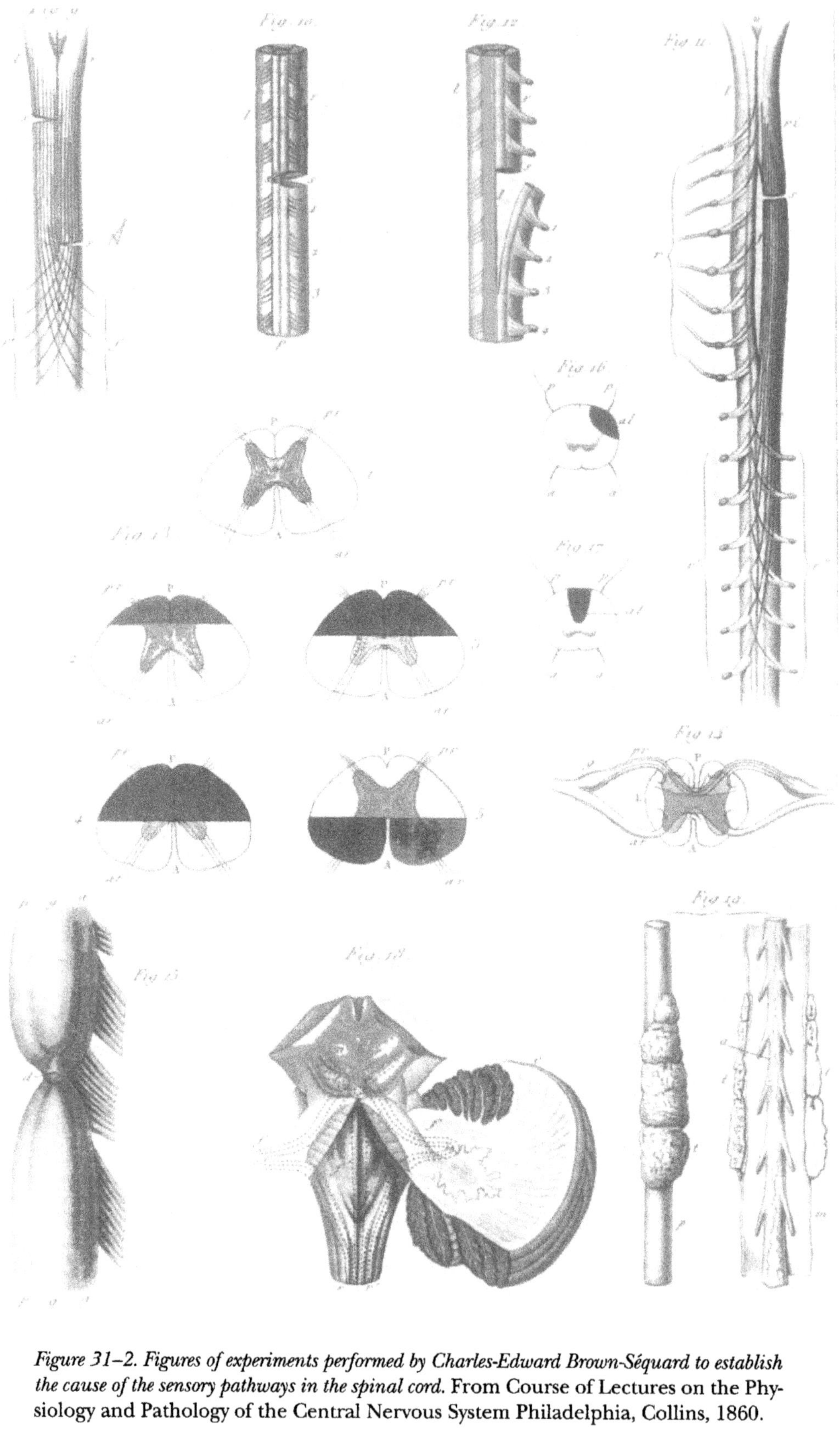

Figure 31–2. Figures of experiments performed by Charles-Edward Brown-Séquard to establish the cause of the sensory pathways in the spinal cord. From Course of Lectures on the Physiology and Pathology of the Central Nervous System Philadelphia, Collins, 1860.

He performed the experiments more than 60 times and concluded:

> La moelle épinière parait donc avoir, au moins en partie, une action croisée, quant à la transmission des impressions sensitives.[13]

[With respect to the transmission of sensory impressions, therefore, the spinal cord at least partly seems to have a crossed action.]

He was able to confirm this theory by clinical observations.

Not until 1855 did Brown-Séquard receive recognition for his neurophysiological work. After the demonstration of a few of his experiments before the Société de Biologie, the society set up a committee (at his request) to examine his findings, which many disputed. Broca, presiding over the committee, of which Claude Bernard and Alfred Vulpian were among the members, reported:

> les premiers travaux de M. Brown-Séquard furent accueillis avec une certaine méfiance, et n'obtinrent qu'une attention passagère . . . Toutes ces contradictions faisaient de la physiologie de la moelle un dédale inextricable et beaucoup d'observateurs, désespérant de débrouiller ces questions épineuses, avaient fini par renoncer à la localisation de la sensibilité et du mouvement, par croire, avec les anciens, que ces deux propriétés étaient uniformement réparties dans les cordons de la moelle, et par répéter cette phrase célèbre de Boerhaave: "Quis dicet: hoc movet, hoc sentit?" . . . Les belles expériences de M. Brown-Séquard viennent de renverser pour toujours cet édifice si bien cimenté dont Longet avait scellé la dernière pierre.[14]

[The first works of Mr. Brown-Séquard were received with a certain distrust, and received only transient attention . . . All these contradictions made an inextricable labyrinth of the physiology of the spinal cord and many observers, despairing of disentangle these knotty questions, had stopped by abstaining from localizing the sensibility and motion, believing, in agreement with the ancients, that both qualities are evenly distributed in the columns of the spinal cord, and by repeating the famous phrase of Boerhaave: "Quis dicet: hoc movet, hoc sentit?" . . . The beautiful experiments of Mr. Brown-Séquard have forever overthrown this well-built edifice, of which Longet laid the last stone.]

With additional experimental findings accumulated over the years, Brown-Séquard later revised his original views. He discovered that in experiments in which unilateral hemisection lesions are made sequentially at two levels of the spinal cord, hyperesthesia may turn to anesthesia, and vice versa. According to him, this "transfert" could be explained only by influences that act on the spinal cord from a distance, in accordance with the mechanism of "inhibition" (causing anesthesia) and "dynamogénie" (causing hyperesthesia). In this way, the changes were not explained by the anatomy of the (crossing) pathways, but solely on the basis of a complex dynamic process. Derek Denny-Brown (1901–1981) demonstrated that ipsilateral hyperesthesia indeed may sometimes be found in man. Moreover, he found that in monkeys, "transfert" from hyperesthesia to anesthesia could result from a second, more complete hemisection in the spinal cord rostrally from the first. He assumed that the anterior columns play an important inhibitory role.[3,15] Patrick Wall, too, emphasized the importance of Brown-Séquard's last article on the subject.

The dynamic balance between tonic inhibiting and exciting influences, in particular, could explain many phenomena.[3,16] In brief, in the words of Brown-Séquard:

> If faut conséquemment admettre un tout autre mécanisme de transmission des impressions sensitives que celui que les anatomistes, comme les physiologistes ont vainement essayé d'établir . . . [pourtant] le type clinique que j'ai décrit . . . reste vrai et peut servir dans la pratique de la médecine, quelles que soient les interprétations physiologiques qu'on donne de ces phénoménes.[17]

[Consequently, one has to admit quite another mechanism of transmission of sensory impressions than those that anatomists and physiologists have tried to establish in vain . . . (however) the clinical syndrome that I described . . . remains true and may help in medical practice, whatever physiological interpretations are given to these phenomena.]

References

1. Koehler P J, Endtz L J. The Brown-Séquard syndrome: true or false? *Arch Neurol.* 1986;43: 921–924.
2. Koehler P J. Het localisatieconcept in de neurologie van Brown-Séquard. Amsterdam: Rodopi; 1989.
3. Aminoff M J. *Brown-Séquard: A Visionary of Science.* New York: Raven Press; 1993.
4. Brown-Séquard C E. *Recherches et expériences sur la physiologie de la moelle épinière.* Paris: Rignoux; 1846.
5. York G K, Steinberg D A, Koehler P J. Brown-Séquard's influence on the young Hughlings Jackson. *Neurology.* 1995;45(suppl):A303.
6. Olmsted JMD. *Charles-Edouard Brown-Séquard: A Nineteenth Century Neurologist and Endocrinologist.* Baltimore: Johns Hopkins Press; 1946:30–31.
7. Koehler P J. Brown-Séquard's spinal epilepsy. *Med Hist.* 1994;38:189–203.
8. Koehler P J. Brown-Séquard and cerebral localization as illustrated by his ideas on aphasia. *J Hist Neurosci.* 1996;5:26–33.
9. Koehler P J, Endtz L J. Between Magendie and Brown-Séquard: Isaäc van Deen's spinal hemisections. *Neurology.* 1989;39:446–448.
10. Van Deen I. Over de voorste en achterste strengen van het ruggemerg. *Tijdsch Natuur Geschied Physiol.* 1838;5:151–186.
11. Van Deen I. *Traités et découvertes sur la physiologie de la moëlle épinière.* Leiden: Luchtmans; 1841.
12. Koehler P J. Isaäc van Deen and Benedikt Stilling: a controversy on the function of the spinal cord in the 19th century. *J Hist Neurosci.* 1992;1:189–200.
13. Brown-Séquard C E. De la transmission des impressions sensitives par la moelle épinière. *C R Séances Soc Biol.* 1849;1:192–194.
14. Broca P P. Propriétés et fonctions de la moelle épinière. Rapport sur quelques expériences de M. Brown-Séquard. (lu à la Soc. Biol. 21 juillet 1855). In *Mémoires,* no 3. Paris: Bonaventura, 1855; and *C R Séances Soc Biol.* 1855;7:23–50.
15. Denny-Brown D. The enigma of crossed sensory loss with cord hemisection. In: Bonica J J, Liebeskind J C, Albe-Fessard D G, eds. *Advances in Pain Research and Therapy.* New York: Raven Press; 1979;3:889–895.
16. Wall P D. The design of experimental studies in the future development of restorative neurology of altered sensation and pain. In: Dimitrijevic M R, Wall P D, Lindblom U, eds. *Recent Achievements in Restorative Neurology.* Basel: Karger; 1990;3:197–205.
17. Brown-Séquard C E. Remarques à propos des recherches du Dr. F. W. Mott sur les effets de la section d'une moitié latérale de la moelle épinière. *Arch Physiol.* 1894;26:195–198.

32

ERB'S PALSY

Richard P. M. Bruyn

Wilhelm Heinrich Erb was born on 30 November 1840 in Winweiler, a small village in the Bavarian Pfalz. His father, a forester, imparted his love of nature to him. Very little is known of his boyhood. From papers commemorating his sesquicentennial[1–2] we know that he loved music and nature and enjoyed intellectual conversation. In general his scientific oeuvre can be divided in two periods: his first Heidelberg period, before his appointment at Leipzig, in which his publications deal with diseases of peripheral nerves and spinal cord; and his second Heidelberg period, mainly dealing with muscular diseases.

He started the study of medicine in Heidelberg at the age of 17, pursued it in Erlangen, and graduated in Munich in 1864, the year in which he also published his first article. From then on, Erb displayed an enormous scientific zeal, which is reflected in his 237 publications.

His first wife, Bertha Karoline Hermann, gave birth to one son and died in 1873. He and his second wife, Anna Gass, were married in 1876 and had three sons.

After graduation in Munich he became *Privat-Dozent* (assistant professor) in internal medicine at Heidelberg in 1865, where he met his teacher Nikolaus Friedreich (see Chapter 48), then Professor Ordinarius of Pathology and Therapy. Friedreich stimulated his interest in neurology and in 1867 Erb's first neurological paper on the pathology and pathological anatomy of peripheral paralysis appeared. He stayed in Heidelberg until 1878, when he was invited by Ernst Wagner to come to Leipzig as chief of the outpatient department. At that time, Erb already was a distinguished clinician and scientist, as shown by milestones such as his *Handbook of Diseases of the Spinal Cord and Medulla* and his pioneering studies on electrotherapy. In Leipzig, he became a good friend of Adolf Strümpell, who said that he knew no physician with greater exactness than Erb.

In 1874 Erb lectured on a peculiar localization of brachial plexus paralysis, later known as Erb's palsy or Erb–Duchenne paralysis; however, his seminal article did not appear until 1877.[3] In 1875, he published a paper on the patellar reflex,[4] illustrated by the following anecdote that he told Strümpell. Assistants and their teachers went to the bowling club on a regular basis, and Erb noted that one of the young doctors was sitting on a table, hitting himself with a heavy key just under his patella, eliciting a knee jerk. Erb went home, thought about this, and practiced this procedure on healthy and ill people. He had to share his fame with Westphal,[5] who independently published on the same topic in the same volume. Carl Westphal was an advocate of the integration of neurology and psychiatry, whereas Erb strongly opposed this and considered neurology a separate part of internal medicine. Because of this controversy, Erb, together with Friedrich Schultze and Ludwig Lichtheim, in 1891 founded the *Deutsche Zeitschrift für Nervenheilkunde.* Other scientific works are his studies on juvenile progressive muscular atrophy, congenital myotonia, and the syphilitic origin of tabes, many years before the discovery of the spirochete in the brain. Famous is his instruction not to ask the patient *if* he has had syphilis, but *when* he acquired syphilis.

Erb remained extraordinary professor until 1883. After Friedreich's death from aortic aneurysm in 1883, Erb succeeded him in Heidelberg, where he remained until he retired in 1907. Even after his retirement he remained productive. Following the foundation of the Society of German Neurologists, Erb was its first president in 1907. He was given the title of Excellency by the Grand Duke of Baden and, as a special honor on the occasion of his seventieth birthday, his bronze statue was unveiled in the park near the Academic Hospital and a street was named after him. His statue now adorns "Erb's Department" of the private Krehl medical hospital (Fig. 32–1).

Two of his sons had died in adult life, one a physician; his third son died in World War I. Erb was a broken man, having lost his will to live. In general he was in good health, although he suffered from tachycardia and arrhythmia, and he underwent an operation for gallstones. The exact cause and place of his death are uncertain; some[6–8] claim that walking home after listening to Beethoven's *Eroica,* he caught a cold, which was followed by pneumonia and death; others[9] claim that during that same performance he collapsed and never regained consciousness, leading to his death on 29 October 1921.

One of Erb's famous studies concerns the upper brachial plexus palsy.[3] In 1877 he described four patients with a typical pattern of paralyzed muscles. The first patient, a 52-year-old ropemaker, after carrying a heavy weight on his head, complained of numbness of his left thumb and index finger and had a paralysis of deltoid, biceps, brachialis, and supinator muscle. Light touch was slightly diminished. All muscles showed atrophy in the course of time, but he completely recovered after seven weeks.

The second patient was a 38-year-old baker, who fell down the stairs and broke his fall with his outstretched left hand, simultaneously hitting his left shoulder on the wall. He then complained of pain in his thumb and numbness of his shoulder, and there was a paralysis of the deltoid, biceps, and brachial muscle. There were no objective sensory abnormalities. Only after six months was there a reasonable improvement.

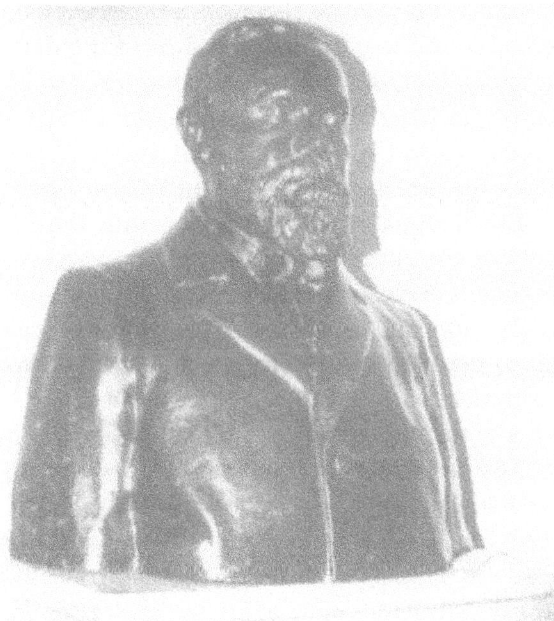

Figure 32–1. Wilhelm Heinrich Erb (1840–1921). Bust situated at the Erb department of the private medical clinic Krehl, Heidelberg. Courtesy of Dr. Erich Kuhn and Dr. W. Kübler.

The third patient, a 17-year-old nailsmith, complained of numbness of his left thumb and index finger for two months, followed by a gradually developing paralysis and atrophy of the left deltoid, biceps, brachialis, and supinator muscles of unknown cause. No objective sensory findings were noted. He recovered after four months.

His fourth patient was a 52-year-old businessman, who complained of weakness of his left arm for six to eight weeks. Simultaneously he had noted enlargement of lymph nodes on the left side of the neck and numbness of his left thumb and index finger. A paralysis of the left deltoid, biceps, and brachialis muscles was found, but no sensory deficit. Several weeks later he developed a paraplegia and died soon after cancer was diagnosed. Erb suggested that in this case the partial brachial plexopathy was caused by pressure of a tumor on the brachial plexus.

After this clinical description, Erb presents an anatomical analysis in an attempt to localize the exact site of the lesion. Erb said that, considering the absence of sensory abnormalities (which in the opinion of the present writer is not completely true, because all patients had sensory symptoms), the lesion had to be sought proximal to the brachial plexus. At that time anatomical research had not yet unraveled the exact innervation of the proximal arm musculature. Erb studied several anatomical preparations and concluded that in his patients the fifth and sixth nerve roots had to be damaged.

A separate category of patients with a similar pattern of paralysis of deltoid, biceps, and brachial muscles, along with the infraspinatus muscle, had been described by Duchenne.[10] Indeed, 20 years earlier, Danyau[11] also had described a paralysis of the upper arm in the newborn in whom the plexus is overstretched during a difficult delivery, or if prolonged traction in the armpit has taken place during delivery. Erb went on to say that he also had examined a baby of two months old who had a very difficult birth; Erb found a paralysis of the deltoid, biceps, brachialis, and probably the supinator and infraspinatus muscles as well. The typical posture consisted of adduction and internal rotation at the shoulder, extension at the elbow, and pronation of the forearm ("waiter's tip") and resulted from loss of abduction and external rotation of the arm and weak forearm flexion and supination.

Erb doubted whether traction with the fingers in the armpit during delivery could be the cause of the paralysis; he suggested that the Prague maneuver, where the fingers enclose the baby's neck like a two-pronged fork and compress the plexus, was the culprit. This maneuver is used for breech delivery, when the back of the fetus fails to rotate to the anterior; it had been described by Pugh as early as 1754,[12] and recommended by Kiwisch of Prague in 1846.[13] According to Erb this may explain also why the infraspinatus muscle frequently is involved in "delivery paralysis."

The Erb–Duchenne palsy nowadays is exceptional in a good obstetric practice. The natural history has a fairly good prognosis. Two of the four adult patients described by Erb had a traumatic partial upper brachial plexopathy; in the third the cause was unknown, while compression was by tumor at the plexus in the fourth. Nowadays, traction injuries are the most common lesions of the brachial plexus, usually caused by motorcycle accidents. The common pattern depends upon the impact of the injury, leading to damage of the upper trunks in milder injuries, while very violent injuries produce avulsion of the whole plexus.[14] The upper three roots C5, 6, and 7 are somewhat more resistant to stretch than the C8 and T1 roots, first because they are anchored to the transverse process by a strong ligament, whereas C8 and T1 are anchored to the spinal cord itself, second because the upper cervical roots run a steeper course than C8 and T1, which run almost horizontal, and finally because the upper four roots are approximately twice as long as T1.

Other causes of brachial plexopathy are direct injuries, such as stabbing or gunshot wounds, and direct pressure, such as carrying heavy loadsover one's shoulder, which in these days is called a *cadet palsy*, but in fact is the same as Erb's palsy. As a matter of fact, Erb's first patient had an upper brachial plexopathy caused by carrying a heavy weight upon his head.

The eponym Erb's palsy today is applied only to the obstetrical complication leading to an upper brachial plexus lesion, despite the earlier descriptions of Duchenne and Danyau. In case of traumatic, nonobstetrical brachial plexus lesion the use of the term Erb's palsy is no longer justified.

Acknowledgments

I wish to express my gratitude to Dr. E. Kuhn of Heidelberg, Dr. W. Zeman for finding the present location of the bust, Dr. P. Voswinckel of Lübeck for several articles, and Dr. G. Wiemers, director of the Leipzig University Archives.

References

1. Kuhn E, Rüdel R. Wilhelm Heinrich Erb (1840–1921). *Muscle Nerve.* 1990;13:567–569.
2. Kuhn E. Wilhelm Erb (1840–1921). *Fortschr Neurol Psychiatr.* 1990;58:405–407.

3. Erb W. Ueber eine eigenthümliche Localisation von Lähmungen im Plexus brachialis. *Verh Naturhist-med Vereins Heidelberg.* 1877;1(new ser):130–136.
4. Erb W. Ueber Sehnenreflexe bei Gesunden und bei Rückenmarkskranken. *Arch Psychiatr Nervenkr.* 1875; 5:792–802.
5. Westphal C. Ueber einige Bewegungs-Erscheinungen an gelähmten Gliedern, II: Ueber einige durch mechanische Einwirkung auf Sehnen und Muskeln hervorgebrachte Bewegungs-Erscheinungen. *Arch Psychiatr Nervenkr.* 1875;5:803–834.
6. Nonne M. Wilhelm Erb. 1840–1921. In: Kurt Kolle, ed. *Grosse Nervenärzte.* 2nd ed. Stuttgart: Thieme; 1970:68–80.
7. Fischer PA. Titelbild. *Nervenarzt.* 1994;65:A4.
8. Viets H R. Heinrich Erb (1840–1921). In: Haymaker W, Schiller F, eds. *The Founders of Neurology.* 2nd ed. Springfield, Ill: Charles C Thomas; 1970:435–438.
9. Torkildsen A, Erickson T. Wilhelm Erb. 1840–1921. *Arch Neurol Psychiatr.* 1935;33:842–846.
10. Duchenne GBA. *De l'électrisation localisée et de son application à la pathologie et à la thérapeutique par courants induits et par courants galvaniques interrompus et continus.* 3rd ed. Paris: Baillière; 1872.
11. Danyau N. Paralysie du membre supérieur chez le nouveau-né. *Bull Soc Chir (Paris).* 1851; 2:148.
12. Pugh A. *Treatise on midwifery chiefly with regard to the operation.* London, 1754.
13. Kiwisch F. H. *Beitr Geburtsk (Würzburg).* 1846;1:69. Cited in: Cunningham F G, Williams J W. *Williams Obstetrics.* Stamford, CT: Appleton & Lange; 1997, 507.
14. Wynn Parry C B. Brachial plexus injuries. In: Vinken P J, Bruyn G W, Klawans H L, eds. *Handbook of Clinical Neurology, 51. Neuropathies.* Amsterdam: Elsevier Science Publishers; 1987:143–155.

33

GILLES DE LA TOURETTE'S SYNDROME

Howard I. Kushner and David Cortes

Tourette syndrome is characterized by an array of sudden, rapid, recurrent, nonrhythmic, and stereotyped motor and vocal tics. The motor tics generally involve head and neck jerking, eye blinking, tongue protrusions, shoulder shrugs, and various torso and limb movements. Vocalizations may include barks, grunts, yelps, coughs, repetition of one's own or other's words (echolalia), uttering obscenities (coprolalia), and blurting out inappropriate remarks. Other associated behaviors may include inappropriate touching of oneself or others. Often these are coupled with compulsive behaviors.[1] Although the syndrome has adopted Georges Gilles de la Tourette's name, it differs in important ways from the disorder described by Gilles de la Tourette.

Georges Gilles de la Tourette was born at Saint-Gervais-les-Trois-Clochers, near Loudun, on 30 October 1857. In 1634 Loudun was the scene of an infamous trial in which Sister Anne de Anges leveled accusations of possession that led to the execution of father Urbain Grandier. Loudun was also the birthplace of Dr. Théophraste Renaudot, an important ally of Richelieu, who advocated medical treatment of the poor. Both Renaudot and Sister Anne de Anges were subjects of biographies written by Gilles de la Tourette.[2]

Completing his medical studies at Poitier, Gilles de la Tourette arrived in Paris in 1877. He impressed his contemporaries as driven, often overexuberant, and extremely combative. Later, one colleague would describe Gilles de la Tourette as an odd-moving and husky-voiced eccentric whose "queer ways . . . got worse and worse and became less and less amusing."[3(p811),2] But more senior physicians at the Salpêtrière, especially Jean-Martin Charcot and Paul Brouardel, under whom he interned, thought Gilles de la Tourette brilliant and exceedingly reliable. In 1887, after finishing his thesis on the diagnostic use of footprints, he was appointed Charcot's *chef*

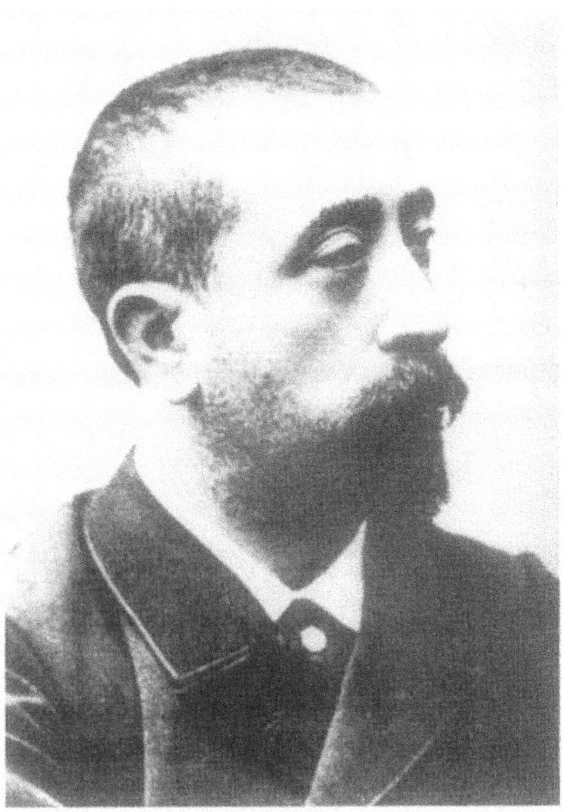

Figure 33–1. Georges Gilles de la Tourette (1857–1904). By permission from Dr. Elaine Shapiro.

du clinique at the Salpêtrière. That same year, he published a study on hypnosis;[4] he also married his cousin Marie Detrois, with whom he would later have four children.

During his tenure at the Salpêtrière Gilles de la Tourette published 16 papers on hysteria, embarked on research into the effectiveness of suspension therapy on locomotor ataxia, and invented a vibrating helmet designed to treat neurasthenia, facial neuralgia, and vertigo. He joined with neurologist Paul Richer and photographer Albert Londe to establish the *Nouvelle Iconographie de la Salpêtrière* in 1888,[2,3] and between 1891 and 1895 he published three volumes on the work of Charcot.[5] In 1893 a former female patient, claiming that Gilles de la Tourette had hypnotized her against her will, fired three bullets into his head and neck.[6] He recovered and accepted appointments as Professeur Agrégé at the Hôpital St. Antoine and chief medical officer to the 1900 World's Fair. In addition to his extensive psychological and physiological works, Gilles de la Tourette also published theatrical and social criticism. He wrote for *La Revue Hebdomadaire,* using the pseudonym Paracelsus.[3,7] In 1901, soon after the publication of his book on bromide treatment of epilepsy, Gilles de la Tourette developed what appeared to be syphilitic dementia. He entered a Swiss psychiatric hospital, where he died in 1904.[3,7]

In 1885, at Charcot's behest, Gilles de la Tourette published a two-part article that identified a combination of multiple motor tics and "involuntary" vocalizations

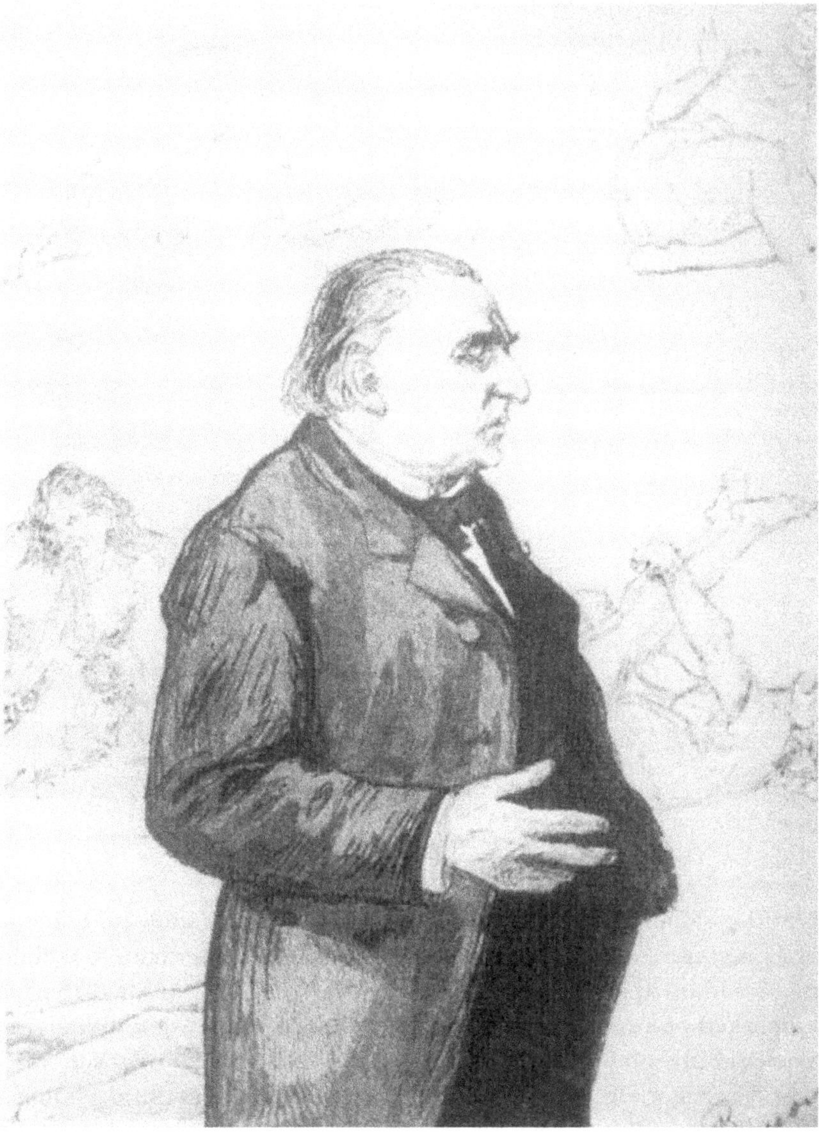

Figure 33–2. Jean-Martin Charcot (1825–1893). Courtesy of the National Library of Medicine, Bethesda, Maryland.

as a distinct disorder that he called *maladie des tics convulsifs avec coprolalie* (convulsive tic disease with coprolalia).[8,9] Charcot had selected Gilles de la Tourette because of the younger man's clinical experience with patients with tics and interest in similar phenomena.[10] In particular, Gilles de la Tourette had been fascinated by jumping and startle behaviors reported in Malaysia, Siberia, and Maine, variously known as "latah," "myriachit," and "jumping." These bizarre behaviors often were accompanied by echopraxia (imitation), echolalia, coprolalia, and copropraxia (sexual touching).[11,12] In a review of these behaviors he drew a parallel between them and similar cases that had presented at Charcot's clinic.[12,13] The next year when Gilles de la Tourette published his two-part study on convulsive tic disease, he included jumping, myriachit, and latah as variations of his typology.[8]

Gilles de la Tourette's 1885 article presented a classification of symptoms and prognosis based on his description of nine patients' case histories. It began with childhood motor and vocal tics, which over time increased in number and variety with the eventual appearance of coprolalia.[8] Unlike choreas and hysterias, *maladie des tics* might wax and wane, but it ultimately resisted all interventions.[14] There was no hope of "a complete cure," argued Gilles de la Tourette, for clinical experience demonstrated that "once a ticcer, always a ticcer."[15(pp155–156),8]

Citing Théodule Ribot,[16] Gilles de la Tourette argued that convulsive tic disease had a "degenerative" hereditary etiology.[8] Advocates of degeneration theory argued that diet and habits such as alcoholism and immoral behavior had a cumulative destructive effect on the nervous system that was inherited by succeeding generations.[17] Thus, Giles de la Tourette concluded:

> Quant à la nature intime de l'affection, que dire en l'absence de toute donné anatome-pathologique? On pourrait, en s'aidant des ressources de la psychologie, essayer d'interpréter quelques symptômes, nous préférons, pour notre part, renvoyer ceux que voudraient tenter cette interprétation au livre si intéressant de M. Ribot, sur les maladies de la volonté.[8(p200)]

[What can we say with respect to the innermost nature of this affliction, in the absence of any anatomical-pathological data? Drawing on the assistance of psychological sources, we could try to interpret some symptoms; on our part, we refer those who would want to attempt this interpretation to the very interesting book on the diseases of the will by Mr. Ribot.]

Charcot concurred with Gilles de la Tourette's assessment, explaining that tic disease was "the direct product of [hereditary] insanity."[14(p61)] As an example of degenerative etiology, Ribot had reported the case of the Marquise de Dampierre, a French noblewoman notorious for publicly shouting out, in the middle of conversations, inappropriate or obscene words, especially "shit and fucking pig."[16] Dampierre's bizarre behavior originally had been reported in 1825 by Jean Itard.[18]

Gilles de la Tourette appropriated Itard's description of the marquise as his first and prototypical example of the progressive course of tic disease and its inevitable obscene outbursts.[8] Although Dampierre lived to be 85 years old, contrary to a variety of assertions since 1885, neither Gilles de la Tourette nor Charcot ever examined or formally met her.[19,(pp238–241)] In contrast, none of Gilles de la Tourette's actual clinical patients fit the symptom course attributed to the Marquise.[9(pp23–26),19(pp241–243)] For instance, Gilles de la Tourette's oldest patient was a 24-year-old clerk, who at 8 years developed facial twitches, followed by arm and leg movements; however, he evidenced no involuntary sounds or coprolalia. In fact, only two of Gilles de la Tourette's clinical observations displayed the range of symptoms that he and Charcot attached to the general syndrome. None, however, fit their assertions that the syndrome was unambiguously progressive and lifelong. In this context, then, the example of the

Marquise de Dampierre was essential as evidence for Gilles de la Tourette's claim that he had described a syndrome that must be distinguished from other seemingly similar disorders.

Because they had identified a set of symptoms, a course of illness, and a predisposing cause, Gilles de la Tourette and Charcot insisted that they had described a *disease,* which Charcot designated *maladie des tics de Gilles de la Tourette.* Gilles de la Tourette's construction of convulsive tic disease was challenged by two of his Salpêtrière contemporaries, Georges Guinon and Edouard Brissaud, who claimed that case histories of their hysteric and choreic patients displayed multiple motor tics, coprolalia, and echolalia.[20–22] As a result of these and other criticisms, Charcot and, to a lesser extent, Gilles de la Tourette refined their claims.[23] They conceded that motor and vocal tics and coprolalia were also symptoms of hysteria, and these symptoms and signs were therefore not unique to Gilles de la Tourette's disease.[14,24] In 1890, with endorsement from Gilles de la Tourette and Charcot, Jacques Catrou distinguished convulsive tic disease from a hysterical illness with similar symptoms by whether or not the *cause* was degenerative and whether or not the symptoms could be eliminated.[25,23]

Although what today is called "Tourette *syndrome*" claims its pedigree from Gilles de la Tourette's 1885 article, the current designation draws only on Gilles de la Tourette's description of symptoms and ignores his and Charcot's attribution of the underlying degenerative causes and progressively deteriorating outcome. In adopting the name "Gilles de la Tourette's syndrome," now shortened to "Tourette syndrome" (TS), Shapiro et al.[26,27] tied the disorder to this nineteenth-century typology, ignoring that Georges Gilles de la Tourette saw the etiology of these symptoms as a degenerative and incurable disease. However, "maladie des tics de Gilles de la Tourette" is not the same as what today is labeled Tourette syndrome.[28,29]

The issue of phenotype is far from settled. Beginning in the 1980s a serious dispute arose among experts over whether obsessive–compulsive behaviors should be included within the Tourette's typology.[30] More recently, a division has emerged among those who believe that conduct disorders are part of TS and those who resist too wide a spectrum of symptoms.[31] In addition, clinicians disagree over the length of time a symptom must be present to be considered for a diagnosis and whether onset must occur before the age of 18.

The revisions of the *Diagnostic and Statistical Manual of Mental Disorders* (DSM-III-R) reveal that there has been no absolute agreement over time about what symptoms are necessary or how long they must persist for a diagnosis of Tourette syndrome.[32] A new effort at a uniform definition was made in the construction of Tourette's categories in the DSM-IV (1994),[1] but dissension over the typology erupted among members of the committee that had been commissioned to write this section, as well as among other experts as soon as the volume appeared.[33] By 1997 a team of experienced Tourette's researchers at Yale University admitted that continuing disagreements over what constitutes the symptoms that are part of the TS phenotype continue to frustrate attempts to locate its etiology.[34,35]

References

1. American Psychiatric Association. *Diagnostic and Statistical Manual of Mental Disorders.* 4th ed, rev. Washington, DC: American Psychiatric Association; 1994.
2. Gilles de la Tourette G P; Rose F C, Bynum W F, eds. *Historical Aspects of the Neurosciences.* New York: Raven Press; 1982:397–415.
3. Lees A J. Georges Gilles de la Tourette: The man and his times. *Rev Neurol.* 1986;142: 808–816.
4. Gilles de la Tourette G P. *L'hypnotisme dans les états analogue au point de vue médico-légal.* Paris: Plon et Cie; 1887.
5. Gilles de la Tourette G P. *Traité clinique et thérapeutique de l'hystérie d'après l'enseignement de la Salpêtrière.* Paris: Plon-Nourrit; 1891.
6. L'Attentat Contre M. Gilles de la Tourette. *La Patrie,* 8 December 1893. In: Bibliothèque Charcot, Salpêtrière, Paris.
7. Gilles de la Tourette. *Nouvelle Iconographie de la Salpêtrière.* 1904;17:265–268. Obituary.
8. Gilles de la Tourette G P. Étude sur une affection nerveuse caractérisée par de l'incoordination motrice accompagnée d'écholalie et de coprolalie (jumping, latah, and myriachit). *Arch Neurol.* 1885;9:19–42, 158–200.
9. Kushner H I. *A Cursing Brain? The Histories of Gilles de la Tourette Syndrome.* Cambridge: Harvard University Press; 1999.
10. Charcot J-M; Goetz C, trans-comm. *Charcot the Clinician: The Tuesday Lessons, Excerpts from Nine Case Presentations on General Neurology Delivered at the Salpêtrière Hospital in 1887–1888.* New York: Raven Press; 1987.
11. Gilles de la Tourette G P. trans. Les Sauteurs du Maine (Etats-Unis) par G. Beard. *Arch Neurol.* 1881;5:146–150.
12. Gilles de la Tourette G P. Jumping, latah, myriachit. *Arch Neurol.* 1884;8:68–84.
13. Lajonchere C, Nortz M, Finger S. Gilles de la Tourette and the discovery of Tourette's syndrome (including a translation of his 1884 paper). *Arch Neurol.* 1996;53:567–574.
14. Charcot J-M. *Leçons du Mardi à la Salpêtrière Policliniques, 1887–1888. Notes de Cours de MM. Blin, Charcot, et Colin. Handwritten and printed.* Paris: Bureaux du Progrès Médical; 1887–1888.
15. Gilles de la Tourette G P. La maladie des tics convulsifs. *Sem Méd.* 1899;19:153–156.
16. Ribot T. *Les Maladies de la Volonté.* Paris: Félix Alcan; 1883.
17. Dowbiggin I R. *Inheriting Madness: Professionalization and Psychiatric Knowledge in Nineteenth-Century France.* Berkeley: University of California Press; 1991.
18. Itard JMG. Mémoire sur quelques fonctions involontaires des appareils de la locomotion, de la préhension et de la voix. *Arch Gén Méd.* 1825;8:385–407.
19. Kushner H I. Medical fictions: the case of the cursing marquise and the (re)construction of Gilles de la Tourette's syndrome. *Bull Hist Med.* 1995;69:224–254.
20. Guinon G. Sur la maladie des tics convulsifs. *Rev Méd.* 1886;6:50–80.
21. Guinon G. Tics convulsifs et hystérie. *Rev Méd.* 1887;7:509–519.
22. Brissaud E. La chorée variable des dégénérés. *Rev Neurol.* 1896;4:417–431.
23. Kushner H I. Freud and the diagnosis of Gilles de la Tourette's illness. *Hist Psychiatry.* 1998;8:1–25.
24. Charcot J-M. Des tics et des tiqueurs. *La Tribune Médicale.* 1888;19:571–573.
25. Catrou J. *Étude sur la maladie des tics convulsifs (jumping—latah—myriachit).* Paris: Faculté de Médecine de Paris, 1890. Thesis.
26. Shapiro A K, Shapiro E. Treatment of Gilles de la Tourette's syndrome with haloperidol. *Br J Psychiatry.* 1968;114:345–350.
27. Shapiro A K, Shapiro E S, Bruun R D, Sweet R D. *Gilles de la Tourette Syndrome.* New York: Raven Press; 1978.
28. Kushner H I, Kiessling L S. The controversy over the classification of Gilles de la Tourette's syndrome, 1800–1995. *Perspect Biol Med.* 1996;39:409–435.

29. Kushner, H I. From Gilles de la Tourette's disease to Tourette syndrome. *CNS Spectrums.* 1999;4:24–35.
30. Shapiro, A K, Shapiro, E S. Evaluation of the reported association of obsessive-compulsive symptoms or disorder with Tourette's disorder. *Comp. Psychiatry.* 1992;33:152–165.
31. Comings D E. Tourette syndrome: a hereditary neuropsychiatric spectrum disorder. *Ann Clin Psychiatry.* 1994;6:235–247.
32. Tourette Syndrome Classification Study Group. Definitions and classifications of tic disorders. *Arch Neurol.* 1993;50:1013–1016.
33. Letters to Editor. DSM-IV criteria for Tourette's. *J Am Acad Child Adolesc Psychiatry.* 1995;34: 400–402.
34. Leckman J F, Peterson B S, Anderson G M, et al. Pathogenesis of Tourette's syndrome. *J Child Psychol Psychiatry.* 1997;38:119–142.
35. Kurlan R. Future direction of research in Tourette syndrome. *Neurol Clin.* 1997;15:451–456.

34

THE GUILLAIN–BARRÉ SYNDROME

Eelco F. M. Wijdicks and Allan H. Ropper

The identification of Guillain–Barré syndrome with an acute polyneuritis has remained unchallenged since its first description. Nearly all cases of Guillain–Barré syndrome follow a typical course. Limb paresthesias are followed by weakness in proximal muscles, sometimes accompanied by cramping pain in the back, buttocks, and thighs. The disorder may follow a viral or bacterial infection, vaccination, or a number of other conditions. Except for facial weakness, cranial nerve involvement is uncommon but may emerge in more severe cases. This includes ophthalmoplegia, oropharyngeal weakness, and, rarely, progression to a "locked-in" state. As a result of impaired baroreceptor function, spontaneous fluctuations in blood pressure and bradycardia may occur. Mechanical ventilation is necessary to support neuromuscular respiratory failure in 30% of patients. The maximal deficit is reached in three weeks, followed by a variable (days to months) interval in which neurologic function does not change. In patients with respiratory failure, weaning from the ventilator can be expected in six to eight weeks, but early weaning (within three weeks) is possible in approximately one in five patients. Ninety percent of patients fully recover, and most walk unassisted, but up to 8% die as a consequence of the complications of longstanding immobilization, mostly when underlying pulmonary disease exists. Relapsing forms are rare, but occasionally the diagnosis needs to be reconsidered and changed to chronic inflammatory demyelinating disease (the term "chronic GBS" cannot be advocated).

Unusual variants causing diagnostic confusion include the Miller–Fisher syndrome (ataxia, ophthalmoplegia, and areflexia) and several regional variants (e.g., pharyngeal-cervical-brachial involvement with ptosis).

The proper pronunciation of the eponym in phonetic spelling is "ghee-len-bharay." It is commonly mispronounced in the United States and Great Britain ("guillian") or simply denoted "GBS."

The risk of diagnostic error in Guillain–Barré syndrome is low, rival disorders are few, and progression to the zenith of the neurologic deficit is predictable. We still do not precisely understand the pathoimmunologic mechanism.

Georges Guillain (1876–1961) was born in Rouen and was an intern under Fulgence Raymond, who succeeded Jean-Martin Charcot as chair of Maladies du Système Nerveux at the Salpêtrière, and under Professors Pierre Marie, Louis Théophite Joseph Landouzy, and Paul Jules Tillaux.[1] At the end of his internship, he visited many prominent American universities, including Columbia, Cornell, and Harvard.[2] After his return from the United States, he became *chef de clinique* of Alix Joffroy at the Sainte-Anne asylum. During World War I, he was stationed in Amiens and worked closely with Professor Jean-Alexandre Barré. He published articles on many neurologic war injuries, which culminated in the text *Travaux Neurologiques de Guerre,* including ischemic contractures, multiple cranial nerve palsies, asphyxia from gases, and traumatic spinal lesions.

After directing *(médecin-chef)* the Centre Neurologique of the 6th Army, he became a member of the Academy of Medicine, and in 1923 he became Professeur de Cliniques des Maladies du Système Nerveux. He attained the chair of the neurology serv-

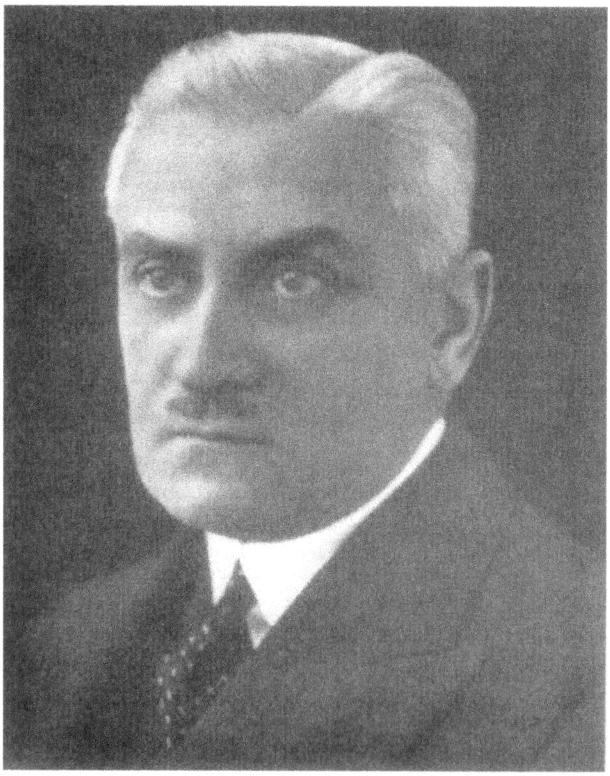

Figure 34–1. Georges Guillain (1876–1961). From Ref. 1 by permission of Masson Editeur Paris.

ice of the Salpêtrière, succeeding Pierre Marie, at the age of 47. He was prolific, and his work included descriptions of hypothalamic syndrome, superior cerebellar artery syndrome, multiple sclerosis, the value of a diagnostic test (*réaction du Benjoin colloidal*), and a syphilis-induced myelopathy carrying the name *Guillain-Thaon syndrome.*[1] After his retirement, he wrote a classic biography of Charcot, published in 1955.

Jean-Alexandre Barré (1880–1967) was born in Nantes and died in Strasbourg. Barré was an intern with Babinski and in 1912 published his medical thesis on *Les ostéoarthropathies du tabès.* After World War I broke out, he joined Guillain at the Centre Neurologique of the 6th Army. There he served with an ambulance unit caring for patients with major traumatic injuries, and these accomplishments won him the Légion d'Honneur, France's most important military distinction. He became a professor of neurology in Strasbourg, at that time unique because only in Paris was such a distinct chairmanship known.[3,4] (A chair was needed in Strasbourg because France reoccupied Alsace-Lorraine after the war ended.)

Barré's work was largely devoted to semiology, which he learned from Babinski. His interests were largely in neuro-otology and vestibular syndromes, and he founded the journal *Revue d'Oto-Neuro-Ophthalmologie.*

In World War II, Barré joined the army again but had to relocate to Clermont-Ferrand in the free zone, "Vichy-France," the seat of the new government.

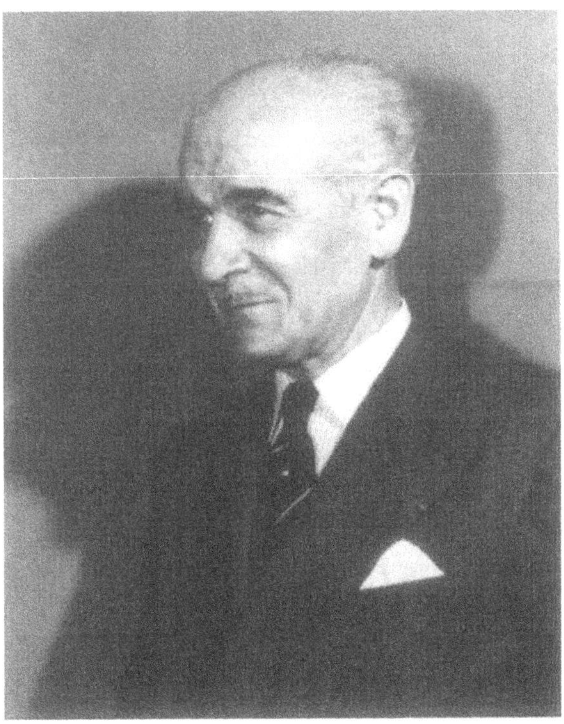

Figure 34–2. Jean-Alexandre Barré (1880–1967). From National Library of Medicine.

The name "Barré" became fixed not only in the Guillain-Barré eponym but also as the Barré test (see Chapter 19) and the "Barré-Liéou syndrome." This controversial syndrome, which has not been settled as a neurologic entity, included occipital headache (*migraine cervicale*), vertigo, ringing in the ears, and blurred vision attributed to "irritation du nerf vertébral par une arthrite cervicale chronique."[3,4]

In 1950, Barré retired and suffered a stroke, which left him with sensory aphasia from which he never recovered.[3,4]

André Strohl (1887–1977) was born in Poitiers, France, but his parents were from Alsace (Alsace, historically, has been governed alternately by Germany and France during a series of wars). His father introduced him to mathematics, but according to Roche,[5] he thought that his fragile health would not allow him to study at the Grandes Ecoles. He went to the Sorbonne and earned a degree in natural science and physical sciences, followed by one in medicine in 1913.[5] He did not have to serve in the army (due to dispensation) but volunteered for service. His mentor later asked him to reorganize the physiology laboratory at Strasbourg, where he became a tenured professor; a position in Algiers (North Africa) followed. In 1925, he became chairman of medical

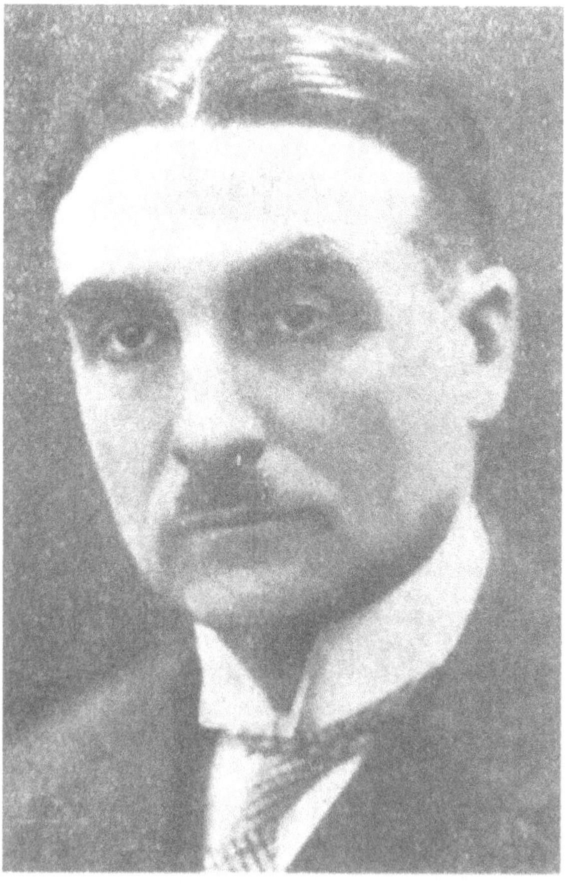

Figure 34–3. André Strohl (1887–1977). From La Vie Médicale (1934), vol. 15, p. 135.

physiology in Paris. He wrote handbooks on medical physics and studied electrical gradients of the skin and neuromuscular excitability. His rather modest accomplishments and diversion from neurology may have led to omission of his name in the eponym, although he performed the electrophysiologic studies in the original patients. His contribution to the paper was not essential to the understanding of the clinical syndrome, merely adding the results of physiologic recording of clinically noted areflexia and retained idiomuscular response after tapping. None of his later work involved electrophysiologic delineation of neurologic disorders. To us, his role remains undetermined.

World War I was at its height in 1916, with the Germans attempting to break the French line at Verdun, trying to end the stalemate of trench warfare. Guillain and Barré were both stationed in Amiens (northwest France in the province of Picardy) and assigned to the Centre Neurologique of the 6th Army. On 20 August and 5 September, two infantry soldiers were admitted with tingling and progressive weakness causing major difficulty with walking.[6] Tingling progressed to the upper extremities and lower part of the face. Guillain and Barré considered the possibilities of syphilis, food poisoning, or alcohol abuse in both patients. On examination, the men had muscles that were tender to pressure; a mild sensory loss of touch, temperature, and pinprick; severe weakness of all four extremities; and notable areflexia. Electrophysiologic studies (by Strohl) confirmed areflexia with retained idiomuscular contraction. One patient recovered strength after two months; the other improved in the first month before he was transferred to another institution. Most notable and arguably unique was a "*hyperalbuminose . . . sans réaction cellulaire*" (albuminocytologic dissociation; Fig. 34–4). Lumbar puncture may have been performed to exclude syphilis or simply because the procedure had become widely applied in neurologic practice.

Initially, the condition became known as "acute febrile polyneuritis," "acute infective polyneuritis," "acute ascending paralysis," and "infective neuronitis." The first confirmatory descriptions after the seminal article were by Pierre Marie and C. Chatelin and Gordon Holmes.[7,8] Several years after the original description, Guillain mentioned it ("*notre syndrome*"; our syndrome) in a paper discussing its criteria.[9] At a symposium in Brussels, however, he proposed four different types, using several more publications, with additional descriptive details and refinements. They were (1) *la forme inférieure* (only paraparesis), (2) *la forme mixte spinale et mésocéphalique* (quadriparesis and cranial nerve involvement), (3) *la forme mésocephalique* (only cranial nerves), and (4) *uniforme de polyradiculonévrite avec troubles mentaux* (prior types but with changes in mental status).[10–12]

A major controversy occurred when the entity was challenged as original in reference to Landry's definition. Guillain tried hard to defend his position that his cases were self-limiting and benign, and he refused to accept fatal cases described earlier by Landry.[13]

The first mention of the eponym was by Baker,[14] who designated it "Guillain–Barré's disease." Why Strohl's name did not become fixed in the eponym remains unclear. Strohl may have been too new in his career to fully appreciate the refined clinical definition of the entity by seasoned neurologists such as Guillain and Barré. Probably the numerous articles by Guillain and Barré in the 1920s without Strohl,

SUR UN SYNDROME DE RADICULO-NÉVRITE AVEC HYPERALBUMINOSE DU LIQUIDE CÉPHALO-RACHIDIEN SANS RÉACTION CELLULAIRE. REMARQUES SUR LES CARACTÈRES CLINIQUES ET GRAPHIQUES DES RÉFLEXES TENDINEUX,

par MM. GEORGES GUILLAIN, J.-A. BARRÉ et A. STROHL.

Nous attirons l'attention, dans la présente note, sur un syndrome clinique que nous avons observé chez deux malades, syndrome caractérisé par des troubles moteurs, l'abolition des réflexes tendineux avec conservation des reflexes cutanés, des paresthésies avec troubles légers de la sensibilité objective, des douleurs à la pression des masses musculaires, des modifications peu accentuées des réactions électriques des nerfs et des muscles, de l'hyperalbuminose très notable du liquide céphalo-rachidien avec absence de réaction cytologique (dissociation albumino-cytologique). Ce syndrome nous a paru dépendre d'une atteinte concomitante des racines rachidiennes, des nerfs et des muscles, vraisemblablement de nature infectieuse ou toxique. Il doit être différencié des radiculites simples, des polynévrites pures et des polymyosites. Des recherches expérimentales par la méthode graphique sur la vitesse des réflexes et leur temps perdu, sur les modalités, la contractilité musculaire, montrent la réalité de la participation, dans ce syndrome, de tout l'appareil moteur neuro-musculaire périphérique. Nous insistons particulièrement aussi sur l'hyperalbuminose du liquide céphalo-rachidien sans réaction cytologique, fait qui, à notre connaissance, n'a pas été mentionné dans des cas semblables.

Figure 34–4. Title page of the original publication. From Ref. 6. English translation: On a syndrome of radiculoneuritis with hyperalbuminosis of the cerebrospinal fluid without a cellular reaction. Remarks on the clinical characteristics and tracings of the tendon reflexes, by G. Guillain, J.-A. Barré, and A. Strohl.

In the present paper, we would like to draw attention to a clinical syndrome observed in two patients that is characterized by motor difficulties, loss of the deep tendon reflexes with preservation of the cutaneous reflexes, paresthesias with slight impairment of objective sensation, muscle tenderness, slight alterations in nerve conduction and electromyographic patterns, and a remarkable increase in cerebrospinal fluid albumin in the absence of a cellular reaction (albumino-cytologic dissociation). This ostensibly infectious or toxic process appears to simultaneously involve nerve roots, peripheral nerves, and muscles. It is distinct from the simple radiculopathies, pure polyneuropathies, and from the polymyositides. Experimental data derived from tracings of the latency and speed of the reflex response and muscular contraction indicate that the entire peripheral neuromuscular motor apparatus is involved. We particularly emphasize the increased cerebrospinal fluid albumin content without cellular reaction, an observation that has not been previously published. From D. A. Rottenberg and F. H. Hochberg, *Neurological Classics in Modern Translation.* New York: Hafner Press, 1977, pp. 309–310. Translated by F. H. Hochberg. By permission of Macmillan Publishing.)

and Guillain's reference to it as "our disease" (Guillain and Barré), initiated and then perpetuated the eponym. A seminal paper by Haymaker and Kernohan from the Mayo Clinic reported the clinicopathologic correlations in 50 fatal cases and introduced the eponym "Landry–Guillain–Barré syndrome."[15] Remarkably, Roche, in an obituary on Strohl, called it the "syndrome neurologique de Guillain, Strohl et

Table 34–1. History of Guillain–Barré Syndrome

1834–1837:	Wardrop and Ollivier describe cases of rapidly progressive paralysis and other features of GBS
1859:	Landry unifies clinical features as "acute ascending paralysis"
1876:	Term "Landry's (ascending) paralysis" first used
1916:	Guillain, Barré, and Strohl note albuminocytologic dissociation in cerebrospinal fluid, a new diagnostic feature of acute paralysis
1920:	Guillain and Barré publish text *Travaux Neurologiques de Guerre,* which links their names and briefly mentions GBS, differentiating it from Landry's paralysis and from nerve gas poisoning; many articles by both follow
1937:	Brussels symposium permanently excludes Strohl from eponym, adds many descriptive details of illness, and clarifies Guillain's definition of the syndrome
Late 1940s:	Development of respiratory intensive care units and use of positive-pressure ventilation reduce mortality from GBS
1949:	Haymaker and Kernohan report on clinicopathologic correlations in a series of 50 fatal cases of "Landry–Guillain–Barré syndrome"
1955:	Experimental autoimmune neuritis, a clinical and pathologic facsimile of human GBS, produced in animals by Waksman and Adams
1956:	Fisher's syndrome described as a variant of GBS
1969:	Pathologic study by Asbury and colleagues shows lymphocytic infiltration in spinal roots and nerves
1975:	Swine flu vaccination program, with increased incidence of the disorder, spurs interest in GBS
1978:	Use of plasma exchange in treatment first reported by Brettle and co-workers
1981:	Symposium on GBS brings immune and pathologic features up to date and proposes modern diagnostic criteria
1985:	North American Plasma Exchange Trial confirms clinical benefit
1992:	First successful trial with intravenous immunoglobulin by Dutch working group led by van der Meché
1997:	Large treatment trial by Hughes and associates confirms that intravenous immunoglobulin is similar in efficacy to plasma exchange

Source: Modified from Ropper et al.[12] By permission of Oxford University Press.

Barré."[5] It is highly likely that the same disorder was noted earlier by James Wardrop, Charles-Prosper Ollivier, Louis-Stanislas Duménil, François Chomel, Robert Graves, and Jean-Baptiste-Octave Landry, and William Osler described it as acute febrile polyneuritis in his textbook *The Principles and Practice of Medicine,*[16–19] but the cerebrospinal fluid served to distinguish it from poliomyelitis. The history of Guillain–Barré syndrome is summarized in Table 34–1.

References

1. Alajouanine T H. Nécrologie: Georges Guillain (1876–1961). *Bull Acad Natl Med.* 1962;146: 18–26.

2. Goetz C G. Georges Guillain's neurologic exploration of America. *Neurology.* 1998;50: 1451–1455.
3. Minkowski M. In memoriam Jean-Alexandre Barré (1880–1967). *Schweiz Arch Neurol Neurochir Psychiatr.* 1968;102:376–379.
4. Thiébaut F J A. Barré (1880–1967). *J Neurol Sci.* 1968;6:381–382.
5. Roche J. André Strohl (1887–1977). *C R Séances Soc Biol Fil.* 1977;171:1161–1162.
6. Guillain G, Barré J A, Strohl A. Sur un syndrome de radiculo-névrite avec hyperalbuminose du liquide céphalo-rachidien sans réaction cellulaire: Remarques sur les caractères cliniques et graphiques des réflexes tendineux. *Bull Soc Méd Hôp Paris.* 1916;40:1462–1470.
7. Chatelin C. Note sur un syndrome de paralysie flasque plus ou moins généralisée avec abolition des réflexes, hyperalbuminose massive et xanthochromie du liquide céphalo-rachidien, évoluant spontanément vers la guérison et de nature indéterminée. *Rev Neurol (Paris).* 1916;23:564–565.
8. Holmes G. Acute febrile polyneuritis. *Br Med J.* 1917;2:37–39.
9. Guillain G, Alajouanine T, Périsson J. Sur le syndrome de radiculonévrite aigue curable avec dissociation albuminocytologique du liquide céphalo-rachidien (deux observations). *Rev Neurol.* 1925;1:492–496.
10. Asbury A K. Guillain-Barré syndrome: historical aspects. *Ann Neurol.* 1990; 27(suppl): S2–S6.
11. Pearce JMS. Octave Landry's ascending paralysis and the Landry-Guillain-Barré-Strohl syndrome. *J Neurol Neurosurg Psychiatry.* 1997;62:495, 500.
12. Ropper A H, Wijdicks EFM, Truax B T. *Guillain-Barré Syndrome.* Philadelphia: F A Davis; 1991.
13. Landry O. Note sur la paralysie ascendante aiguë. *Gaz Hebd Méd.* 1859;6:472–474.
14. Baker A B. Guillain-Barré's disease (encephalo-myelo-radiculitis): a review of 33 cases. *Lancet.* 1943;63:384–398.
15. Haymaker W, Kernohan J W. Landry-Guillain-Barré syndrome: clinicopathologic report of 50 fatal cases and critique of literature. *Medicine.* 1949;28:59–141.
16. Cosnett J E. Wardrop-Landry-Guillain-Barré-Strohl. *Lancet.* 1987;1:861–862.
17. Duménil L. Paralysie périphérique du mouvement et du sentiment portant sur les quatre membres: Atrophie des rameaux nerveux des parties paralysées. *Gaz Hebd Méd.* 1864;1: 203–206.
18. Chomel A-F. De l'épidémie actuellement regnante à Paris. *J Hebd Méd.* 1828;1:333.
19. Graves R J. *Clinical Lectures on the Practice of Medicine.* London: New Sydenham Society; 1884: 579–580.

35

HORNER'S SYNDROME

George W. Bruyn and William Gooddy

The year 1869 has something of a neuro-ophthalmological vintage: Argyll Robertson described "his" pupil and Johann Friedrich Horner (1831–1896) reported his symptom triad.[1] Parallels between the two men can be extended: both trained further in ophthalmology in Albrecht von Graefe's clinic in Berlin during their *Wanderjahr,* a popular customar following graduation in those times; both became attached to von Graefe by ties of lifelong friendship; both initiated (in their respective countries) teaching of ophthalmology; both were the first to introduce Lister's antisepsis in their operating theaters. Neither published many papers, but what they published was to the point, exemplifying the old *multum, non multa.*

Johann Friedrich Horner, born on 27 March 1831 in Zurich, was the second child in a large Protestant family. He had an older brother and four younger sisters. His father, an overburdened, conscientious general physician, subject to bitter moods, found himself hard put to make ends meet. Primary school and Gymnasium in Zurich provided Johann Friedrich with thorough knowledge of the classics, mathematics, and natural history, so that after completing his military service, the student life at Zurich's university (1849–1854) promised to be a pleasant one. This was not to be: his brother Konrad, who studied classic philology in Bonn, died of endocarditis in 1851; his father, coming home from patient rounds, developed a fatal apoplexy in January 1852; his mother died in December of that year. As the household dissolved, Johann Friedrich moved in at his grandfather's house. Despite the shocking events, he took the M.D. degree with highest honors with a thesis on the curvature of the spinal column.

The customary *peregrinatio academica* took him to Vienna, where Friedrich von Jaeger taught him the use of the ophthalmoscope invented by Helmholtz two years earlier and alerted him to the new *Archiv für Ophthalmologie,* founded by his pupil von

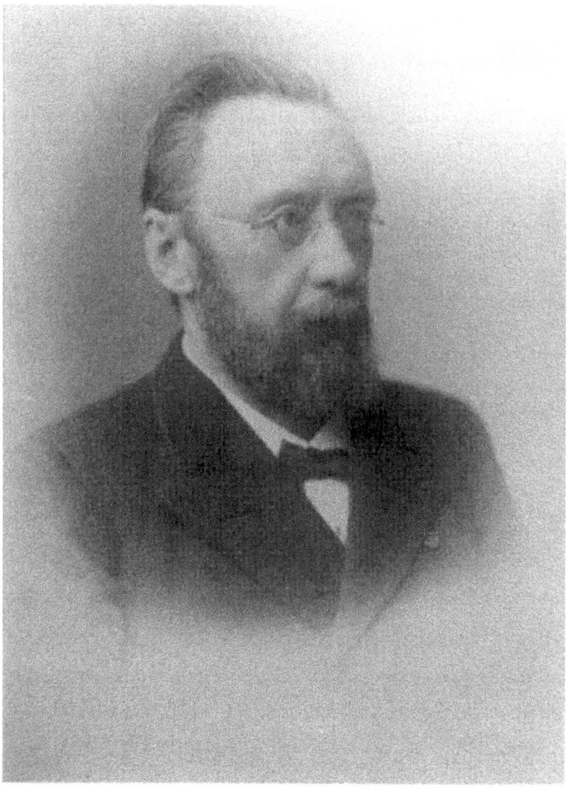

Figure 35–1: Johann Friedrich Horner (1831–1886) Courtesy Medizinhistorisches Institut Zurich, Switzerland.

Graefe. After the Viennese sojourn, he studied as assistant to von Graefe (October 1854–May 1855) in Berlin. A close and lifelong friendship developed. In Paris (May–December 1855) he practiced ophthalmology, in particular cataract extractions, under Louis-Auguste Desmarres.

On return to Zurich, he established a general and ophthalmological practice, in 1856 he read his *Habilitation* (Thesis required for the position of *Privat-Dozent*) and, on the emphatic recommendation of von Graefe, he was appointed Professor Extraordinarius in Ophthalmology in 1862. He married Anna Louise Henggeler, and their marriage was blessed with the births of a daughter (Anna Louise, 1866) and a son (Konrad Friedrich, 1869). The latter, who also became a physician and collected most details on his father, donated this material to Zurich University after his death in 1942. These *Horneriana* first went to the Ophthalmological Clinic but ultimately came to rest in the Institute of Medical History.

From 1873 on, Horner mainly worked in the private ophthalmological clinic, the Hottinger Hof, he had established. This clinic, which commanded 44 beds and up-to-date facilities, was visited by about 5000 patients per year, who went there because of Horner's reputation of diagnostic thoroughness, his fabulous memory of patients, his operative skills, and his principle of keeping the patient the focus of all activities.

Also in 1873 he was appointed ordinary professor and acquired additional fame for his rhetoric. He refused to call himself a "specialist," as he was convinced that an ophthalmological disease, wherever and whenever possible, ought to be related to other somatic dysfunctions of the patient. He did an estimated 5000 cataract extractions, with a failure rate of only 1%, a record low in those days when a rate of 6%–7% prevailed.

As early as 1861, on his fiftieth birthday, Horner was offered a *Festschrift,* organized by his pupil Prof. Marc Dufour of Lausanne. In 1862, the University Ophthalmology Clinic remained a controversial subject: the surgeon Christian Albert Theodor Billroth did not want ophthalmology to become autonomous and had kept the surgery and ophthalmology departments in his own hand, against the wish of the faculty council. The government finally ordered the separation and appointed Horner to the chair. Horner succeeded surprisingly well in getting this department going; next he initiated the foundation of a children's hospital, the improvement of hygiene at schools, and care for the vision and learning capacities of schoolchildren. If this were not enough, he was an active and successful advocate of the foundation of the Burghölzli Psychiatric Clinic (later made famous by Eugene Bleuler and Carl Gustav Jung), founded the Zurich Cantonal Medical Assocation, became city councillor, inspector of public health, member of diverse university committees, and he sustained an extensive exchange of letters with colleagues abroad and at home. These letters were published by the ophthalmologist A. Bader.[2] He presented his famous technique of iridectomy for glaucoma at the International Congress of Ophthalmology in Brussels in 1857. Horner prepared his lectures meticulously and read them at high speed.

Twenty-eight dissertations were composed under his guidance, among them five by women pupils, testifying to his (in those times "progressive") attitude. Also among his Ph.D. students were von Muralt and Albert Kölliker. Five of his pupils ultimately chaired Swiss university ophthalmology clinics as Professor Ordinarius: August Siegrist (Bern), Marc Dufour (Lausanne), Karl Mellinger (Basel), Otto Haab (Zürich), and Georges Haltenhoff (Geneva).

Horner's plan to write a textbook of practical ophthalmology was not achieved because of the disease that wrecked most of his last years. Part of his manuscript was published as a chapter in Gerhardt's *Handbuch der Kinderkrankheiten* (1879/80). He also began to write his autobiography in 1885, but it had to be completed after his death by his pupil and friend Edmund Landolt.[3]

The papers he wrote dealt with retinal tumors, foreign bodies of the iris, keratoconus, corneal herpes, mycotic keratitis, pterygium, congenital myopia, and refraction improvement. He made an excuse for the modest size of his professional *oeuvre* by observing that prolific writers are bad clinicians because they see diseases instead of the diseased, and he claimed he gave the best he had to his pupils for elaboration in theses (which, even if true, carries a holier-than-thou ring). He lamented that his overcrowded daily schedules left no room for a proper meal at leisure, and that only too late in life could he use the microscope. The obvious motive—that he preferred praxis to theory, the scalpel to the fountain pen—apparently was anathema to his conscience.

Horner was a humane, good man. The extraordinary lengths he went to in order to help a friend at his own expense has been eloquently documented by Schleich.[4]

Progressive atherosclerosis of heart and kidney, with labored breathing and pleural exudates, forced him to resign his position in 1885. While at home, during a merry conversation in the family circle, he developed an apoplexy with aphasia during the evening of 15 December 1886. His life expired five days later.

> Many of my colleagues are familiar with longstanding cases of incomplete ptosis in adults, lacking the usual accompanying signs of oculomotor paralysis but exhibiting the striking symptoms of myosis of the pupil on the same side. This clinical picture was not new to me when at the end of last November a woman, 40 year of age, presented herself with these symptoms . . . the upper lid covers the right cornea to the upper edge of the pupil . . . The pupil of the right eye is considerably more constricted than that of the left, but reacts to light . . . During the clinical discussion of the case, the right side of her face became red and warm . . . while the left side remained pale and cool . . . The patient thereupon told us that the right side had never perspired.[1,8]

Horner examined his patient meticulously.[1] He noted the miosis and ptosis; he suspected the slight enophthalmos to be apparent merely because of the ptosis, but he verified its presence by repeated measurements; he noted as well the tonometrically proven hypotonia of the bulbus, the conjunctival injection, the hyperthermia of the axilla and facial half, and the hemifacial anhidrosis, all ipsilaterally. He inferred that the symptoms were the result of a lesion of the cervical sympathetic nerve.

His was a concise, fact-based paper, though a mere anecdote without mention of previous literature, a task he left to his pupil Nicati,[5] who did a thorough review. Horner intentionally left many of his observations to his pupils for elaboration. That he did so on purpose is confessed in his autobiography:

> Ich habe später, als Lehrer, alles Mögliche getan, um meine Schüler zur literarischen Arbeit anzuleiten, und gerade deshalb *mein* Bestes in Dissertationen usw. niedergelegt.[3]

[Later, as a teacher, I did all I could to stimulate my pupils to write papers, and therefore I just put down *my* best in dissertations, etc.] Nearly 30 theses written under his guidance testify to the veracity of this statement.

According to Stiegler's law,[6] scarcely any eponym honors the *auctor intellectualis,* the *princeps observator.* Conscientious historical search will invariably hit upon someone who made the observation or did the experiment earlier. Whether Nicati presaged Stiegler or not, he dug up most sources on Horner's syndrome, beginning with Pourfour du Petit.[7] Fulton,[8] Bonnet,[9] Ott,[10] and Ogle[11] might qualify for the pre-Hornerian laurels of priority, so that long list of candidates included not only experimental (neuro-)physiologists, but also a few clinicians. Ogle reviewed animal experiments as well as human disease.[11]

John W. Ogle's namesake William Ogle—assistant physician to St. George's Hospital, like the first-named Ogle—who was the first to describe agraphia (1867) and also translated the first text on physiology, Aristotle's *De partibus animalium* (1882), referred to the princeps case of Mitchell–Morehouse–Keen (see below) and presented a personal case with miosis, ptosis, enophthalmos, hyperthermia, hyperaemia, and anhidrosis. He recalled the macabre experiment by Prof. R. Wagner:

> In 1859 a female criminal aged 28 was beheaded at Würzburg. As soon as the axe had fallen, the head was wrapped in hot cloths and carried off to the neighbouring theatre of anatomy, where Prof. Wagner with a number of physiologists and students was [*sic*] awaiting it. Only 18 minutes had elapsed since the moment of decapitation, when a magneto-electric current was applied to the left cervical sympathetic . . . exposed by the axe, an inch and a quarter below the superior ganglion . . .

After 4.5 seconds, the left eye slowly opened and its pupil was seen to dilate widely. Wagner had conducted a similar experiment on another criminal's head a year earlier, with similar results.[12,13]

The clinicians included F. Arnold (1831), E. S. Hare (1838), John Reid (1839), S. Biffi (1846), J. L. Budge and A. V. Waller (1851)—who received for their impeccable experiments the coveted Prix Montyon of the Institut de France, and who still are eponymously known by most neurologists today for the "Budge–Waller ciliospinal center" and "Wallerian degeneration"—(see Chapter 10) F. Bidder (1852)— eponymously known for "Bidder's ganglion" in the frog's heart—Claude Bernard (1852), W. T. Gairdner (1855), R. Remak (1855)—good for five neurological eponyms—C. G. Ruete (1847), and S. Weir Mitchell, G. R. Morehouse, and W. W. Keen (1864).

As Ogle[11] and Fulton[8] argued, the majority of these otherwise illustrious colleagues either described only part of the constituent symptoms of the syndrome or failed to grasp its significance, and therefore they are not "really" qualified. The brilliant Edward S. Hare, who died lamentably young from typhus one day before his paper was published on 11 September 1838, came within a hairs breadth of being a contender for eponymic fame, having observed all the pertinent symptoms, but he failed to attribute them to involvement of the cervical stellate ganglion by carcinoma (Pancoast tumor?) in his patient.[8] The same obtains for John Reid (1809–1849), Chandos Professor of Anatomy at St. Andrews.[14] Only Claude Bernard, experimentally,[15] and Mitchell–Morehouse–Keen, clinically,[16] fully meet the criteria of priority, completeness, and interpretation. As it is, the French national medical literature successfully defended the term *syndrome de Claude Bernard*—which is largely correct—or at best, in a fit of generosity, *syndrome de Claude Bernard–Horner*, but the three American authors lost the eponymic acknowledgment race. As a telltale, if rather intransigent, example of chauvinism, Bonnet's paper defending the eponym "Pourfour du Petit syndrome" instead of Horner's, carries the first prize.[9] He begins:

> Il n'est pas possible de tolérer plus longtemps que, dans la littérature anglosaxonne, le syndrome paralytique du sympathique cervical soit designé sous le nom de syndrome de Horner.

[It is not possible to tolerate any longer that the name of Horner's syndrome is designated to the paralytic syndrome of the cervical sympathetic in the Anglo-Saxon literature.] Following a historical review which emphasizes the experimental work of Pourfour and of Bernard, he continues:

> Le tableau clinique qui traduit la paralysie du sympathique cervical devrait légitimement porter le nom du Pourfour du Petit.

[The clinical picture that expresses paralysis of the cervical sympathetic should rightfully carry the name of Pourfour du Petit.] He concludes:

> Il est temps que le nom de Horner—tout au moins en ce qui concerne le syndrome paralytique du sympathique—rentre dans l'ombre, d'òu il n'aurait jamais dû sortir.

[It is time that the name of Horner—at least with respect to the paralytic syndrome of the sympathetic—returns to the shade which it should never leave again.] Chauvinism appears prone to vanquish civility, courtesy, and grace.

Today's definition of Horner's syndrome includes most of the features specified in Horner's 1869 paper, although quite a few clinicians tend to deny the presence of enophthalmos. Otherwise, Horner's syndrome, being due to ipsilateral interruption of the sympathetic efferent system to head and neck, is not amenable to localizing. One can determine the sympathetic denervation hypersensitivity in the first, second, or third order (pre-postganglionic) fibers with the aid of cocaine and adrenaline instillations. Associated neurological symptoms and radiological examination invariably indicate the way to ultimate diagnosis. Even the combination of Horner's syndrome with either Ross's syndrome[17] or harlequin syndrome[18] calls for advanced diagnostic techniques.

References

1. Horner J F. Über eine Form von Ptosis. *Klin Monatsbl Augenheilkd.* 1869;7:193–198.
2. Bader A. Weitere unbekannte Ophthalmologenbriefe der Jahre 1856–1885 aus dem Hornerschen Nachlass. *Klin Monatsbl Augenheilkd.* 1936;97:787–812.
3. Horner J F. *Ein Lebensbild geschrieben von ihm selbst, ergänzt von Dr. E. Landolt.* Frauenfeld; 1887.
4. Schleich C L. *Besonnte Vergangenheit.* Berlin: Rowohlt Verlag; 1924:133.
5. Nicati W. La paralysie du nerf sympathique cervical Lausanne: Mignot H & Delahaye A; 1873.
6. Stiegler S M. A law of eponymy. In: Gieryn T F, ed. *Science and Social Structure: A Festschrift for Robert K. Merton.* New York: New York Academy of Science; 1980.
7. Pourfour du Petit P. Mémoire dans lequel il est démontré que les nerfs intercostaux fournissent des rameaux que portent les esprits dans les yeux. *Hist Acad Roy Sci (Paris).* 1727:1–19.
8. Fulton J F. Horner and the syndrome of paralysis of the cervical sympathetic. *Arch Surg.* 1929;18:2025–2039; also (on Hare) *Proc R Soc Med.* 1930;23:152–154.
9. Bonnet P. L'histoire du syndrome de Claude Bernard. Le syndrome paralytique du sympathique cervical. *Arch Ophthalm (Paris).* 1957;17:121–138.
10. Ott E. *Friedrich Horner 1831–1886: Leben und Werk.* Zurich: Juris Druck; 1980.
11. Ogle J W. On the influence of the cervical portion of the sympathetic nerve and spinal cord upon the eye and its appendages. *MedicoChir Trans (London).* 1858;41:397–340.
12. Ogle W. A case illustrating the physiology and pathology of the cervical portion of the sympathetic nerve. *MedicoChir Trans (London).* 1869;52:152–177.

13. Wagner R. Note sur quelques expériences sur la partie du nerf grand sympathique, chez une femme décapitée. *(Brown-Séquard's) J Physiol.* 1860;3:174–176. This paper is a translation of Wagner's article in: Z. *Ration Med.* 1859;5 (3rd ser).
14. Reid J. On the effects of lesion of the trunk of the ganglionic system of nerves in the neck, etc. *Edinb Med Surg J.* 1838;51:132–139; 1839;52:36–43.
15. Bernard C. Sur les effets de la section de la portion céphalique du grand sympathique. *C R Séances Soc Biol* 1852;4:155, 168–170.
16. Weir Mitchell S, Morehouse G R, Keen W W. *Gunshot Wounds and Other Injuries of Nerves.* Philadelphia: Lippincott: 1864:40ff.
17. Morrison D A, Bilby K, Woodruft G. The harlequin syndrome and Horner's syndrome. *J Neurol Neurosurg Psychiatry.* 1997;62:626–628.
18. Ten Holter J B, Visser A. Harlequin syndrome. *Ned Tijdschr Geneeskd.* 1997;141:2495–2499.

36

KORSAKOFF'S SYNDROME

Ben A. Blansjaar

The name of Sergei Sergeivich Korsakoff* (1854–1900) is associated with the amnestic syndrome which he defined between 1887 and 1891. Korsakoff is also known as the principal founder of Russian psychiatry. He was born on 23 February 1854 in Guss-Chrustallny, south of Moscow, where his father managed a glass and crystal factory. He received his education at home, until he entered secondary school in Moscow at the age of ten. After he completed his secondary school education with honors, he studied medicine at the University of Moscow. After his studies, he worked for a year as a physician at the psychiatric Preobrazhensky Clinic and from 1876 to 1879 in Alexei Yakovlevich Kozhevnikov's (1836–1902) neurology clinic. He then returned to the Preobrazhensky Hospital until he was appointed managing director of the newly established psychiatric clinic of Moscow University.

Korsakoff's work in many fields was meritorious. He investigated psychiatric syndromes, developed the concept of paranoia, and refined the prevailing classification of mental illness. He was largely instrumental in founding the Society for Neuropathologists and Psychiatrists in Moscow in 1890, organizing the Twelfth International Medical Congress in Moscow in 1897 and founding the Russian Association for Psychiatry and Neurology, which was established shortly after his death. Korsakoff was a notable advocate of nursing care without physical restraint for psychiatric patients and was a staunch supporter of improved public health and of democratic reform. He transferred psychotic patients from psychiatric institutions to family care on farms, under close hospital supervision.

Notwithstanding his humanitarianism Korsakoff tried to explain psychopathology largely on a physiological, biological basis, like most of his medical contemporaries. With respect to Emil Kraepelin's nosology and classification he remarked:

*In his German publications, Korsakoff spelled his name with a double *f* at the end, consistent with the Russian custom at the time of spelling names phonetically.

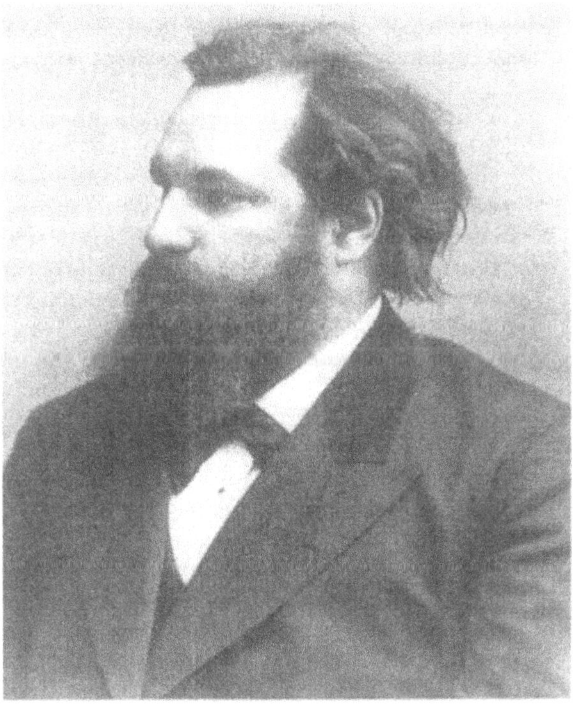

Figure 36–1. Sergei Sergeivich Korsakoff (1854–1900). From Ref. 1 with permission from Thieme Verlag, Stuttgart, Germany.

> There is no doubt that there are diseases in which diagnosis defines prognosis. In many cases, however, the outcome is also dependent on the circumstances of the patients, the treatment, the severity of the disease, and the background against which the disease evolves. This general pathological rule also relates to mental diseases, whilst Kraepelin is not sufficiently considering these individual particularities in every single case.[1(p90)]

Korsakoff is lauded in biographies both as an educator and as a physician.[1,2] The lecture hall was always packed when he lectured; his surgery often went on after midnight. According to Snjeshnewski,[1] Serbski wrote the following passage concerning his efforts on behalf of his colleagues:

> Whether we needed counsel in our work, whether we required a scientific explanation or a rare book, whether we were in need of money, or there was question of misunderstandings in family matters, if we required advice on a difficult medical case, we could always call on Sergei Sergeivich without hesitation, without having to worry about whether he had time for us, and he always found time for us.

Sergei Sergeivich Korsakoff died from a cardiac illness on 14 May 1900 at the age of 46.

Korsakoff described the amnestic syndrome in alcoholics, which was later named after him in a series of six articles published between 1887 and 1891. The third article in particular extensively and precisely described the disease symptoms of the central and peripheral nervous system. The article appeared in 1889 in Russian,[3] and in the following year in two German versions.[4,5] The comprehensiveness of Korsakoff's findings is clear from the following excerpts:

> The disturbed state of consciousness is almost always accompanied by a serious loss of memory, although a disturbed state of consciousness sometimes occurs by itself. In such cases the loss of memory often manifests as an extremely singular amnesia whereby recent events in particular are forgotten, while events from the distant past are usually well remembered. . . Amnesia of this kind usually develops after a state of agitation associated with a disturbed state of consciousness. This state of agitation persists for several days, whereupon the patient calms down. His state of consciousness improves and he gradually begins to recover his mental capacities. His memory, however, remains seriously impaired. The mental defect is initially difficult to detect in conversation. The patient gives the impression of someone in full possession of his faculties. The patient speaks with great deliberation and draws proper conclusions from given assumptions, plays chess or cards, in short, behaves as a mentally healthy person. Only after prolonged conversation does it become noticeable that the patient occasionally confuses issues and does not recall anything which he has had in mind. He does not recall whether or not he has eaten, or risen from his bed. The patient often promptly forgets what has transpired; someone has approached him and addressed him, has left him alone for a few moments and when they return he has no idea that anyone has been with him. It is notable that, while the patient has forgotten everything which has just occurred, he remembers earlier incidents which transpired prior to his illness. Usually that which has occurred during the illness or immediately preceding it disappears from memory. This is typical of most cases. In other cases, the memory of earlier events is also lost. Besides these mental symptoms, other symptoms appear, as previously mentioned, which correspond with multiple degenerative neuritis expressed as paralysis of the lower extremities, but also of the upper extremities. However, the fact must be emphasized that the symptoms are not always clearly manifest. In many cases there is only insignificant pain in the legs and an aimless gait. Neither are the knee reflexes always absent, but are often intensified or remain normal. For that matter, a thorough examination will almost always reveal signs of neuritis which thus facilitate diagnosis of a mental aberration.

Other authors had described memory loss associated with chronic alcoholism prior to Korsakoff. Korsakoff himself cited Magnus Huss as the first. However, none of these authors "could correlate the mental aberrations with neuritis. All regarded the psychosis as a complication affected by alcohol." Korsakoff justly assumed that the mental symptoms as well as peripheral neuropathy in the ailments he described are caused by a common pathogenic mechanism. For this reason, he proposed calling the ailment he described "psychosis polyneuritica." The concept of disease resulting from deficiency was unknown in his time and Korsakoff believed that intoxication of the central nervous system was the basic cause of an ailment with such diverse etiology. Later on, he therefore preferred the term "cerebropathia psychica toxemica." The term psychosis polyneuritica was deemed as less appropriate because "cases of such a mental aberration can occur in those whereby the symptoms of multiple degenerative neuritis are extremely slight and can therefore be overlooked."

Korsakoff's articles and lectures inspired a number of studies and publications in Western Europe. In 1897, the psychiatrist Friedrich Jolly[6] from Berlin proposed replacing the term cerebropathia psychica toxemica with "Korsakoff's syndrome" and to reserve this name solely for this particular amnestic condition. This concept became widespread, with the terms Korsakoff's psychosis, Korsakoff's syndrome, and Korsakoff's disease have been used interchangeably since. In the first half of the twentieth century the etiology (thiamine deficiency), the pathological-anatomical abnormalities, and the relation of Korsakoff's syndrome to Wernicke's disease have been more explicitly defined by a number of researchers.[7–13] Whether Korsakoff's disease is preceded in all cases by Wernicke's disease has been open to discussion throughout several decades. Victor, Adams, and Collins were the most widely known advocates of the view that Wernicke's disease and Korsakoff's syndrome are consecutive stages in the course of the same pathological process. Victor and his colleagues reported that of the patients they examined, only 4% presented amnesia as the only symptom of an illness which they in these cases termed Korsakoff's psychosis.[14] Victor et al. propagated the name "Wernicke–Korsakoff syndrome" in their cogent monograph because these afflictions appeared together in the majority of their patients. We can, however, note in this respect that Victor et al. collected their patient data largely during the 1950s and 1960s in large North American hospitals. Most patients were admitted in very poor health, with serious malnutrition; 96% suffered from symptoms of Wernicke's disease, 15% suffered from delirium tremens, and 17% died within three weeks.

More recent Dutch research indicates that 75% of a group of 44 Korsakoff patients, some of whom were examined retrospectively and some prospectively, had shown no symptoms of Wernickes disease—that is, a disturbed state of consciousness, eye movement disorders, and ataxia.[15] A possible explanation for this "mild" course of the illness is that most of these patients had a previous history of periods of alcohol abuse and malnutrition, alternating with periods of treatment in which they also received vitamin B supplements. It is possible that the Korsakoff syndrome developed in these patients because of repeated periods of thiamine deficiency. These deficiencies were, however, not serious enough to cause Wernicke's disease. Needless to say, an amnestic disturbance in patients lacking other neurological symptoms could better be termed Korsakoff's syndrome than a Wernicke–Korsakoff syndrome. Both these syndromes and those they were named after deserve recognition.

References

1. Snjeshnewski A W. Sergej Sergejewitsch Korsakow (1854–1900). In: Kolle K. *Grosse Nervenärzte, 3.* Stuttgart: Thieme; 1963.
2. Katzenelbogen S. Sergei Korsakov (1853–1900). In: Haymaker W, Schiller F, eds. *The Founders of Neurology.* 2nd ed. Springfield, Ill: Charles C. Thomas; 1970.
3. Korsakoff S S. Psychosis polyneuritica seu Cerebropathia psychica toxaemica. *Med Obozrenije.* 1889; 31, (no 13).
4. Korsakoff S. Eine psychische Störung combinirt mit multipler Neuritis (Psychosis polyneuritica seu Cerebropathia psychica toxaemica). *Allgem Z Psychiatr.* 1890;46:475–485.
5. Korsakoff S S. Ueber eine besondere Form psychischer Störung combinirt mit multipler Neuritis. *Arch Psychiatr.* 1890;21:669–704.

6. Jolly F. Ueber die Psychiatrischen Stoerungen bei Polyneuritis. *Charité Ann Berlin.* 1897; 22:580–612.
7. Wernicke C. *Lehrbuch der Gehirnkrankheiten fuer Aerzte und Studierende.* Kassel: Theodor Fisher; 1881;2:229–242.
8. Bonhoeffer K. *Die akuten Geisteskrankheiten der Gewohnheitstrinker.* Jena: G. Fisher; 1901.
9. Bonhoeffer K. Der Korsakowsche Symptomenkomplex in seinen Beziehungen zu den verschiedenen Krankheitsformen. *Allgem Z Psychiatr.* 1904;61:744–752.
10. Gamper E. Zur Frage der Polioencephalitis haemorrhagica der chronischen Alkoholiker: Anatomische Befunde beim alkoholischen Korsakow und ihre Beziehungen zum klinischen Bild. *Dtsch Z Nervenheilkh.* 1928;102:122–129.
11. Kant F. Die Pseudoencephalitis Wernicke der Alkoholiker (Polioencephalitis haemorrhagica superior acuta). *Arch Psychiat Nervenkrankh.* 1932–1933;8:702–768.
12. Bowman K M, Goodhart R. Joliffe N. Observations on the role of vitamin B_1 in the etiology and treatment of Korsakoff psychosis. *J Nerv Ment Dis.* 1939;90:569–575.
13. Joliffe N, Wortis H, Fein H D. The Wernicke syndrome. *Arch Neurol Psychiatry.* 1941; 46:569–597.
14. Victor M, Adams R D, Collins G H. *The Wernicke-Korsakoff Syndrome and Related Neurologic Disorders Due to Alcoholism and Malnutrition.* 2nd ed. Philadelphia: Davis; 1989.
15. Blansjaar B A, Van Dijk J G. Korsakoff minus Wernicke syndrome. *Alcohol Alcohol.* 1992; 27:435–437.

37

PARINAUD'S SYNDROME

Ernst H. Koppejan

Parinaud's syndrome is an eponym that keeps alive the memory of a very modest man, who was outstanding not only for his achievements as a neuro-ophthalmologist, *avant la lettre,* but also for his courage and philanthropy, shown on many occasions.

The first of May, 1844, Henri Parinaud was born in Bellac (Haute-Vienne), a small village in the Limousin region of France.[1] His father, a locksmith, died in 1863, leaving the family in poverty. Only by accepting the job of private teacher in two families was Henri able to start his study at the Medical School of Limoges in 1865. As an intern, he received an award for excellent progress in 1868. The following year, he moved to Paris to continue his medical training but the outbreak of the Franco-Prussian War in 1870 interrupted his career. Parinaud enrolled in the first field hospital of the Red Cross on its way to Metz, the first stop of what proved to become a very long and demanding journey. Parinaud's extraordinary courage in fulfilling his tasks drew the attention of many. In one of his tales about the war, the writer Ludovic Halévy described Parinaud's dedication and brave behavior during the evacuation of the wounded citizens of Châteaudun, and the French prime minister Léon-Michel Gambetta (1838–1882) awarded Parinaud a decoration to commemorate these deeds.

After the war, Parinaud returned to Paris and resumed his training. In 1877, during his term in a pediatric hospital (Hôpital des Enfants-Malades), he wrote his thesis: *Etudes sur la névrite optique dans la méningite aigue de l'enfance* [Studies on neuritis of the optical nerves in acute meningitis of childhood].[2] Its most remarkable statement was that papilledema of infantile meningitis is caused by obstructive hydrocephalus and not by inflammation of the optic nerves, as had been supposed previously. The thesis drew the attention of Jean-Martin Charcot (1825–1893), who appointed Parinaud as ophthalmologist to the neurological clinic of the Salpêtrière. In the famous painting *Une leçon clinique à la Salpétrière* (1887), André Brouillet depicted Parinaud sitting in the first row between Raymond Vigouroux and Paul Berbez.

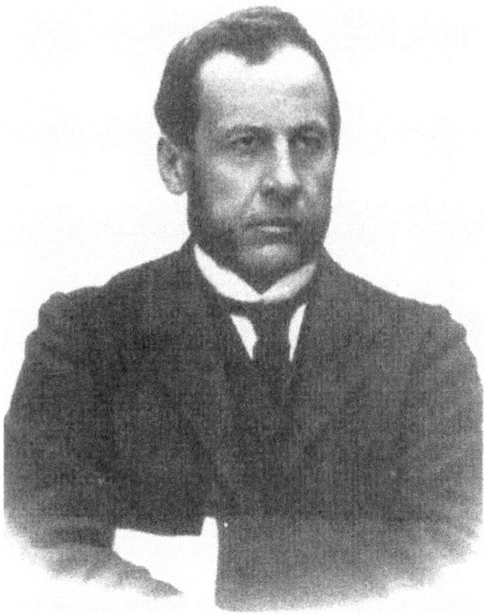

Figure 37–1. Henri Parinaud (1844–1905). Courtesy Bibliothèque Interuniversitaire de Médecine, Paris.

Seriously hindered by delicate health from his very youth, but with great perseverance, Parinaud wrote two more books and 77 articles, especially on disturbed binocular vision, hysteria and vision, strabismus as a neurological sign, nyctalopia, and color vision. Together with Pierre Marie (1853–1940), he described the syndrome that later was termed *migraine ophtalmoplégique* by Charcot. Moreover, he was active in ophthalmological and neurological scientific societies and did some research in these fields. In ophthalmology, his name is attached to *"Parinaud's conjunctivitis,"* a rare syndrome including conjunctivitis and enlargement of the parotid gland, and to "Parinaud's oculoglandular syndrome".[3] Notwithstanding his scientific achievements, Parinaud never held a chair or any other influential position, first because he lacked the ambition to compete for such a position, but his low birth could also have been an obstacle. As a consequence, it often took him great pains to convince the scientific world of the importance of his work.

Parinaud was a sincerely modest and philanthropic man. He gave expression to his philanthropy by supporting a free medical clinic for the poor people of Paris for many years. His modesty was even reflected in the way he furnished his house, as visitors noticed. In his scarce leisure hours, Parinaud was an enthusiastic composer of music, using his pseudonym of Pierre Erick. His music was published by Ricordi in Paris.

The death of his wife in the autumn of 1904 was more than he could bear; his health deteriorated and shortly after, on 23 March 1905, Henri Parinaud died from bronchopneumonia.

In 1883, Parinaud published his landmark article, "Paralysie des mouvements associés des yeux" [Paralysis of associated eye movements].[4] He rejected the prevailing concept of lesions of peripheral nerves or the nuclei of these nerves as the sole and adequate explanation of disturbed conjugated eye movements. Clinical practice taught him that this concept was not sufficient to understand the observed features of eye movements. Based on anatomical, physiological, and clinical observations, Parinaud supposed that central lesions could also cause disorders of eye movements:

> Dans l'étude des paralysies motrices de l'oeil, on semble admettre que la lésion est toujours périphérique . . . Mais, le plus souvent, la lésion est centrale.[4]

[In the study of motor paralysis of the eye one seems to assume that the lesion is always peripheral . . . But, more often, the lesion is central.]

To support this theory, he referred to the work of Foville, Millard and Gubler, Henoch, Wernicke, and Féréol. Achille Louis Foville (1799–1878) had published a paper of a case of facial paralysis and conjugate gaze palsy to the left and paresis on the right side 25 years earlier.[5] He postulated a center for conjugate eye movements to the left in the left pontine half, near the abducens nucleus. Foville referred to Edmé-Felix-Alfred Vulpian (1826–1887), who proposed an ascending tract in the contralateral pons to the oculomotor nucleus. Carl Wernicke (1848–1905) had demonstrated a patient suffering from a slowly progressive lesion in the pons and medulla oblongata, showing conjugate gaze preference to the right (and gaze palsy to the left) and peripheral facial paralysis on the left, without pyramidal involvement. At postmortem the lesion appeared to be due to tuberculosis. Meticulous localization was possible. As the oculomotor nucleus and nerve were intact, Wernicke reasoned that some other cause should result in the "paralysis" of the internal rectus muscle of the right eye. The abducens and facial nuclei were both destroyed. Only in this case a circumscribed lesion was present, while the oculomotor nucleus and nerve were demonstrated to be intact. The center, Wernicke reasoned, has to be present bilaterally, and is localized near the abducens nucleus.[6]

Summing up arguments in favor of the existence of central systems for the coordination of eye movements, Parinaud expressed his firm belief that the abducens nerve and the contralateral oculomotor nerve must have a connection in humans, as was demonstrated in cats in 1879, though he did not mention the medial longitudinal fasciculus.

Parinaud distinguished two classes of central disorders of eye movements: first, the so-called partial or dissociated paresis of both oculomotor nerves, which he did not discuss in the article, and second, the conjugated eye movement disorders, subdivided in disturbed horizontal and vertical movements, the group of the parallel movements, and on the other hand disorders of convergence and divergence, the nonparallel movements:

> Les mouvements associés des yeux sont de plusieurs espèces; ils sont parallèles ou non parallèles. Dans les mouvements parallèles, les yeux se déplacent dans le même sens, par rapport à l'axe du corps . . . Les mouvements non parallèles ont pour but de modifier les rapports des axes entre eux, de manière à produire leur rencontre sur des objets fixés à des distances différentes.[4]

[The associated eye movements are of many kinds; they are parallel or non-parallel. In the parallel movements the eyes move in the same direction in relation to the axis of the body . . . The aim of the non-parallel movements is to modify the relation of the (eye) axes to one another in such a way that they come together on fixed objects at different distances.]

Ten case histories were added to illustrate the clinical relevance of the presented classification. Parinaud described convergence disorders more extensively in a well-known article in *Brain:* " Paralysis of the Movements of Convergence of the Eyes".[7] Of the ten presented patients, "observation IV" and "observation V" are particularly interesting: a 67-year-old man could not look upward or downward except for a slight movement upward with the right eye, resulting in diplopia; and a 20-year-old woman was unable to look upward, becoming nauseated and complaining of headache when she tried to do so. Convergence was nil in both patients and, as mentioned, the pupils did not react to light. Horizontal eye movements were normal. Combining these observations with the description by Priestly Schmidt of a patient who could not look downward or make convergent eye movements, Parinaud presented a simple scheme to bring together these clinical findings. He considered three varieties of the same paralysis: (1) paralysis of downward movements, (2) paralysis of upward movements, and (3) paralysis of all vertical movements, all three in combination with convergence paralysis. Parinaud was rather reticent to localize the underlying lesion, referring to the lack of anatomical knowledge of his time.

Since the 1930s, the eponym "Parinaud syndrome" is accepted in the Anglo-Saxon literature to indicate the occurrence of vertical eye movement disorders—particularly for upward gaze—in combination with absent convergence, but many authors have criticized its use.[8–10] In their opinion, Parinaud was not sufficiently clear in his description of the syndrome (which cannot be denied, as he did not intend to establish a new syndrome), he was not the first one to report on these clinical signs (a point Parinaud immediately would agree upon), and he was not aware of the anatomical localization of the syndrome (which is not very different from the situation in many other eponyms). Moreover, Parinaud did not mention that vestibulo-ocular reflexes are intact, his description of the reaction of the pupils to light and convergence was wrong, and he did not provide information about lid retraction, Bell's phenomenon, or skew deviation. Without a definite description of the syndrome, its use in clinical practice is not unequivocal: some clinicians restrict its use to the extensive clinical syndrome, others use it in cases of paralysis of upward gaze only. Other names have been proposed, like pretectal syndrome, aquaduct syndrome, dorsal midbrain syndrome, and Koerber–Salus–Elschnig syndrome.[11] Nowadays, commissura posterior syndrome could be added to these alternatives for Parinaud's syndrome.

In spite of all these criticisms, right or wrong, and in spite of possibly more appropriate names, Parinaud's syndrome is not supplanted yet. It continues to pay tribute to an astute observer, a pioneer in the field of neuro-ophthalmology, but first of all to an exemplary colleague.

References

1. H. Parinaud (1844–1905). *Ann Ocul (Brux).* 1905;133:321–337. Obituary, with a summary of thesis and list of medical publications.

2. Parinaud H. *Etudes sur la névrite optique dans la méningite aigue de l'enfance.* Thèse de Paris, Faculté de Médicine, no. 19, 1877.
3. Parinaud H, Galezowski X. Conjonctivite infectieuse transmise par les animaux. *Ann Oculist (Brux).* 1889;101:252.
4. Parinaud H. Paralysie des movements associés des yeux. *Arch Neurol.* 1883;5:145–172.
5. Foville ALF. Note sur une paralysie peu connue des certains muscles de l'oeil et sa liaison avec quelques points de l'anatomie et la physiologie de la protubérance annulaire. *Bull Soc Anat.* 1858;33:393–405.
6. Wernicke C. Ein Fall von Ponserkrankung. *Arch Psychiatr (Berl).* 1877;7:513–538.
7. Parinaud H; Juler H, trans. Paralysis of the movements of convergence of the eyes. *Brain.* 1886;9:330–341.
8. Wilkins R H, Brody I A. Parinaud's syndrome. *Arch Neurol.* 1972;26:91.
9. Ouvrier R. Henri Parinaud and his syndrome. *Med J Austr.* 1993;158:711–714.
10. Keane J R. The pretectal syndrome: 206 patients. *Neurology.* 1990;40:684–690.
11. Leigh R J, Zee D S. *The Neurology of Eye Movements.* 2nd ed. Philadelphia: Davis, 1991.

38

WERNICKE'S APHASIA

Annelies J. E. Dalman and Paul Eling

Carl Wernicke was born on 15 May 1848 in Tarnowitz, Upper Silesia.[1,2] His father worked as a secretary of a mining company's main administration. Wernicke's childhood was not easy; there were constant worries about money and he suffered from poor health. He attended the Gymnasia in Oppeln and Breslau. Subsequently, he studied medicine at the University of Breslau and took the doctoral degree in 1870. He spent six months as assistant to the ophthalmologist R. F. Foerster (1825–1902), not to be confused with the neurologist and neurosurgeon Otfrid Foerster (1873–1941), one of Wernicke's students. During the Franco-German War of 1870–1871, he assisted a surgeon named Fischer on the battlefields. After the war he became a registrar at the All Saints Hospital in Breslau, where Heinrich Neumann acted as his superior.

In 1871 Wernicke joined Theodor Meynert (1833–1892) in Vienna to practice brain anatomy. He worked there for six months and held Meynert in great admiration for the rest of his life. Back in Breslau, Wernicke wrote *Der aphasische Symptomencomplex: Eine psychologische Studie auf anatomischer Basis* (1874).[3] It earned him a lectureship in 1875, and work as a registrar under Carl Westphal (1833–1890) in the psychiatric and neurological department of the Charité in Berlin from 1876 till 1878. His stay there came to an untimely end because of a personal conflict with the board of directors of the Charité. Up to 1885 he had to earn his living in a neuropsychiatric private practice and as *Privat-Dozent* without a clinical position.[2] These years without steady employment were difficult, but he found satisfaction in his scientific work and wrote his *Lehrbuch der Gehirnkrankheiten* (1881–1883), containing the description of the clinical syndrome of "polioencephalitis superior haemorrhagica," also known as "Wernicke's encephalopathy."

Wernicke was appointed extraordinary professor in Breslau in 1885, succeeding Heinrich Neumann. He became full professor of psychiatry and neurology in 1890 as well as head of department of the city's mental hospital. Consequently, he had the

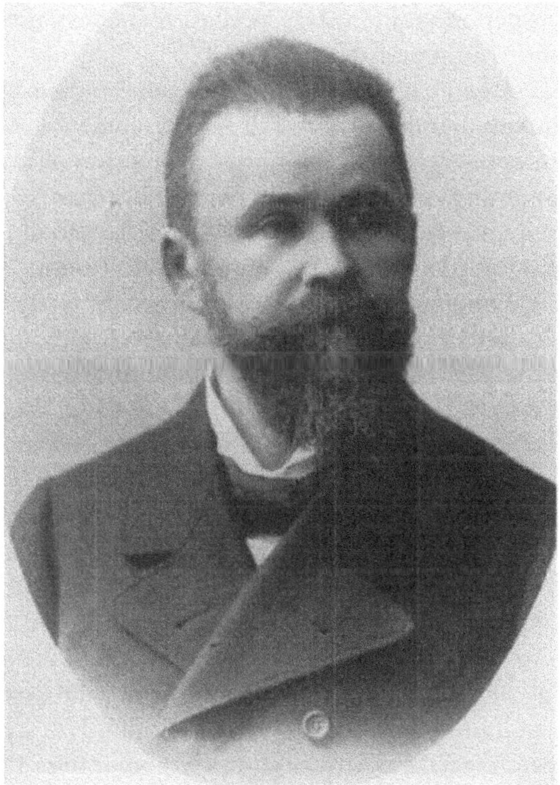

Figure 38–1. Carl Wernicke (1848–1905). Courtesy of Medizinhistorisches Institut, Zurich, Switzerland.

opportunity to observe many neurological and psychiatric patients. Wernicke wanted to create a new psychiatry based on the principle of localization, whose merit he had proved in the theory of brain diseases.[4] Hugo Liepmann (1863–1925) characterized Wernicke's psychiatry as follows: "The essence of his psychiatry is the attempt to conceive of the mental disorders as neurological phenomena." This has to be considered against the background of the German neuropsychiatry movement of the period and the well-known remark *"Geisteskrankheiten sind Nervenkrankheiten"* (mental diseases are brain diseases) of Wilhelm Griesinger (1817–1868), professor of psychiatry in Berlin from 1865 to 1868. Wernicke's ideas were laid down in his *Grundriss der Psychiatrie,* published in 1894. In this period, Wernicke influenced and inspired many students, and several achieved a good reputation in the field of neurology and psychiatry. Among these are distinguished men such as Hugo Liepmann, Heinrich Lissauer, Karl Heilbronner, Otfrid Foerster, Karl Kleist, and Kurt Goldstein. Wernicke's psychiatric views were soon ignored because of the increasing influence of Kraepelin's clinical approach.

The authorities of the city's mental hospital refused to fund a new building for the university psychiatric clinic, and this put Wernicke in an awkward position. The university authorities declined Wernicke access to the clinic and he was without a university affiliation for a year. This came to an end when he went to Halle in 1904. He worked as director of the psychiatric and neurological clinic in Halle for only a short period. In June 1905 he died, a few days after an accident during a bicycle tour in the Thüringer forest.

Presumably, Wernicke's personality played an important role in the conflicts mentioned above. According to Liepmann his resoluteness was the essence of his personality.[2] He would not hear of any compromise and pursued his aims unrelentingly and resolutely. If someone did not please him, he would show this and get into dispute. He could be merciless, which caused much animosity. He could be a warm and loyal friend as well as an implacable enemy.

Patients suffering from disorders of language as the result of brain lesions had been described several times before the nineteenth century, for example, by Schenck von Grafenberg (1530–1598) in 1558, Johann Jakob Wepfer (1620–1695) in 1727, Carl Linnaeus (1707–1778) in 1745, and by Johann Ludwig Buxtorf in 1758. Franz Joseph Gall (1758–1828) gave a new impetus to the search for a biological basis of psychological functions. He localized the language center in the supraorbital lobe. In general he determined the site of faculties by feeling "bumps" on the skull. Despite the fact that he produced a rather complete case description of an aphasic patient,[4] he showed no direct interest in such cases. Jean-Baptiste Bouillaud (1796–1881) popularized this method in France. In 1861 Pierre Paul Broca (1824–1880) described two cases with aphasia and claimed that the faculty of articulating words is localized in the inferior frontal gyrus (see Chapter 30). It appears that the notion of aphasia at that time primarily referred to problems of language production. Problems with comprehension were usually regarded as intellectual deficits (dementia) or disorders of memory, since words were stored in memory according to the classical psychological views.

The situation changed after Wernicke's study, *Der Aphasische Symptomenkomplex* (1874).[3] Wernicke argued that the aphasia described by Broca was only one form of aphasia, motor aphasia:

> Wenn nun schon a priori, nach der gegebenen Entwickelung des Sprachvorganges als einer spontanen Bewegung, die Annahme durchaus unwahrscheinlich war, dass die im Stirntheil des beschriebenen I. Windungsbogens gelegene Broca'sche Stelle das einzige Sprachcentrum sei, so führt die Berücksichtigung der beschriebenen anatomische Verhältnisse, der zahlreichen dafür sprechenden Sectionsbefunde, endlich der Verschiedenheit in dem klinischen Bilde der Aphasie in zwingender Weise zu folgender Auffassung des Sachverhaltes. Das ganze Gebiet der I., die Fossa Sylvii umkreisenden Windung im Verein mit der Inselrinde dient als Sprechzentrum; und zwar ist die I. Stirnwindung, weil motorisch, das Centrum der Bewegungsvorstellungen, die I. Schläfenwindung, weil sensorisch, das Centrum für die Klangbilder; die in der Inselrinde confluirenden Fibrae propriae bilden den vermittelnden psychischen Reflexbogen.[5(pp102–103)]

[In harmony with the preceding review, which considers speech development from the standpoint of conscious movement, a priori reasoning would view restriction of the speech center to a single area, namely Broca's gyrus, as highly improbable. A consideration of the anatomic structure as described above, the support of numerous necropsy findings, and finally, the variability in the clinical picture of aphasia, all strongly lead us to the following interpretation of the data. The entire region of the first primordial convolution, the gyrus surrounding the Sylvian fossa in association with the island cortex, serves as a speech center. The first frontal gyrus (Leuret), which is motor in function, acts as a center of motor imagery; the first temporal gyrus, which is sensory in nature, may be regarded as the center of acoustic images; the fibrae propriae, converging into the island cortex, form the mediating reflex arc.]

He attempted to apply Meynert's brain anatomy to normal language production and to aphasia. The book consists of three parts. First, Wernicke provides a general introduction on the psychological functions of the brain, as well as the localization of these functions in the cerebral cortex. In the second part, he applies this general theory to speech and language disorders, leading to a classification of several forms of aphasia. In the third part, he illustrates his theory with case histories and provides an elaborate account of a patient with sensory aphasia.

Wernicke shared Meynert's ideas that conduction pathways in the brain can be divided into projection and association systems. The *projection pathways* connect the sensory impressions and the musculature with specific sites of the cerebral cortex, the so-called projection fields. The cells of these projection fields undergo permanent change resulting from stimuli, resulting in mental images of sensory impressions and mental images of motor forms. The *association pathways* connect these mental images into a mosaic, and thus become the anatomical substrate for the conceptualization of ideas and thoughts.

Wernicke described the speech process, using the notion of the psychological reflex arc (Fig. 38–2). He applied Meynert's ideas to the psychophysics of speech: every word evokes an auditory and a motor image. A spoken word produces an *auditory perception* (in *a*). This induces an auditory image of the word and through association the meaning of the word is evoked. This becomes the *input representation* (in a_1). Through the representation chain, which represents the line of thought, the resulting *object representation* appears (in *b*). The object representation evokes the representations of *speech movements* (b_1). These are the so-called motor images, by which the object representation is expressed. Accordingly, there are two language centers in the human brain: the center for motor language, that is, the center for motor representations, and the

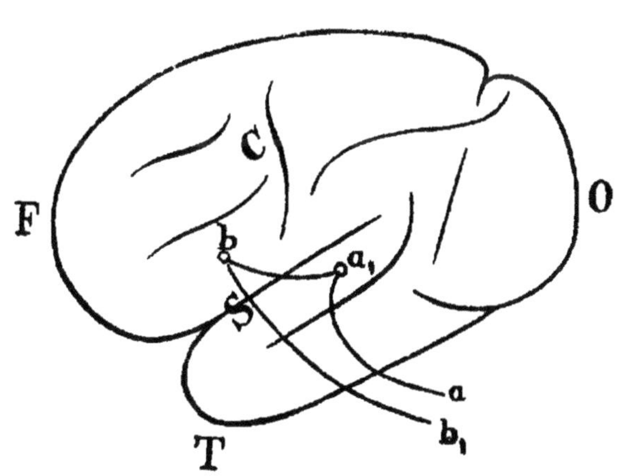

Figure 38–2. Psychological reflex arc applied for language and speech. From Ref. 3.

sensory language center, representing the center for auditory images. The site of the lesion within this reflex arc determines the clinical picture of aphasia. He demonstrated that a lesion of the superior temporal gyrus manifests itself clinically as sensory aphasia. Sensory aphasia may be interpreted as the loss of auditory images. Motor aphasia results from damage to the motor images. Wernicke also described a form of aphasia in which the sensory and motor images remain intact, but the connections between them are interrupted. This later became known as conduction aphasia *(Leitungsaphasie)*.

Ludwig Lichtheim (1845–1920) later deduced theoretically the existence of different forms of aphasia and substantiated them with clinical observations. He distinguished cortical aphasias (motor and sensory aphasia), subcortical aphasias (caused by interruption of projection systems of the speech center), and transcortical aphasias (caused by interruption of the association systems) and a new syndrome, which he refered to as "isolated speech deafness." Wernicke adopted Lichtheim's views in 1885 and provided a nomenclature for the whole range of aphasia syndromes, based on pathological-anatomical findings.[6]

Wernicke was not the first to describe the clinical picture of language comprehension problems. Henry-Charlton Bastian (1837–1915) argued in 1869 that there should be a disturbance in language comprehension, paralleling the speech production deficit of Broca. Adolf Baginsky (1843–1918) argued along the same lines in 1871, but both authors failed to supply autopsy evidence. It has been argued by Whitaker and Etlinger[7] that Meynert's case description of 1866 should be regarded as the first in which language comprehension disorders were correlated to anatomical and pathological findings. Eling,[8] however, demonstrated that Meynert, to the extent that he was interested in language at all, wrote about language production problems. As Wernicke claimed, he was the first to describe clinical cases of language comprehension problems and providing neuroanatomical support for the syndrome.

The symptoms have barely changed through the years. Wernicke's characteristic description—a rapid flow of voluble speech (logorrhea), paraphasias, lack of language comprehension, inability to repeat words, agraphia and alexia without hemiplegia—is still acknowledged today. In this sense, sensory aphasia is rightly referred to as "Wernicke aphasia." The classification of aphasia he developed in his monograph has undergone several changes through the years, but there are still some obvious similarities with the present classification. Nowadays, a distinction is often made between fluent and nonfluent aphasia. Within the nonfluent aphasias, Broca aphasia, mixed transcortical aphasia, transcortical motor aphasia, and global aphasia can be distinguished.[9] Fluent aphasia embraces Wernicke's aphasia, conduction aphasia, transcortical sensory aphasia, and anomic aphasia.

Wernicke's book has also been important for the development of theories concerning language representation in the brain. He not only provided new evidence for the localization of the aphasias, but also developed a theory that connected the phenomena with contemporary neurological knowledge.[10] This theory implied the existence of unknown syndromes. It was consistent with associationist psychology and contemporary neurophysiological reflex action theory. In his book *Neurolinguistics and Linguistic Aphasiology*, Caplan described Wernicke as a representative of the classical "connectionist" model.[11] The connectionist theories have played an important role in the development of theories on language representation in the brain.

For Wernicke, aphasia was particularly important for the development of his ideas on psychiatric disorders. The language model, based on the psychological reflex arc, served as the paradigm for all psychological processes, and thus for a theory of mental disorders. His pupils, Liepmann and Lissauer, for example, applied the model for describing and explaining apraxia and agnosia. Henry Head condemned them as "diagram makers" and the approach became less attractive in the first half of the twentieth century. Norman Geschwind revived the interest in Wernicke's methodological approach in the 1960s: the decomposition of a psychological function in terms of centers and connections. Since his seminal paper on disconnections in 1965, many new diagrams have been developed illustrating views of how the brain performs cognitive functions such as language, vision, and memory. It should be noted, however, that Wernicke probably took this approach from Baginsky[12] without giving him proper credit for it.

References

1. Kolle K. *Grosse Nervenaerzte, 2.* Stuttgart: Thieme; 1970.
2. Liepmann H. Carl Wernicke (1848–1905). In: Kirchhoff T, ed. *Deutsche Irrenaerzte, II.* Berlin: Springer; 1924.
3. Wernicke C. *Der aphasische Symptomencomplex; eine psychologische Studie auf Anatomischer Basis.* Breslau: Cohn & Weigert; 1874.
4. Dalman J. *Carl Wernicke en de localisatie van het herinneringsbeeld. Een wijsgerige analyse van het werk van de neuroloog/psychiater Carl Wernicke, scriptie filosofie/ Wetenschappelijke stage geneeskunde.* University of Nijmegen, 1989.
5. Eggert G. *Wernicke's Works on Aphasia.* The Hague: Mouton; 1977.
6. Wernicke C. Einige neuere Arbeiten über Aphasie, Kritisches Referat. In: Wernicke C. *Gesammelte Aufsätze und kritische Referate zur Pathologie des Nervensystems.* Berlin: Fischer's Medizinische Buchhandlung; 1893.
7. Whitaker H, Etlinger S. Theodor Meynert's contribution to classical 19th century aphasia studies. *Brain Lang.* 1993; 45:560–571.
8. Eling, P. Meynert on aphasia. Third annual meeting of the International Society for the History of the Neurosciences. Annapolis, Maryland, June 1998. Abstract in: *J Hist Neurosci.* 1999; 8.
9. Devinsky O. *Behavioral Neurology.* London: Arnold; 1992.
10. Geschwind N. *Selected Papers on Language and the Brain.* Boston: Riedel; 1974.
11. Caplan D. *Neurolinguistics and Linguistic Aphasiology: An Introduction.* Cambridge: Cambridge University Press; 1987.
12. Baginsky, A. Aphasie in folge schwerer Nierenerkrankungen-Uraemie. *Berl Klin Wochenschr.* 1871;8:428–431, 439–442.

39

WALLENBERG'S SYNDROME

Henry J. M. Barnett and Heather Meldrum

Wallenberg's name has been a household word in neurology for the last century. His observations were made close to the zenith of the hundredth anniversary of descriptive neurology's birth and epitomized the best skills of neurologists of this epoch. His careful honing of the art of history taking and neurological examination, knowledge of neuroanatomy, and resolute pursuit of bedside studies to the postmortem room were exemplary.

Adolf Wallenberg was born in Stargard (near Danzig, in Prussia, the present Gdansk in Poland) on 10 November 1862. His father was the district's physician, Samuel Wallenberg; his grandfather was a rabbi. Samuel died when Adolf was six years old. He and his three brothers received an academic education but were also given music lessons. Adolf learned to play the violin, which he practiced for many years. He formed a trio with his brother Georg (cello), who became a mathematician, and Theodor (piano), who became an ophthalmologist. He also played music with his friend Heinrich Lissauer, also from Danzig.

Wallenberg studied medicine in Heidelberg, where Wilhelm Erb was among his teachers, and in Leipzig, where he was a student of Adolf Strümpell and Carl Weigert. He wrote a dissertation on poliomyelitis. He moved back to Danzig, where he worked as a physician at the city hospital. After two years he started a private practice. Max Nonne wrote about him: "As a human being, Wallenberg was characterized by a rare modesty and he was unusually warmhearted and helpful."

In his spare time Wallenberg studied birds, bonefish, and mammals, because of interest in comparative neuroanatomy. In 1891 he suffered from a skull base fracture when the horse of his carriage bolted. Apart from diplopia, he suffered from loss of smell, and he believed his character became weaker and compulsive.

The publication in 1895 of a case history of a patient with the eponymous syndrome was an important turning point in his life. Victor von Weizsäcker commented:

Figure 39–1. Adolf Wallenberg at age 82, Illinois, 1944. Photograph Courtesy of Dr. Louis Caplan.

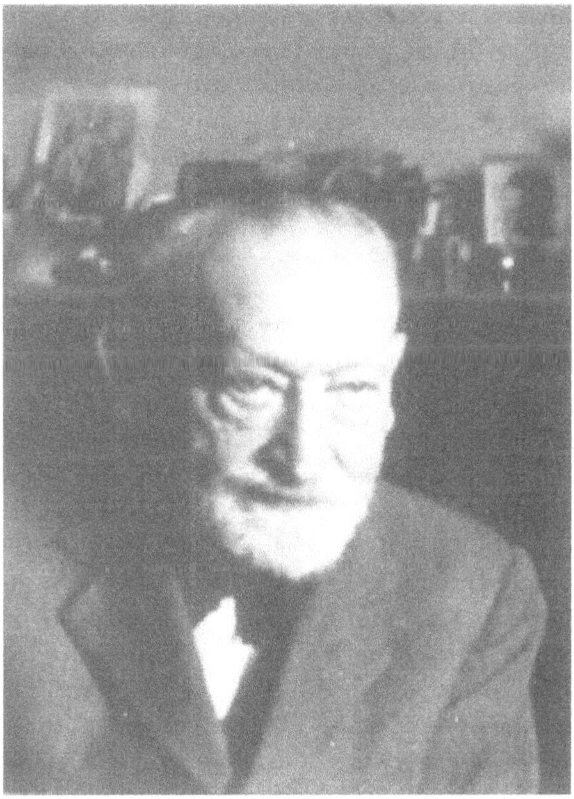

"Such mastery is only conferred on him who works with endless patience and renouncement, with a proud conscience." Ludwig Edinger corresponded with Wallenberg and they became lifelong friends. They also cooperated scientifically and published the biannual *Fortschritte in der Anatomie des Nervensystems,* as well as papers on comparative neuroanatomy. Edinger once said to Max Nonne: "Wallenberg is my anatomic conscience"

He was offered chairs several times, but preferred to stay in his native country. In 1907 he was appointed chief physician to the internal and psychiatric department of the city hospital. During World War I, he acted as adviser for the 17th Army. He received the Erb Commemorative Medal in 1929, "for his merits in the field of anatomy, physiology, and pathology of the nervous system." Between 1895 and 1915 he published 47 papers.

At the age of 66, he gave up his work as chief physician at the hospital. He was given a room in the basement to continue his scientific work. In 1938, the German occupation forced him to finish his career as a physician in Danzig. He moved to a gloomy house and his neuroanatomic collection was accommodated in the storerooms of a fur trader. The collection perished during the war. Wallenberg rejected many offers to flee to other countries as he remained reluctant to leave his native country. Only after prolonged insistence from his wife did they flee via Holland to Oxford, just two days before Hitler's invasion of Danzig. There he pursued clinical neurology and worked with the eminent neuroanatomist LeGros Clark. In 1943 he received a visa for the United States and accepted a residency at a state mental hospital near Chicago. He presented lectures for the asylum physicians. He also gave a lecture in Chicago, after which he became an honorary member of the Chicago Neurologic Society.

Wallenberg died from coronary heart disease in 1948, aged 86. His daughter, Marianne Wallenberg-Chermak, wrote a biographical essay, which formed the source of this biographical sketch.[1,2]

The earliest known description of the clinical syndrome of the lateral medulla is not Wallenberg's but came from an account given in 1810 to the Medical and Chirurgical Society of London. A Geneva physician, Gaspard Vieusseux, was persuaded to describe his dramatic symptoms, later recorded by the overseas secretary of this society.[3] Vertigo, unilateral facial numbness, loss of sensation and temperature appreciation in the opposite limbs, dysphagia and hoarseness, minor tongue involvement, hiccups ("cured by taking up the habit of a morning cigarette"), and a drooped eyelid were related to the meeting. It was described as "a peculiar nervous affliction, and that the brain was not originally affected as is the case in paralytic attacks." Despite this earlier account, Wallenberg deserves to have his name attached to the syndrome. He was the first to marry the clinical symptoms with accurate speculation about the localization of the lesion in a single case report. More important, six years later he proved his hypothesis at autopsy.

Wallenberg wrote four papers on the lateral medullary syndrome (LMS). The first publication (1895) described the clinical findings in the index patient. Based on the anatomical observations published by Duret in 1873,[4] Wallenberg proposed that the lesion was in the lateral medulla supplied by the posterior inferior cerebellar artery (PICA).[5] The second paper (1901) described the postmortem findings of the original patient, confirming an old infarction and stenosis at the origin of the PICA with total occlusion 2 cm distally (Fig. 39–2).[6] The third paper reported another single case[7] and after 27 years Wallenberg described the clinicopathologic correlations in his fifteenth patient.[8]

Wallenberg's "recapitulation" of the clinical picture of the first patient is worth repeating:

> A 38-year-old man, with poor vision caused by a preexisting ocular condition (cataract on the left side, corneal scarring and anterior synechia on the right side. . .) . . . suffered an attack of vertigo without loss of consciousness. At the same time he developed pain and hyperesthesia on the left side of the face and body, hypoesthesia of the right half of the face, and loss of pain and temperature sensitivity in the right extremities and the right half of the torso, with retention of the sense of touch. There was paralysis of swallowing; impaired sensation on the mucosa of the mouth, throat and palate; disturbed motility of the soft palate (on the first day bilateral, later left-sided); total paralysis of the left recurrent laryngeal nerve, and paresis of the left hypoglossal muscle . . . with no disturbance in the innervation of the facial muscles. He also had ataxia of the left extremities without impairment of gross strength, and he fell to the left side . . . The pulse became slower (from 96 to 76–82).

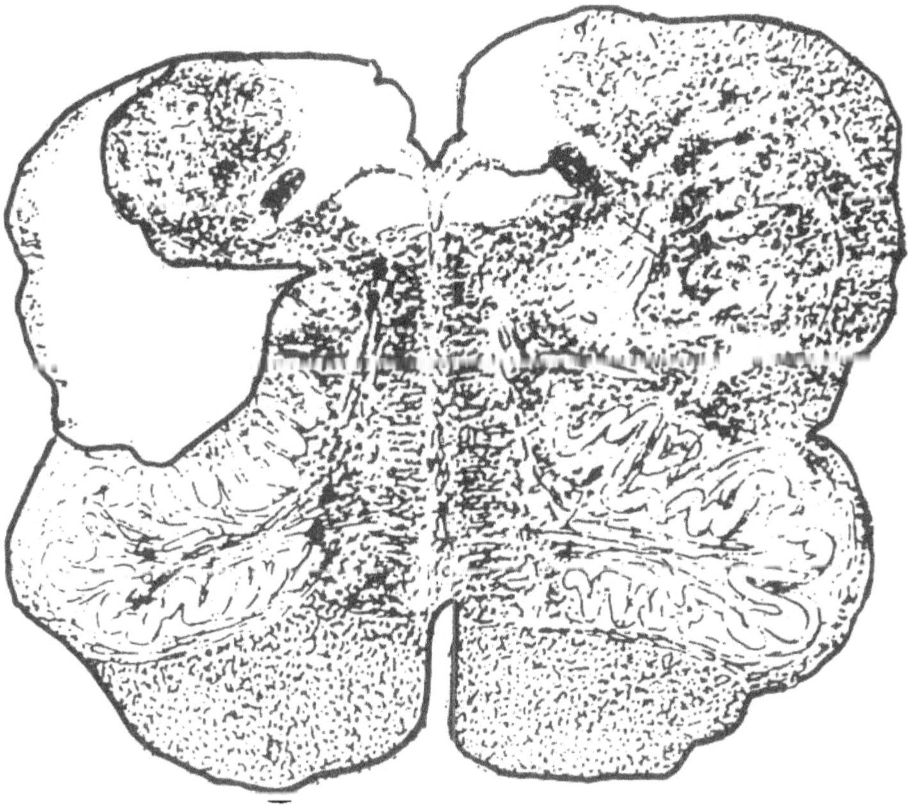

Figure 39–2. (a) Copy of the original drawing taken from the cross section of the medulla of Wallenberg's first patient. The white area represents the infarction in PICA territory. From L. Caplan, *Posterior Circulation Disease: Clinical Findings, Diagnosis, and Management.* Cambridge, Mass.: Blackwell Science, 1996, by permission of Louis Caplan.

During the ensuing days the sensitivity of the right half of the face returned to normal. The hyperesthesia of the left half of the body disappeared, and that of the left trigeminal region changed to anesthesia predominantly for pain and temperature (less for proprioceptive and electrocutaneous sensations), with suppression of the corneal and conjunctival reflexes . . . The pulse quickened again, but the other disturbances remained. On the eighth day an herpetic eruption appeared on some of the analgesic areas: the left face (including nasal mucosa; the sensitivity of the mouth and throat had returned), right shoulder, and right inguinal region . . .

Two to three months after the attack, the patient's status was as follows:

a. Subjective symptoms
   1. Vertigo and a sense of falling to the left.
   2. Numbness on the left half of the face and the right half of the body.
   3. Difficulty in swallowing (very slight).
   4. Pain in the nape of the neck and occasionally in the left eye.
b. Objective signs
   1. Unsteadiness of gait, with veering toward the left.
   2. Ataxia of the left extremities.
   3. Paresis of the left half of the soft palate.

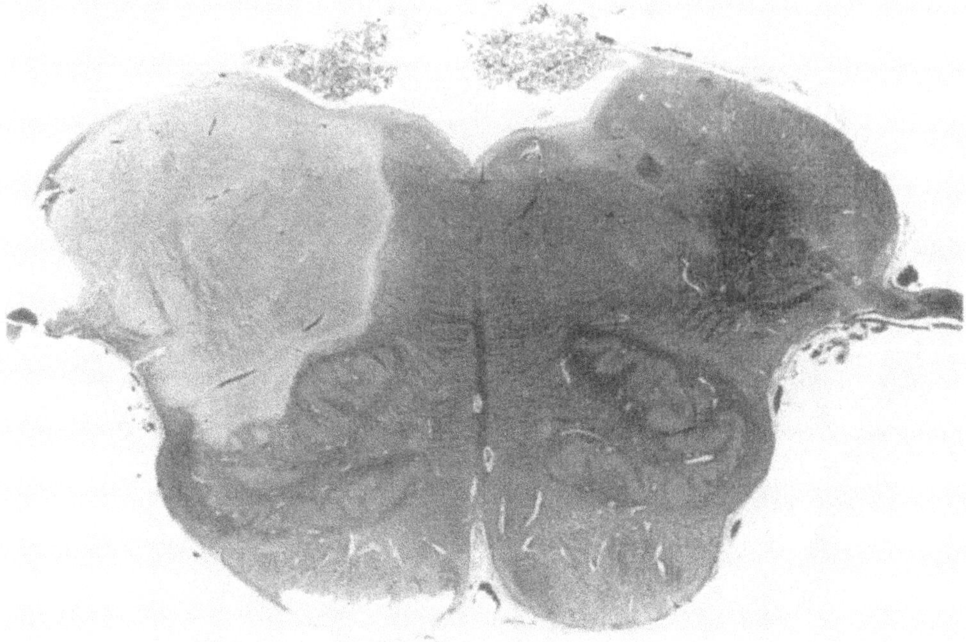

Figure 39–2. (Continued) (b) Cross section with hematoxylin and eosin stain of contemporary lateral medullary infarction with some area of involvement but with considerable ventral extension. Photograph courtesy of Dr. David Munoz.

4. Paralysis of the left vocal cord; followed by paresis, suggesting atrophy.
5. Greater volume of the left half of the tongue while resting in the mouth.
6. Disturbance of sensation in the first and to a lesser degree, in the second divisions of the left trigeminal nerve, especially affecting the eyes, eyelids, bridge of the nose and nasal mucosa . . . The impairment mainly affects pain and temperature, but localization, electrocutaneous and pressure sensations are also involved to some extent.
7. Absence of the left corneal and conjunctival reflexes.
8. Disturbance of pain and temperature sensitivity on the right side of the body . . .
9. Slight alteration of the other sensations (i.e., localization, faradocutaneous and pressure sensations) . . .

In the following weeks, the difficulty swallowing, the falling to the left, and the ataxia gradually disappeared. The other phenomena . . . remained unchanged.[9]

This description includes clinical features observed by modern neurologists, verified by magnetic resonance imaging. The Horner's syndrome was overlooked because the patient had a cataract in one eye and corneal scar in the other. The familiar diagram (Fig. 39–3) explains the main components of the symptoms and signs confirming the accuracy of Wallenberg's examination. Attention is directed to the sparing of the medial medullary components. Wallenberg noted the normality of limb strength and

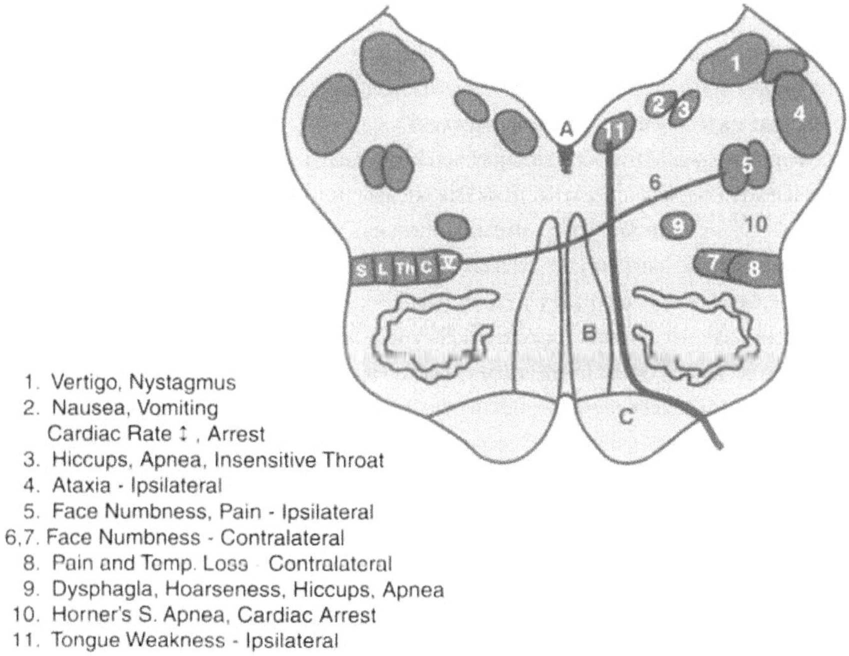

Figure 39–3. Sketch of medulla oblongata with numbered structures (1–11) involved in LMS and their clinical features: 1, vestibular nucleus; 2, DMNX; 3, nucleus solitarius; 4, restiform body; 5, nucleus and descending tract V; 6, 7, quintothalamic decussation and tract; 8, spinothalamic tract; 9, nucleus ambiguus; 10, rostral ventrolateral medulla; 11, 12th nerve; structures A, B, C generally not in PICA supply: A, medial longitudinal fasciculus; B, medial lemniscus; C, corticospinal tract.

the sparing of proprioception and touch. Some impairment of sensibility was noted on both sides of the face. We account for this bilaterality because of involvement of the descending trigeminal tract plus the decussating quintothalamic fibers carrying sensation from the other side of the face to join the spinothalamic tract.

Contributions to this syndrome since the days of Wallenberg fall into three areas. First, variations in the clinical picture have been described. Second, accurate imaging of the medulla, cerebellum, and the responsible arteries is feasible. Finally, we may soon be able to offer treatment for patients with brainstem infarction.

Several large studies detailing the prevalence of symptoms have emerged from experienced clinical centers.[10–16] Sacco's compilation from all the large reported series notes that in order of frequency the majority of patients experience ataxia, numbness, vertigo, dysphagia, nausea–emesis, headache, and dysarthria. Lesser degrees of involvement occur. Symptoms may be confined to minor ataxia, transient vertigo, a Horner's syndrome, and possibly a reduced corneal reflex. Other patients will have only minor unsteadiness, some vertigo, and minor hoarseness. Confirmation of the diagnosis of these subtle manifestations of ischemia relies on magnetic resonance imaging. Lesions confirmed by MRI may reflect more ischemia than infarction.[14,16]

Wallenberg's original autopsy specimen and many MR images depict quite a narrow lesion. Cephalad extension produced signs from the lower pons: partial lower motor neuron facial palsy or diplopia from involvement of the sixth nerve. More medial or ventral extensions are also observed.

Recovery from LMS is commonly striking and may be complete. Functional independence has been the rule for the majority of the survivors with long-term follow-up.[15,17,18] A number of potential causes of early mortality face patients with LMS: thromboembolism to the basilar artery and its branches;[13] myocardial infarction due to coexisting coronary artery disease; fatal nocturnal apnea from involvement of one of the areas concerned with expiratory control in the nucleus retroambiguus or of the inspiratory part of the nucleus solitarius;[15,19] sudden death from cardiac arrest either from involvement of the vagal input to the heart from the nucleus ambiguus or from involvement of the premotor area to all sympathetic output located in the rostral ventrolateral medulla;[20] pneumonia related to bulbar palsy and gastrointestinal hemorrhage. Some patients develop a "thalamic" or "central" type of pain in the appropriate trigeminal territory or in areas of the opposite limbs and trunk.

Imaging of posterior fossa structures has sharpened our understanding of Wallenberg's syndrome. Abnormalities are seen in MRI of more than 90% of patients and vary greatly in size and extent.[13,21] The arterial lesions of the LMS are identified as atherothrombotic, dissections, and less frequently due to cardioembolism.[14] In Wallenberg's original description he attributed the LMS to a presumed cardiac embolus to the PICA. In the postmortem examination cardiac enlargement was present but so too was extensive atherosclerosis of the vertebral and basilar arteries and within PICA.

Fisher, whose work on the carotid artery in the 1950s changed the usual focus of assignment of hemisphere strokes away from middle cerebral artery disease, challenged the concept that the LMS was usually a primary lesion of PICA. In his postmortem series of 16 patients who had experienced LMS, the vertebral artery was the site of occlusion in 12, PICA in 2, no obstruction in 2. Including 22 cases from the literature, his conclusion was that 75% of LMS resulted from occluded vertebral arteries.[12] A later series identified 66% of patients with lateral medullary infarcts as due to vertebral artery occlusion, only 6% to PICA occlusion.[15] Of 29 patients of a series with vertebral artery dissections following chiropractic manipulations, presented with LMS (John Norris, written personal communication August 7, 1999).

Spontaneous and traumatic dissections of the vertebral artery, with or without complete vertebral artery occlusion, were not identified in Wallenberg's day. In 1947 three young patients were described who died as a consequence of basilar and vertebral artery occlusions following chiropractic manipulation.[22] Today these occlusions would be attributed to vertebral artery dissections. In 1956 two more patients were described with symptoms following neck manipulation, one of whom had LMS,[23] probably the first description of the syndrome related to traumatic dissection. Fisher's 1961 postmortem series included an LMS after neck manipulation.[12] With increased use of angiography confirmations of many dissections have appeared.[24]

Lateral medullary syndrome has emerged as the most frequent single manifestation of vertebral artery dissection.

Until recently there was no therapy for individuals with brainstem infarction beyond general measures including risk factor management and antithrombotic agents. The introduction of tissue plasminogen activators (tPA) used intravenously or intra-arterially has raised hopes for an exciting new strategy.

Wallenberg described a distinct syndrome which helped open many doors. The combination of detailed neurological examination followed by careful postmortem study led to considerable understanding of functional brainstem anatomy. His original work remains unchallenged after 100 years. We remain in his debt.

Acknowledgments

We are indebted to Fern Livingstone and Cathy Wild for their careful attention to the preparation of this manuscript and to George Moogk for his very talented artistic contribution.

References

1. Wallenberg A. Beiträge zur vergleichenden Anatomie des Zentralnervensystems. With biographical notes from J. Gerlach. *J Hirnforsch.* 1964;7:275–300.
2. Wallenberg-Chermak M. Adolf Wallenberg (1862–1939). In: Kolle K, ed. *Grosse Nervenärzte.* Stuttgart: Thieme; 1963;3:190–196.
3. Marcet A. History of a singular nervous or paralytic affection attended with anomalous morbid sensations. *Medico-Chir Trans.* 1811;2:215–233.
4. Duret H. Sur la distribution des artères nourricières du bulbe rachidien. *Arch Physiol Normale.* 1873;5:97–114.
5. Wallenberg A. Akute Bulbäraffektion (Embolie der Arteria cerebelli post. inf. sin.?). *Arch Psychiatr.* 1895;27:504–540.
6. Wallenberg A. Anatomischer Befund in einen als "acute Bulbäraffection" (Embolie der Art. cerebellar post. sinistr.?) beschriebenen Falle. *Arch Psych Nervenkrankh.* 1901;34:923–959.
7. Wallenberg A. Verschluss der arteria cerebelli inferior posterior sinistra. *Neurol Zentralbl.* 1915;34:236–247.
8. Wallenberg A. Verschluss der arteria cerebelli inferior posterior dextra (mit sektionbefund). *Dtsch Z Nervenheilk.* 1922;73:189–212.
9. Wilkins R H, Brody I A. Wallenberg's syndrome. *Arch Neurol.* 1970;22:379–382.
10. Currier R D, DeJong R N. The lateral medullary (Wallenberg's) syndrome. *Univ Mich Med Bull.* 1962;28:106–113.
11. Peterman A F, Siekert R G. The lateral medullary (Wallenberg) syndrome: clinical features and prognosis. *Med Clin North Am.* 1960;44:887–896.
12. Fisher C M, Karnes W E, Kubik CS. Lateral medullary infarction: the pattern of vascular occlusion. *J Neuropath Exp Neurol.* 1961;20:323–379.
13. Caplan L R. *Posterior Circulation Vascular Disease: Clinical Findings, Diagnosis, and Management.* Boston: Blackwell; 1997.
14. Sacco R L, Freddo L, Bello J A, Odel J G, Onesti S T, Mohr J P. Wallenberg's lateral medullary syndrome: clinical-magnetic resonance imaging correlations. *Arch Neurol.* 1993;50:609–614.
15. Norrving B, Cronqvist S. Lateral medullary infarction: prognosis in an unselected series. *Neurology.* 1991;41:244–248.
16. Kim J S, Lee J H, Lee M C. Patterns of sensory dysfunction in lateral medullary infarction: clinical-MRI correlation. *Neurology.* 1997;49:1557–1563.
17. Nelles G, Contois K A, Valente S L, et al. Recovery following lateral medullary infarction. *Neurology.* 1998;50:1418–1422.

18. Graf K F, Pessin M S, DeWitt L D, Caplan L R. Proximal intracranial territory posterior circulation infarcts in the New England Journal Medical Center posterior circulation registry. *Eur Neurol.* 1997;37:157–168.
19. Bogousslavsky J, Khurana R, Deruaz J R, et al. Respiratory failure and unilateral caudal brainstem infarction. *Ann Neurol.* 1990;28:668–673.
20. Loewy A D, Spyer K M. *Central Regulation of Autonomic Functions.* New York: Oxford University Press; 1990.
21. Kim J S, Lee J H, Choi CG. Patterns of lateral medullary infarction: vascular lesion-magnetic resonance imaging correlation of 34 cases. *Stroke.* 1998;29:645–652.
22. Pratt-Thomas H R, Berger K E. Cerebellar and spinal injuries after chiropractic manipulation. *JAMA.* 1947;133:600–603.
23. Ford F R, Clark D. Thrombosis of the basilar artery with softenings in the cerebellum and brain stem due to manipulation of the neck: a report of two cases with one post-mortem examination. Reasons are given to prove that damage to the vertebral arteries is responsible. *Bull Johns Hopkins Hosp.* 1956;98:37–42.
24. Fisher C M, Ojemann R G, Roberson G H. Spontaneous dissection of cervico-cerebral arteries. *Can J Neurol Sci.* 1978;5:9–19.

V

Diseases and Defects

40

ALZHEIMER'S DISEASE

Nicolaas J. M. Arts

Alzheimer's disease is one of the most widely known eponymous diseases. Nevertheless, its status as a nosological entity has always been uncertain.[1–4] Alois Alzheimer himself was the first to doubt the validity of the concept of "Alzheimer's disease,"[5] and a clear-cut definition is still beyond reach. These problems have even led to allegations that the patients described by Alzheimer may have been suffering from some other disease. However, German scientists[6] have recently retrieved the original brain samples from Auguste D., the patient in Alzheimer's original paper,[7] and Johann F., the second patient he described.[5] A fresh look at these samples confirmed that both brains displayed the classic signs of Alzheimer's disease.

Alois Alzheimer was born on 14 June 1864 in Marktbreit, a small town near Würzburg, where his father was a notary.[8–10] He had four brothers. After his secondary school education in the district capital, Aschaffenburg, he studied medicine in Berlin, Würzburg, and Tübingen. He completed his studies in 1887 and qualified as a doctor a year later. For a short period he conducted research at Albert Köllikers histological laboratory in Würzburg. From 1888 until 1895 Alzheimer worked as an assistant medical officer; from 1895 until 1902 he worked as a senior medical officer at the municipal mental asylum in Frankfurt-am-Main. Emil Sioli (1852–1922) had become the director a year earlier. Shortly after Alzheimer, Franz Nissl (1860–1919) accepted a post as assistant in Frankfurt. They were ideal partners for scientific research and became close friends. Alzheimer took on the postmortems and analyzed the histopathological findings of the patients, while Nissl was more interested in experiments and in the methodological aspects of neuropathology; he developed several new methods for fixing and staining microscopic preparations of the nervous system. Between 1891 and 1895, Alzheimer published his first papers on progressive paralysis and on cerebral arteriosclerosis. These disorders held his interest for the rest of his life.

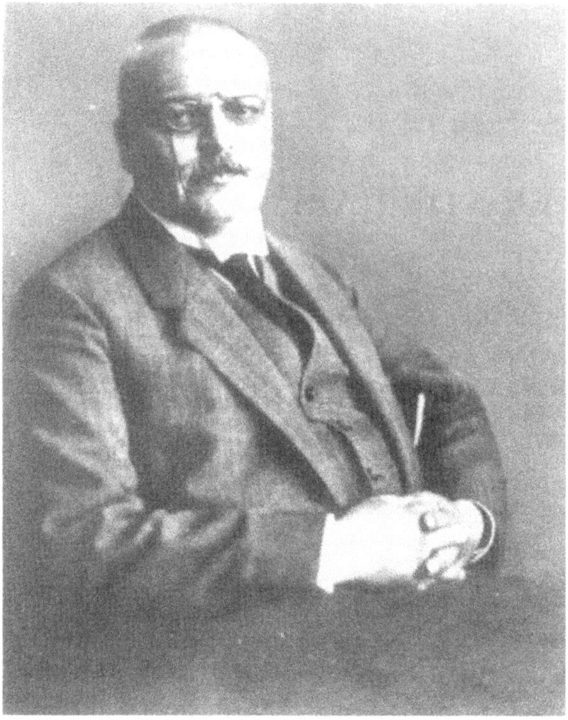

Figure 40–1. Alois Alzheimer (1864–1915). From K. Kolle, ed., *Grosse Nervenaerzte.* Stuttgart: Thieme Verlag, 1970, pp. 32–38; Permission of Thieme Verlag, Stuttgart, Germany.

In 1894, Alzheimer received a telegram from his colleague and close friend Wilhelm Erb (1840–1920). He was accompanying Otto Geisenheimer, one of the directors of Hoechst Chemical–Pharmaceutical Industries, on a scientific expedition in northern Africa. Geisenheimer was suffering from progressive paralysis and became very ill in Algeria. Because Alzheimer had become a generally recognized expert on this disease, Erb asked him to come to Africa. Although he could not save Geisenheimer, he proved to be more than a source of comfort to the widow, Cecile Geisenheimer-Wallerstein, who, within weeks after her husband's death, asked Alzheimer to marry her. They married in April 1894 and had two daughters and a son.

Nissl left the Frankfurt asylum in 1895, because Emil Kraepelin (1856–1926) had offered him a position in Heidelberg. Alzheimer followed in 1902. For a short time the friends were reunited. However, when Kraepelin moved to Munich in 1903, Nissl remained in Heidelberg and became director there, whereas Alzheimer followed Kraepelin and became head of the neuroanatomical laboratory at his clinic.

In Munich, Kraepelin was closely involved in the planning and building of the new psychiatric clinic. He emphasized the importance of a continuous flow of new patients toward the university clinic to ensure sufficient new cases, and the possibility of referring chronic cases to asylums, where they could remain permanently. Records were kept on each individual patient, including an admission diagnosis and reports of the observations made during the subsequent stay. Owing to his good contact with the asylums in the region, Kraepelin was able to obtain data on a large number of the patients while in his clinic as well as the autopsy findings.

Kraepelin's well-thought-out system of psychiatric care was—in hindsight—a major foundation for the flowering period of German neuropathology and psychiatry. The other prerequisite was the high level of histological and neuropathological research in Germany, which was made possible by the development of the apochromatic microscope by Zeiss and the development of new staining and dyeing methods by the large and prosperous German chemical industries.

In short, the facilities offered to Alzheimer were unique and could not be found elsewhere in the world at that time. As a result, his laboratory had an enormous impact on the development of neuropathological research in psychiatry. Alzheimer was the first to reliably describe the histological alterations in Alzheimer's disease, Pick's disease, Binswanger's disease, Huntington's chorea, and metachromatic leucodystrophy. Friederich Lewy (1885–1950) discovered Lewy bodies while working in Alzheimer's laboratory; and both Hans Creutzfeldt (1885–1964) and Alfons Jakob (1884–1931) had been trained as neuropathologists by Alzheimer (see Chapter 43).

Cecile Alzheimer died from an infection in 1901. As a result of his marriage with the wealthy Cecile, Alzheimer had gained considerable financial independence. This enabled him to work at his Munich laboratory from 1903 until 1912 without ever receiving a salary. After the death of his wife, he had an uneventful life. He lived close to his laboratory and never went on vacation because he did not want to delay his scientific work. According to Kraepelin, he was interested only in nature and natural sciences, had no understanding of music or the arts, and disapproved of politics. He preferred a homelike, steady, and consistent way of life, and carefully avoided any change, either in his personal life or in his scientific work. Although he spent little time with his children, he seems to have been a warm and loving father, always willing to support them.

In 1908 the University of Munich offered Alzheimer an assistant professorship. He had become a universally esteemed researcher and a popular teacher. His laboratory attracted a large number of pupils from all over the world. Nevertheless, he wanted to have his own clinic. In 1912, he was appointed full professor and director of the psychiatric hospital in Breslau. Kraepelin suspected that the abilities he had to offer our science would be lost in such a position, but he deferred to Alzheimer's decision. Unfortunately, Alzheimer became ill with infectious tonsillitis, accompanied by nephritis and arthritis. He never fully recovered and died of rheumatic endocarditis and uremia in Breslau on 19 December 1915, at the age of 51 years.

In November 1901, Alzheimer examined a 51-year-old woman who had been admitted to the psychiatric hospital in Frankfurt. She presented with an "unusual" picture of neuropsychological disturbances and behavioral problems. When she died in 1906, Sioli sent her brain to Alzheimer, who in the meantime had moved to Munich. Alzheimer discovered unusual histological changes in her brain and presented his findings at a conference for psychiatrists in Tübingen in November 1906. An abstract of this report was published in 1907:

> A. reports on a patient observed in the insane asylum in Frankfurt am Main, whose central nervous system had been sent to him for investigation by Director Sioli. Clinically the patient presented such an unusual picture that the case could not be

categorized under any of the known diseases. Anatomically the findings were different from all other known disease processes.

A woman, 51 years old, showed jealousy toward her husband as the first noticeable sign of the disease. Soon a rapidly increasing loss of memory was noticed. She could not find her way around in her own apartment. She carried objects back and forth and hid them. At times she would think that someone wanted to kill her and she would begin to shriek loudly.

In the institution her behaviour bore the stamp of utter perplexity . . . Periodically she was totally delirious, dragged her bedding around, called her husband and her daughter, and seemed to have auditory hallucinations . . . During her subsequent course, the phenomena that were interpreted as focal symptoms were at times less noticeable. But they were only slight. The generalized dementia progressed however . . .

After 4½ years of the disease death occurred. At the end, the patient was completely stuperous; she lay in her bed with her legs drawn up under her . . .

The autopsy revealed a generally atrophic brain without macroscopic lesions. The large brain vessels were altered by arteriosclerosis.[7, p.109–110]

In the brain of this woman, Alzheimer found "peculiar changes of the neurofibrils . . . [which] are eventually seen clustering together in thick bundles which emerge at the surface of the cell" and "miliary foci distinguishable by the deposit in the cerebral cortex of a peculiar substance which can be recognized without stain and is, in fact, very refractory to staining." Later these changes were called "neurofibrillary tangles" and "amyloid plaques."

Alzheimer did not claim that he had found a new disease. All he had wanted to do was to emphasize the variety of as yet unknown neuropathological processes. He also wished to point out the potential of modern histological techniques for psychiatry. To him, the case of Auguste D. represented just one of the numerous forms of "atypical" senile dementia.

A year after Alzheimer's report, his Italian co-worker Francesco Bonfiglio (1883–1966) described a second patient,[11] and two years later another Italian co-worker, Gaetano Perusini (1879–1915), published a long paper in which he redescribed the patients of Alzheimer and Bonfiglio and added two new cases.[12] Like Alzheimer, these co-workers believed that they had described a special form of senile dementia.

Kraepelin introduced the eponymic term "Alzheimer's disease" in the eighth edition of his textbook on psychiatry (1910).[13] Only the cases of Alzheimer and Bonfiglio had actually been published, but Kraepelin also knew of the two new cases that Perusini was about to publish. Alzheimer did not agree with Kraepelin's proclamation of "Alzheimer's disease." In 1911, he presented a case that did not show any neurofibrillary tangles, and he interpreted the plaques as phenomena of secondary importance. He also noticed that the changes could be slight, even in patients with severe disturbances.[5]

Kraepelin's statement that Alzheimer's disease was a disease *sui generis* seems peculiar. Why did he deviate from Alzheimer's opinion? He probably relied on two arguments: the age of the patients and the peculiar clinical picture, with severe dementia, restlessness, and a number of focal signs, such as language disturbances, "fits," and spastic movements.

Several modern authors have suggested that Kraepelin had other reasons for the statement of this disease as an entity. Some have argued that he intended to show the superiority of his own school over that of Pick's neuropathological laboratory in Prague or over Freud's psychoanalytical theories. Others have contended that he wanted to reward his loyal and selfless co-worker by naming a disease after him. However, the arguments to support these hypotheses are far from convincing.[4,14]

The new eponym "Alzheimer's disease" was generally accepted in neuropsychiatric literature, but Kraepelin's claim that it was a disease *sui generis* was contested promptly. A controversy started that was to last until the 1980s. It focused on two questions.[1,2] First, is Alzheimer's disease identical to—or a variant of—senile dementia, or is it a disease *sui generis*? Second, is senile dementia a disease or is it the result of aging? As early as 1911, Simchowicz argued that there was no essential difference between senile dementia and aging.[15]

Between 1920 and 1960, few researchers showed interest in Alzheimer's disease. Most research efforts were focused on the plaques and the neurofibrillary tangles.[16] Specifically, researchers sought to understand the relevance of these features in Alzheimer's disease and senile dementia, as well as their pathological significance. It rapidly turned out that plaques and tangles were not specific to Alzheimer's disease. Moreover, some cases with presenile and senile dementia were not found to have any signs of either plaques or tangles. In the 1930s, it became clear that the majority of all nondemented individuals over the age of 65 years had some senile plaques and tangles. In 1962, Corsellis recognized the identity of "Alzheimer's disease" at a presenile age, and "senile dementia."[17]

Neither the source nor the significance of the plaques could be clarified in this period, but research into the tangles fared somewhat better and seemed to confirm what Alzheimer and others had long suspected: that these tangles were probably normal cytoskeletal elements that had developed an abnormal, twisted structure, and were undoubtedly interfering with the proper functioning of the neuron and ultimately led to its death. In 1963, Kidd described the ultrastructure of the tangles with electron microscopy.[18]

The meager correlation of clinical with neuropathological phenomena, and the impossibility of distinguishing Alzheimer's disease from senile dementia on neuropathological grounds, led some researchers to the conclusion that plaques and tangles were of minimal diagnostic value and that the diagnosis had to rely on clinical criteria. However, to distinguish Alzheimer's disease and senile dementia reliably on clinical grounds proved to be impossible as well. Contrary to what Kraepelin had asserted, neither restlessness nor focal symptoms were unique to Alzheimer's disease.

In the 1970s it became evident that the Kraepelinian approach had to be discarded. All attempts to formulate clinical and neuropathological criteria to delineate Alzheimer's disease as a unique disease entity, separate from senile dementia, had failed. The only tangible distinction which remained was age. In 1978, as a consequence of these insights, the clinical distinction between Alzheimer's disease and senile dementia was dismissed completely. Instead the terms "senile dementia of the Alzheimer's type (SDAT)" for patients older than 65 and "Alzheimer's disease" for patients younger than 65 were recommended.[19] Kraepelin's naturalistic conception of Alzheimer's disease as a separate disease entity was replaced by a syndrome concept. However, the discovery of a selective loss of central cholinergic neurons in Alzheimer's disease by Davies and Maloney[20] in 1976 favored the development of a new disease concept based on the hypothesis that Alzheimer's disease is a disorder of cortical cholinergic innervation.

In the 1980s, public interest in Alzheimer's disease grew quickly.[21] Government officials in many countries recognized that as the number of elderly was rapidly increasing, the incidence of dementia would also increase, creating a need for massive additional resources. The research efforts expanded accordingly.

Since then, inflammatory mechanisms, oxidative damage, and inappropriate apoptosis have been identified as factors contributing to the pathogenesis of Alzheimer's disease. Neuropathologists showed that the neuropathological alterations, especially the tangles, occur first in highly characteristic locations, specifically in the entorhinal and perirhinal cortex, parts of the hippocampus, and the amygdala. They also occur frequently in the nucleus basalis of Meynert, the temporal isocortex, and the dentate gyrus. Neuronal loss, decreased synapse density, and the intra- and extracellular deposition of abnormal proteins constitute the histological hallmark lesions.

The intraneural accumulation of the microtubule-associated protein tau in a hyperphosphorylated state has been identified as the cause of the formation of neurofibrillary tangles. As a result, the normal cytoskeleton is disrupted and synapses and neurons are lost. The widespread distribution of these lesions in the neocortex correlates with the patient's cognitive decline. A similar correlation could not be found for the extracellular beta protein–loaded senile plaques, but nevertheless there is a consensus that amyloid beta-protein contributes to the characteristic neurodegeneration.

It has also become evident that the clinical and histopathological phenotypes of the disease are caused by heterogeneous genetic and probably also by environmental factors. Although the majority of the cases are late in onset, lack an obvious genetic etiology, and are characterized as sporadic, a small percentage is early in onset and seems to have a genetic etiology. In 1993, Saunders et al. reported the strong association between apolipoprotein E genotypes and sporadic and late-onset familial forms of Alzheimer's disease.[22] Subsequently, three genes have been identified that together appear to cause most of the early onset familial forms of the disease.

The neuropathological diagnosis of Alzheimer's disease still rests on semiquantitative and not on qualitative criteria, because the disease is heterogeneous, there are no specific markers, and the neuropathology overlaps the morphology in nondemented elderly individuals.

The antemortem diagnosis still relies on a clinical diagnosis of dementia in combination with the exclusion of all causes of dementia other than Alzheimer's disease. Nowadays, in specialized centers, the antemortem diagnosis of Alzheimer's disease is confirmed neuropathologically in 80%–90% of the cases, as a result of the refinement of clinical diagnostic criteria. Research on antemortem biomarkers for Alzheimer's disease has yielded the first results.

The identification of extensive disruption of cholinergic input to the forebrain in Alzheimer's disease has led to the development of anticholinesterase drugs that have proved to be of modest benefit.

In conclusion, while the abundant new data are pieces of a puzzle that is still difficult to put together and the exact pathogenesis of Alzheimer's disease remains elusive, while the clinical and neuropathological diagnoses remain problematical, and while a rational therapy remains a remote prospect, progress has definitely been made since the 1980s in identifying possible pathogenic mechanisms and promising therapeutic approaches.

References

1. Dillmann RJM. *Alzheimer's Disease: The Concept of Disease and the Construction of Medical Knowledge.* Amsterdam, 1990. Thesis (Free University).
2. Dillmann RJM. Alzheimer's disease: epistemological lessons from history? In: Whitehouse P J. Maurer K. Concepts of Alzheimer Disease. Baltimore: Johns Hopkins University Press; 2000.
3. Bick K L, Amaducci L A, Pepeu G. *The Early Story of Alzheimer's Disease.* Padova: Liviana, 1987.
4. Arts NJM, ed. Das schwindende Hirn: *Alzheimer und die Anfänge der Demenzforschung.* Nijmegen: Sylvius, 2000.
5. Alzheimer A. Über eigenartige Krankheitsfälle des späteren Alters. *Z Ges Neurol Psychiatr.* 1911;4:34–57. Reprinted in: Arts.[4] Translated in: *Hist Psychiatry.* 1991;2:71–101.
6. Graeber M B. No man alone: the rediscovery of Alois Alzheimer's original cases. *Brain Pathol.* 1999;9:237–240.
7. Alzheimer A. Über eine eigenartige Erkrankung der Hirnrinde. *Allgem Z Psychiatr Ger Med.* 1907;64:146–148. Reprinted in: Arts.[4] Translated in: Bick;[3] also in: Wilkins R H, Brody I A. Alzheimer's Disease *Arch Neurol.* 1969;21:109–111.
8. Hoff P. Alzheimer and his time. In: Berrios G E, Freeman H L. *Alzheimer and the Dementias.* London: Royal Society of Medicine; 1991.
9. Weber M M. Aloys Alzheimer, a coworker of Emil Kraepelin. *J Psychiat Res.* 1997;31: 635–643.
10. Maurer K, Maurer U. *Alzheimer: Das Leben eines Arztes und die Karriere einer Krankheit.* München: Piper; 1998.
11. Bonfiglio F. Di speciali reperti in un caso di probabile silfilide cerebrale. *Riv Sperim Freniat.* 1908;34:196–206. Translated in: Bick.[3]
12. Perusini G. Über klinische und histologisch eigenartigen, psychischen Erkrankungen des späteren Lebensalters. *Histologische und histopathologische Arbeiten über die Grosshirnrinde.* 1911;3:297–358. Reprinted in: Arts.[4] Translated in: Bick.[3]
13. Kraepelin E. *Psychiatrie.* 8th ed, vol 2, pt 1. Leipzig: Barth; 1910.
14. Berrios G E. Alzheimer's disease: a conceptual history. *Int J Geriatr Psychiatry.* 1990;5: 355–365.
15. Simchowicz T. Histologische Studien über die senile Demenz. Histol histopathol Arb Grosshirn. 1911;4:267–444.
16. Berchtold N C, Cotman C W. Evolution in the conceptualization of dementia and Alzheimer's disease: Greco-Roman period to the 1960s. *Neurobiol Aging.* 1998;19:173–189.
17. Corsellis JAN. *Mental Illness and the Aging Brain.* London: Oxford University Press; 1962.
18. Kidd M. Paired helical filaments in electron microscopy in Alzheimer's disease. *Nature.* 1963;197:192–193.
19. Katzman R, Terry R D, Bick K L. Recommendations on the nosology, epidemiology, and etiology and pathophysiology of the workshop-conference on Alzheimer's disease, senile

dementia and related disorders. In: Katzman R, Terry R D. *Alzheimer's Disease.* New York: Raven Press; 1978.

20. Davies P, Maloney AJF. Selective loss of central cholinergic neurons in Alzheimer's disease. *Lancet.* 1976; ii:1403.
21. Rabins PV. Science and medicine in the spotlight: Alzheimer's disease as an example. *Perspect Biol Med.* 1988;31:161–170.
22. Saunders AM, Strittmatter WJ, Schmechel D. Association of apolipoprotein E allele epsilon4 with late-onset familial and sporadic Alzheimer's disease. *Neurology.* 1993;43:1467–1472.

41

CHARCOT'S DISEASE: AMYOTROPHIC LATERAL SCLEROSIS

Christopher G. Goetz

Primary amyotrophy, primary lateral sclerosis, amyotrophic lateral sclerosis (ALS), and the concept of motor neuron disease are of significant input in contemporary neurology. They have been widely discussed in the United States under the rubric "Lou Gehrig's disease," after the famous baseball hero who succumbed to the condition. Most commonly, ALS is referred to as Charcot's disease, in recognition of Jean-Martin Charcot's major nosographic contributions and his recognition of the two distinct lesions seen in the disease. These observations set the foundation for the understanding of the organization of the normal motor system and represent in its most complete form the fruit of Charcot's anatomoclinical technique in neurology.

In the history of neurology, few leaders have had the scientific and personal impact of Jean-Martin Charcot.[1] Born in Paris in 1825, the son of a carriage maker, he studied medicine after wavering between careers in art and science; he received his medical degree in 1853, and spent part of his internship at the Salpêtrière, where he would return as a faculty member in 1862 and remain for the rest of his career. In 1872, he received the post of professor of pathologic anatomy; in 1882, a new chair was specifically created for him, professor of diseases of the nervous system, the first neurologic professorship in Europe. He died unexpectedly during his summer vacation in 1893 during a trip in rural France with his students. Charcot left behind him the first school of neurology, a younger generation of international students devoted to neuroscience, and a framework for thinking about the nervous system both clinically and anatomically. This heritage persists in contemporary neurology.

Charcot's work can be divided into three large categories: general medicine,[2,3] diseases of the brain and spinal cord,[4,5] and hysteria/hypnotism.[6] Curiously, the last is often remembered more than the other two, although Charcot's long-term contributions to general medicine and neurology remain incontestably more important than his psychiatric work. In regard to general medicine, he studied rheumatism and gout, endocarditis, tuberculosis, syphilis, and pneumonia as well as diseases of the liver and kidneys. These subjects occupied his early career, and because the Salpêtrière was largely a nursing home for elderly destitute women, he was exposed to the gamut of diseases affecting the geriatric population.[2]

In the realm of clinical and neuroanatomical neurology, Charcot's contributions are numerous. He differentiated the clinical picture of multiple sclerosis from Parkinson's disease, two conditions predominated by tremor and heretofore confused;[7,8] he differentiated epilepsy from pseudoepilepsy;[6] he graphically described the trophic changes that occur in spinal and cerebral diseases; he extensively studied and defined the lesions of numerous spinal cord and cortical/subcortical syndromes; with his students, he studied tic disorders (Gilles de la Tourette's syndrome), hereditary neuropathies, miliary aneurysms and cerebral hemorrhage, aphasia and tabetic syndromes.[1] In his later works with hysteria, he established the important point that the disease affects both men and women, although perhaps with different specific presentations.

Charcot was a dominant figure, difficult to work with, highly authoritarian, and intolerant of views different from his own.[1,9] He was a friend to such writers as Victor Hugo and Alphonse Daudet, and a close associate of political figures such as Léon-Michel Gambetta. He was physician to many of the royal families, and a social, political, and scientific figure of his time.

His talents covered areas beyond medicine: he was an accomplished sketcher and ceramist, and he understood and read numerous languages. His marriage to a wealthy widow and his successful career provided a sumptuous life with an exquisite mansion in central Paris and a villa in the nearby country village of Neuilly. His power, however, probably alienated many of the people who survived him, and as a consequence, many of the elements of his heritage have survived poorly.[10] The Charcot Museum has disappeared, and the Bibliothèque Charcot houses only a fraction of his manuscripts, notes, and scientific book collection. Thanks largely to the efforts of D. M. Bourneville (1840–1909), Charcot's primary lectures were published worldwide in several languages during Charcot's lifetime and have remained part of standard reading for contemporary neurologists.[3–8] Wide availability of his texts and lessons permit students to appreciate the many contributions made by Charcot and the important role he has played in the evolution of neurology as it is practiced more than a century after his death.

At the centenary celebration of Charcot's birth in 1925, Pierre Marie cited the words of one of Charcot's students (possibly Marie himself) who had said of amyotrophic lateral sclerosis, "Like a certain goddess of antiquity, it sprang fully armed from the head of its creator."[11] Indeed, Charcot's famed presentation in 1874 was, and remains compelling in its style of concise delivery and its anatomoclinical exactitude. Marie's allusion, however, conjures the image of a single and explosive discovery, whereas, in fact, Charcot's description of amyotrophic lateral sclerosis did not evolve in this dramatic way. Rather, this work represented the synthesis of a large series of previous studies, each a small contribution to the "fully armed creation."[1]

Substantial clinical material for studies of weakness and muscle wasting existed among the thousands of patients at the Salpêtrière. As chronic inhabitants of the hospital, these patients provided clinical material and later autopsy material for Charcot's eventual analyses. At the core of Charcot's neurological work was the technique known as the "anatomoclinical method." Adapted from Laennec's earlier discipline, Charcot adopted a two-part method to determine the correlation between clinical signs and anatomical lesions. He first tried to identify the prototypic patients where only weakness occurred without the complications of other neurological or medical problems. With rudimentary strategies based on careful observation, and tenaciously disciplined documentation, he identified weak patients without sensory difficulties, epilepsy, or other involuntary movements. Whereas all were weak, some were spastic with contractures, and some were amyotrophic. He followed these patients clinically, documenting the findings and progressive decline of function in full detail. Some of these case histories or *observations* are still available in folders in the Charcot library, showing clearly Charcot's method of scientific inquiry. Alongside the handwritten notes, Charcot accumulated pictorial diagrams of patients and their deformities, and finally autopsy drawings and pictures of microscopic observations. In addition to his own notes, Charcot completed the patient file with pictures and articles on similar or contrasting cases from the international medical literature (Fig. 41–1).

The second step of the clinicoanatomic method involved autopsy-based anatomic correlation of signs with lesions. A large postmortem anatomy and histology department developed under Charcot's surveillance, and patients' neurological systems were systematically examined after death in order to link type and location of lesions with specific clinical signs. The discipline of clinicoanatomic correlation in contemporary neurology can be directly traced to Charcot's work.

Using the anatomoclinical method, Charcot separated cases of acute weakness from those with slowly progressive courses and chronic disability.[12] As the physician in charge of a chronic care hospital, he concentrated primarily on chronic and progressive forms of weakness. Charcot did not restrict himself to diagnostic categories established by others but reviewed cases independently. In this context, he made his first major discovery of anatomoclinical significance to amyotrophic lateral sclerosis in 1865.

He presented to the Société Médicale des Hôpitaux de Paris a case report of a young woman diagnosed as hysteric who had developed slowly progressive but profound weakness and showed increased muscle tone, with contractures of all extremities during life.[13] At her death, Charcot found specific and isolated lateral column degeneration in the spinal cord:

> On careful examination of the surface of the spinal cord, on both sides in the lateral areas, there are two brownish gray streak marks produced by sclerotic changes. These grayish bands begin outside the line of insertion of the posterior roots and their anterior border approaches, but do not include the entrance area of the anterior roots. They are visible throughout the thoracic region and continue, though

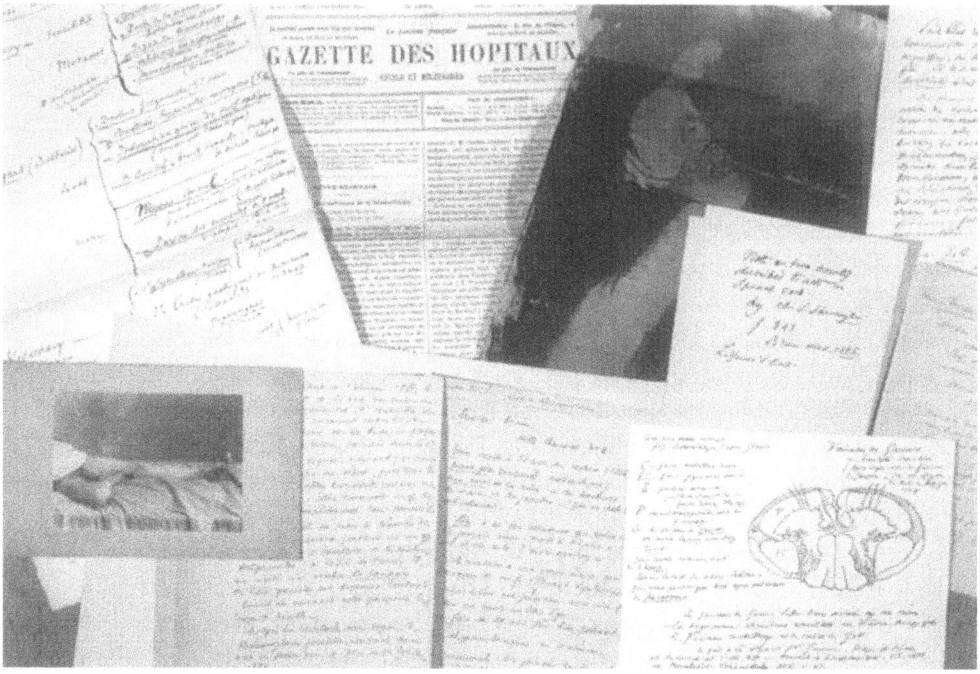

Figure 41–1. The anatomoclinical method of Charcot. In this photograph, numerous medical documents concerning a patient are assembled. Charcot first collected handwritten notes on the patient and monitored the clinical disease progression over time. Photographs, drawings, and footprints of the patient helped to characterize the clinical features of the illness. After death, autopsy material was collected in the same patient file. Clinical–anatomic correlations were suggested based on these combined data. In addition, Charcot, who read several languages, kept pertinent articles from the medical literature in the folder to complement his own material. Courtesy of Bibliothèque Charcot, M VIII, No. 6.

> greatly thinning out, up to the widening point of the cervical cord. Below, they are barely visible in the thoracolumbar region. Transverse sections taken at different levels allows one to see that the lateral columns have in their most superficial and posterior regions a gray, semitransparent appearance, rather gelatinous . . . At no point does the diseased tissue penetrate the gray matter, which remains unaffected.[13]

An early second observation concerned weakness in patients without contractures. In 1869, while working with his colleague Alix Joffroy (1844–1908), Charcot encountered pediatric cases of infantile paralysis and noted that "the spinal lesions are systematically limited to the anterior horns of the gray matter."[14]

The two seemingly unrelated observations from 1865 and 1869—(1) lateral column degeneration in the patient with chronic progressive paralysis and (2) contractures without atrophy of muscles and anterior horn degeneration in patients with infantile paralysis with atrophy of muscles—became the reference points for Charcot's motor system analyses. He returned to the Salpêtrière wards to find additional patients to test his hypothesis that the motor system in the spinal cord was organized into this two-part division, and whereas weakness linked the two, each clinical division had a different anatomical lesion.

Charcot was careful to select only the most typical cases with motor problems to ensure that they were "freed from all the extraneous elements that are unrelated."[15] In some, he noted that clinical and pathological features resembled the 1865 case, and in others the findings were those of his 1869 observations. These corroborative findings strengthened his concept of the two-part motor system organization. More perplexing and exciting, however, he found that even with careful selection, some cases had amyotrophy as well as spasticity and contractures. At autospy, he found both the anterior horn cell lesion typical of acute amyotrophy and also the distinctive bilateral and symmetric sclerosis of the lateral spinal cord columns. These cases became the third essential element to support his thesis and represented the first diagnosed cases of amyotrophic lateral sclerosis as a specific clinical disorder with a specific pathological correlate.[16,17]

As a result of these tenacious studies, Charcot suggested with conviction that specific clinical signs predictably occurred when certain spinal cord lesions were present and predictably did not occur when the signs were absent. As such, he established for the first time a clear medical paradigm for a direct correlation between a neuroanatomical lesion and a patient's neurological signs and symptoms. In opening the horizons for the study of direct relationships between clinical and anatomically pathologic states, Charcot presented the revolutionary concept that a precise anatomic diagnosis could be made before death. Charcot recounted:

> In the beginning, it was a matter of studying a series of cases primarily from an anatomic perspective. Nonetheless, the clinical characteristics of the patients had always been recorded carefully. Eventually among these different cases, it became possible to delineate a certain number of fundamental features, characteristics that permitted us later to recognize the condition clinically during life.[16]

With the success of the spinal cord research, Charcot and his student team expanded his work to confirm that comparable lesions in the brainstem were associated with weakness of the muscles controlling the face, mouth, and tongue. In 1871–1872, Charcot's student Albert Gombault (1844–1904) published "Symmetrical Sclerosis of the Lateral Spinal Columns and the Anterior Pyramids of the Lower Brainstem: Progressive Muscular Atrophy: Glossolaryngeal Paralysis."[18]

The clinical description of bulbar signs in amyotrophic lateral sclerosis actually dated back to earlier research by G.B.A. Duchenne de Boulogne (1806–1875) from over a decade earlier. Charcot commented that many investigators had previously tried without success to correlate a primary lesion of the gray matter of the medulla in the brainstem with the clinical signs known as labioglossolaryngeal paralysis. Now, with his anatomic study, and his appreciation of the anatomic parallels between the anterior horn of the spinal cord and the nuclear regions of the brainstem, he finally confirmed this early hypothesis that previously had been only suggested.[12] His conclusions became pillars of modern neurology—when gray matter motor nuclei are damaged, weakness is associated with muscular atrophy in the body areas supplied by those cells; when white lateral column damage occurs, weakness is associated with progressive contractures and spasticity.

Whereas all the essential descriptions of the motor neuron diseases were developed in early works, the term "amyotrophic lateral sclerosis" was not offered by Charcot until 1874 in his two lectures (12 and 13) gathered in Volume 2 of his *Oeuvres Complètes*.[16,17] These lectures synthesized the prior studies and were enormously successful in their succinct and compelling logic. They drew attention nationally and internationally to the condition, and simultaneously to Charcot and the Salpêtrière.

The name "amyotrophic lateral sclerosis" incorporated the two aspects of gray matter involvement causing amyotrophy and white matter damage (lateral sclerosis) (Fig. 41–2). The designation was anatomic and steered away from clinical terminology of the earlier years; as such, weakness and paralysis were not part of the name. Charcot's own later description of the importance of the work is not overinflated:

> I do not think that elsewhere in medicine, in pulmonary or cardiac pathology, greater precision can be achieved. The diagnosis as well as the anatomy and physiology of the condition "amyotrophic lateral sclerosis" is one of the most completely understood conditions in the realm of clinical neurology.[10,19]

Amyotrophic lateral sclerosis is still referred to as Charcot's disease in many parts of the world, although in the United States, as a reflection of the power of sports culture in society, "Lou Gehrig's disease" is a far more common name. Even during

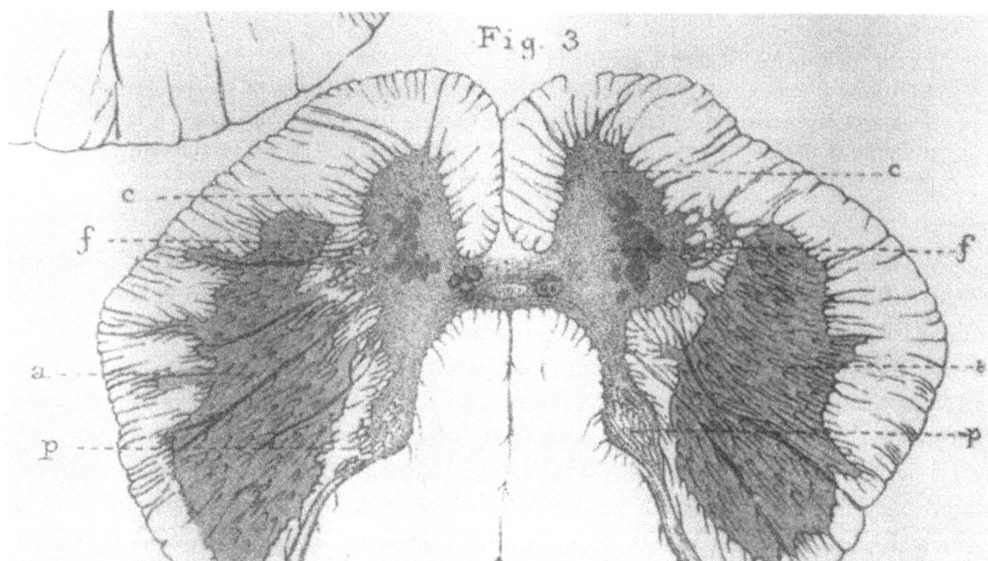

Figure 41–2. Cross section of the spinal cord in the superior cervical region in a patient with amyotrophic lateral sclerosis. From Charcot and Joffroy's 1869 report in the Archives de Physiologie Normale et Pathologique. f represents intermittent cells or debris in the anterior horn; a represents sclerosis of the lateral columns.

Charcot's time, however, there was ambiguity in the meaning of Charcot's disease, partly because he was so celebrated that multiple discoveries were linked to his name. The most important of these was the neuroarthropathy of locomotor ataxia, often called "Charcot's joints." At the International Medical Congress in London in 1881, Charcot presented his findings on locomotor ataxia and brought with him photographs, wax casts of deformed joints, and even a patient's entire skeleton. In a multimedia spectacle, he displayed these specimens along with microscopic sections of the spinal cord, joints, and bones. The international audience acclaimed his presentation with ovations and fanfare. The summary of Charcot's presentation from the *Transactions* of the Congress ended with these words:

> This disease is, in fact, a distinct pathological entity and deserves the name, by which it will be known, of "Charcot's disease."[20]

Since the death of Charcot in 1893, major additional discoveries have been made in the molecular and genetic understanding of amyotrophic lateral sclerosis. Few additions and revisions, however, have been made to Charcot's original clinical and anatomical descriptions. Charcot's contributions remain fundamental, and issues that puzzled him continue to challenge contemporary researchers. In this context, Charcot wrestled with the putative relationship between the two pathological features of amyotrophic lateral sclerosis, the white matter (lateral sclerosis) lesion and the gray matter (anterior horn cell degeneration) lesion. Did the two degenerative processes occur independently or was one component in fact secondary to the other? In a rare instance of physiological speculation, Charcot suggested that the anterior horn cell degeneration in amyotrophic lateral sclerosis was a result of the lateral column degeneration and that "the propagation is effected by means of the nerve filaments, which, you are aware, normally establish a communication between the lateral columns and the anterior horn cells."[16] This hypothesis unleashed a debate between Charcot and Gowers, who argued that the degeneration was a uniform and single event. More than a century later, the cause of amyotrophic lateral sclerosis, its earliest manifestations, and the relationship between the two prototypal lesions in the gray and white matter remain debated.

References

1. Goetz C G, Bonduelle M, Gelfand T. *Constructing Neurology: Jean-Martin Charcot.* New York: Oxford University Press; 1995.
2. Lellouch A. *Jean Martin Charcot et les origines de la gériatrie.* Paris: Payot; 1992.
3. Charcot J-M, *Maladies des vieillards: goute et rhumatisme.* Paris: Progrès Médical; 1876.
4. Charcot J M. Troubles trophiques consecutifs aux lesions des nerfs. In: *Oeuvres Complétes.* Paris: Bureaux du Progrès Médical; 1880;1:1–32. In English: Disorders of nutrition consequent on lesions of the nerves. In: Sigerson G, trans. *Clinical Lectures on the Diseases of the Nervous System.* London: New Sydenham Society; 1887:3–27.
5. Charcot J M. Du tabes dorsal spasmodique. In: *Oeuvres Complètes.* Paris: Bureaux du Progrès Médical; 1894;2:301–322. In English: On spasmodic tabes dorsalis. In: Sigerson G, trans. *Lectures on Diseases of the Nervous System.* London: New Sydenham Society; 1887:233–248.

6. Charcot, J M. De l'hystéroépilepsie. In: *Oeuvres Complètes.* Paris: Bureaux du Progrès Médical; 1890;1:367–386. In English: Sigerson G, trans. *Hysteroepilepsy, Lectures on the Diseases of the Nervous System.* Philadelphia: HC Lea; 1879:247–260.
7. Charcot, J M. De la paralysie agitante. In: *Oeuvres Complètes.* Paris: Bureaux du Progrès Médical: 1892; 1155–189. In English: On paralysis agitans. In: Sigerson G, trans. *Lectures on the Diseases of the Nervous System.* Philadelphia: HC Lea; 1879:105–127.
8. Charcot, J M. Tremblements et mouvements choreiformes. In: *Oeuvres Complètes.* Paris: Bureaux du Progrès Médical, 1890;9:215–228. In English: Choreiform movements and tremblings. In: Hurd E P, trans. *Clinical Lectures on the Diseases of the Nervous System.* Detroit: G S Davis; 1888.
9. Charcot, J M. Leçon d'ouverture. In: *Oeuvres Complètes.* Paris: Bureaux du Progrès Médical; 1889; 3:1–23. In English: Opening lesson. In: Savill T, trans. *Clinical Lectures on the Diseases of the Nervous System.* London: New Sydenham Society; 1889:1–20.
10. Goetz, C G. *Charcot the Clinician: The Tuesday Lessons.* New York: Raven Press; 1987.
11. Marie P. Eloge de J-M Charcot. *Rev Neurol.* 1925;5:736–745.
12. Charcot, J M. Des amyotrophies chroniques—atrophie musculaire progressive spinale prototypique. In: *Oeuvres Complètes.* Paris: Bureaux du Progrès Médical; 1874;2:221–233. In English: Chronic spinal amyotrophies: protopathic spinal progressive muscular atrophy. In: Sigerson G, trans. *Lectures on Diseases of the Nervous System.* London: New Sydenham Society; 1887:163–191).
13. Charcot J-M, Sclérose des cordons latéraux de la moelle èpiniére chez une femme hystérique atteinte de contracture permanente des quatre membres. *Bull Soc Méd Hôp Paris.* 1865:24–35.
14. Charcot J-M, Joffroy A. Deux cas d'atrophie musculaire progressive avec lésions de la substance grise et de faisceaux antérolatéraux de la moelle épinière. *Arch Physiol Norm Pathol.* 1869;1:354–67; 2:628–649; 3:744–757.
15. Charcot, J M. Révision nosographique des amyotrophies. In: *Oeuvres Complètes.* Paris: Bureaux du Progrès Médical; 1885;3:1–22. In English: Nosographic revision of the amyotrophies. In: Hard E P, trans. *Clinical Lectures on Certain Diseases of the Nervous System.* Detroit: G S Davis; 1888:1–20.
16. Charcot, J M. Sclérose latérale amyotrophique In: *Oeuvres Complètes.* Paris: Bureaux du Progrès Médical; 1874;2:234–248. In English: Amyotrophic lateral sclerosis. In: Sigerson G, trans. *Lectures on Diseases of the Nervous System.* London: New Sydenham Society; 1887: 192–204.
17. Charcot, J M. Amyotrophies deuteropathiques de cause spinale. In: *Oeuvres Complètes.* Paris: Bureaux du Progrès Médical; 1874;2:267–300. In English: Spinal induced amyotrophies. In: Sigerson G, trans. *Lectures on Diseases of the Nervous System.* London: New Sydenham Society: 1887:205–232.
18. Gombault A. Sclérose symétrique des cordons latéraux de la moelle et des pyramides antérieures dans le bulbe: atrophie des cellules descornes antérieures de la moelle et atrophie musculaire progressive paralysie glossolaryngée. *Arch Physiol Norm Pathol.* 1871–1872; 4:509–518.
19. Charcot, J M. *Les Leçons du Mardi: policlinique.* Paris: Bureaux du Progrès Médical; 1887–1888.
20. *Transactions of the International Medical Congress.* 3 vol. London, 1881.

42

THE CHIARI MALFORMATION

Peter J. Koehler and Samuel H. Greenblatt

Rachischisis, including spina bifida, meningomyelocele, and encephalocele, is usually treated by the pediatrician (or pediatric neurologist) and neurosurgeon. The neurologist will have a greater chance of observing associated conditions such as tethered cord, syringomyelia, and Chiari malformation, since these may first present in late childhood, adolescence, or adult life. The Chiari malformation, also called Arnold–Chiari malformation, comprises a syndrome of abnormalities at the base of the brain, particularly extension of the cerebellar tonsils into the cervical spinal canal caudal to the medulla oblongata. It is sometimes accompanied by displacement of the medulla oblongata into the spinal canal.[1] In modern literature, the term "hindbrain herniation" is sometimes applied. Many articles on the Chiari malformation, mostly case reports, are added to the already extensive literature every year. The etiology is still unknown. Chiari type I, with or without syringomyelia, is distinguished from Chiari type II. Although the latter clearly is a malformation, it is still uncertain whether the same is true for type I.

Hans Chiari was born on 4 November 1851 in Vienna.[2–4] His father, Johann Baptist, was a gynecologist at the Viennese University Women's Clinic and subsequently professor of gynecology at the University of Prague. Hans studied medicine and graduated in Vienna in 1875. His brother was the rhinolaryngologist Ottokar Chiari (1853–1918). Hans became second assistant to the famous pathologist Karl Freiherr von Rokitansky (1804–1878), who worked at the Institute of Pathology in Vienna (and had also been an important protector of Theodor Meynert; see Chapter 5), and subsequently first assistant to his successor, Richard Heschl (1824–1881). He was appointed prosector at the large Viennese St. Anna Children's Hospital in 1878, the year in which he finished his thesis on tuberculosis of the thyroid gland. In 1882 he was called to succeed Edwin Klebs (1834–1913), following a short interregnum of Hans Eppinger (1846–1916), as

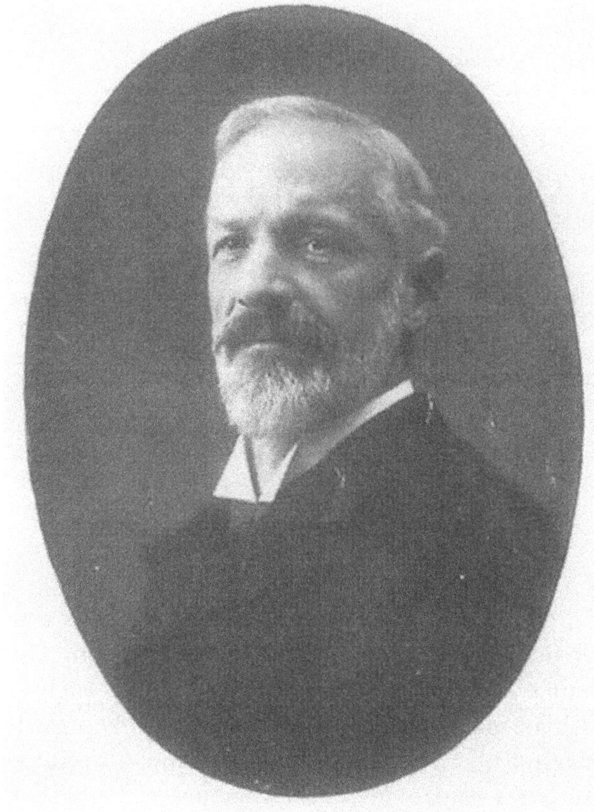

Figure 42–1. Hans Chiari (1851–1916). Courtesy of Institut für Geschichte der Medizin der Universität Wien.

professor of pathology at the University in Prague, which was a part of Prussia at that time.

> His intention was to shape the tuition in pathological anatomy into an observational instruction as much as possible, to provide the opportunity of independent work at the institute and consider the different sections of pathological anatomy, including macroscopic and histological, as well as bacteriological research for all those who were interested in pathological anatomy.[2]

During his stay in Prague, the intensifying internal political problems in Bohemia resulted in a partition of the university, including the department of pathology. By negotiation with colleagues at other hospitals, Chiari succeeded in limiting the loss of demonstration material. He guided his institute with a tight fist and demanded full dedication of his assistants, offering himself as an example. At exactly 8 A.M. the autopsies were distributed among the assistants, and at 11 A.M. the *Referierstunde* (lecture) started. As an inexhaustible *Fundgrube* (repository) of knowledge, he possessed an extensive experience and knowledge of the medical literature, partly because he understood many foreign languages. He became an important teacher for regional as well as foreign students, including American and Japanese.

During the political riots of 1898, which also affected the student circles, rioters entered his laboratory and destroyed a number of showcases. Ultimately, when he was called to become the successor of Friedrich von Recklinghausen (1833–1910) as professor in Strassburg in 1906, he did not hesitate to accept, despite the fact that he had worked in Prague for 24 years and had even been rector of the university in 1902–1903. During his stay in Strassburg, he traveled to the United States, invited by the Herter Foundation, on a lecture tour to Baltimore, Chicago, and New York (1910).

Following a short illness, Chiari died on 6 May 1916.

Chiari produced more than 200 publications on many different subjects. In addition to his work on cerebellar ectopy, he worked on syphilitic diseases of the aorta[5] and stomach,[6] and he published the first report on choriocarcinoma.[7] His work on the pathology of the pancreas, including the concept of self-digestion, was of great importance. He also wrote a chapter on the history of pathology.[8] More important for neurology is the fact that Chiari was the first to relate arteriosclerosis, or "endarteritis chronica deformans" of the carotid bifurcation, to cerebral embolism.[9]

Chiari's first article on cerebellar ectopia was published in 1891.[10] English translations of the original German article appeared in 1971[11] and 1987.[12] Important translation errors were found in the latter article.[13] As is obvious from the title of the 1891 paper, Chiari assumed that the changes in the cerebellum and brainstem resulted from chronic congenital hydrocephalus. He had never observed it in acute or late-onset hydrocephalus. He admitted that such abnormalities had been published before, but without discussing the causative relationship between the two phenomena.

Chiari distinguished three types of malformations. In type I, there was "elongation of the tonsils and medial parts of the inferior lobes of the cerebellum into cone-shaped projections, which accompany the medulla oblongata into spinal canal."[10] On pathological examination, the elongated parts of the cerebellum appeared to be occasionally normal, but in many cases sclerosis or softening was found. The fourth ventricle was normal or only slightly elongated. The medulla oblongata was flattened in some cases. The clinical symptoms and signs were unknown, but Chiari assumed that bulbar symptoms had been present.

Displacement of parts of the cerebellum within the elongated fourth ventricle into the widened spinal canal was found in type II malformation. He demonstrated this type of abnormality by a six-month-old child who had suffered from paraplegia and paralysis of the bladder and had died from pneumonia. The pons descended into the spinal canal over a distance of 6 mm and the medulla oblongata reached the level of the third cervical vertebra. Hydrocephalus was found, as well as a "cylindrical hole 6 mm in width, filled with clear serum" in the dorsal side of the spinal cord extending from the first to the seventh segment. A second cavity, "hydromyelie," was found a few segments lower. There were diastematomyelia, myelomeningocele, and the conus medullaris was located at the sacral level. Only one case of type III was observed. A five-month-old child with spina bifida, enlarged skull, strabismus, and cervical "hydromyelocele." The tentorium was missing at autopsy and the cerebellum had herniated into the spinal canal. The hydromyelia communicated with the fourth ventricle.

Chiari considered the 1891 article to be a preliminary report and provided more material in a study published in 1896.[14] In this paper, he described 63 cases of congenital hydrocephalus, collected from 4276 autopsies performed between 1889

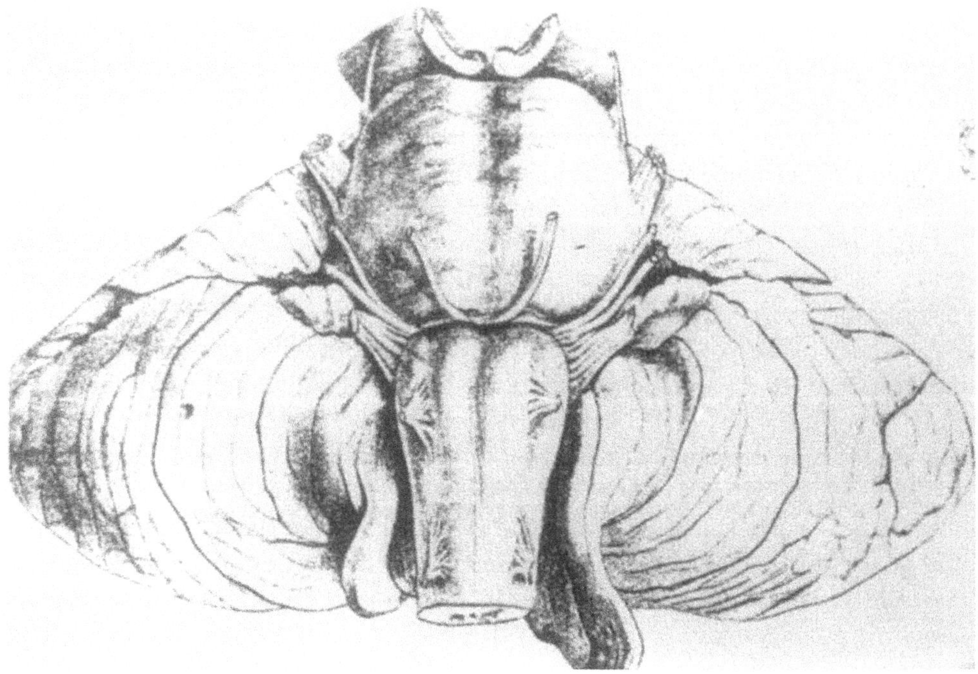

Figure 42–2. Cone-shaped elongation of cerebellar tonsils and inferior lobi in type I Chiari malformation. From Ref. 14.

and 1892. Fourteen cases had type I (Fig. 42–2) and seven had type II malformations. The first type was found in children and adults, the second type only in infants of a few days old. All seven patients with type II malformation had rachischisis. Chiari acknowledged the description of these abnormalities by other authors, including Arnold and Cleland (see below).

Interestingly, in this publication he theorized about a second etiological mechanism in addition to the hydrocephalus. He had noticed that the grade of hydrocephalus did not correlate with the extent of the cerebellar abnormalities. Insufficient growth of bone and inadequate enlargement of parts of the skull, resulting in increased intracranial pressure, were now supposed to play an important part. The description of type II malformation (seven cases) in this paper was different from that in the first paper. Whereas parts of the cerebellum were said to be displaced *within* the elongated fourth ventricle in the previous report, parts of the inferior vermis, pons, and medulla oblongata were displaced *together with* the elongation of the fourth ventricle in the present report. Chiari assumed that there is a gradual transition from cases in which cerebellar tissue descends *within* the fourth ventricle to cases where it descends *dorsal to* the fourth ventricle.[13] Although no cases of type III malformation were described in this paper, Chiari added the description of two patients with a type IV, consisting of hypoplasia in the cerebellar region assumed to be caused by hydrocephalus.

As Chiari admitted, the abnormalities had been described previously by other authors, including Cleland in 1883[15] and Arnold in 1894.[16] John Cleland (1835–1925) studied in Edinburgh, Scotland, and succeeded his teacher Allen Thomsen as professor of anatomy in Glasgow in 1877. He described an infant with spina bifida and hydrocephalus. The cerebellar nodulus was displaced into the elongated fourth ventricle, and the cerebellar lobes were completely divided. The anomaly corresponded to the first case of type II malformation that Chiari described in 1891. Chiari commented that in contrast to his own publications, Cleland had dealt only briefly with the findings. He considered the illustration of the case not sufficiently distinct to judge the anatomical relationships. Moreover, the case was investigated macroscopically only.[14]

Julius Arnold (1835–1915) studied under Rudolf Virchow (1821–1902) and Nikolaus Friedreich (1825–1882; see Chapter 48). He graduated in Heidelberg in 1859 and became professor of pathological anatomy there in 1866. In his 1894 paper he described an infant with spina bifida, without hydrocephalus.[16] The hindpart of the cerebellum was elongated, covered the fourth ventricle, and extended into the spinal canal. The paper concentrated on spina bifida and its possible cause. Arnold only briefly mentioned that abnormalities higher up in the nervous system may accompany it. In his 1896 paper, Chiari stated that this case corresponded to his type II cases, although Arnold had not found hydrocephalus. Chiari assumed it may have been present originally, causing the malformation, but disappeared aftwards.[14] The name Arnold was added to type II Chiari malformation by Arnold's pupils in the laboratory at Heidelberg, Schwalbe and Gredig, in 1907. Moreover, they wrongly distinguished between the cerebellar malformation (Arnold's deformity) and the medullary malformation (Chiari's deformity).[17]

Although Cleland and Arnold published on abnormalities of the hindbrain in cases of spina bifida, they discussed them only briefly as side issues. It was Chiari who described a considerable number of cases, provided accurate descriptions, and presented a theory of their pathogenesis. The eponym "Arnold–Chiari malformation" is still sometimes used, but we believe that neither Cleland's nor Arnold's name should be added to Chiari's. Fortunately, the American neurosurgical literature[18,19] exhibits a strong trend in this direction, at least since Gardner's chapter in Youman's textbook,[20] where Chiari's papers are cited directly.

Currently, the common classification is Chiari I, consisting of herniation of the cerebellar tonsils into the foramen magnum and upper cervical spinal canal (some authors include descent of the medulla oblongata); and type II, consisting of descent of the inferior vermis, as well as the inferior tonsils, and in some cases the elongated fourth ventricle, below the foramen magnum. Type III and Type IV malformations are rare afflictions.

References

1. Adams R D, Victor M, Ropper AH. *Principles of Neurology*. 6th ed. New York: McGraw-Hill; 1997:1006–1007.

2. Dürck H. Hans Chiari. *Münch Med Wochenschr.* 1916;63:1080–1082.
3. Gruber G B. Hans Chiari. *Zentralbl Allg Pathol Pathol Anat.* 1916;27:289–294.
4. Gruber G B. Hans Chiari. *Dtsch Med Wochenschr.* 1916;42:982–983.
5. Chiari H. Ueber die syphilitischen Aortenerkrankungen. *Verh Dtsch Path. Ges.* 1904;6: 137–163.
6. Chiari H. Ueber Magensyphilis. *Int Beitr Wiss Med.* 1891;2:295–321. Festschrift für R Virchow.
7. Chiari H. Über drei Fälle von primärem Carcinom im Fundus und Corpus des Uterus. *Med Jahrbuch.* 1877:364–368.
8. Chiari H. Geschichte der pathologischen Anatomie des Menschen. In: Puschmann T. *Handbuch der Geschichte der Medizin.* 1903;2:473–559.
9. Chiari H. Ueber das Verhalten des Teilungswinkels der Carotis communis bei der Endarteriitis chronica deformans. *Verh Dtsch Path Ges.* 1905;9:326–330.
10. Chiari H. Ueber Veränderungen des Kleinhirns infolge von Hydrocephalie des Grosshirns. *Dtsch Med Wochenschr.* 1891;17:1172–1175.
11. Wilkins R H, Brody I A. the Arnold-Chiari malformation. *Arch Neurol.* 1971;25:376–379.
12. Chiari H. Concerning alterations in the cerebellum resulting from cerebral hydrocephalus. *Pediatr Neurosci.* 1987;13:3–8.
13. Koehler P J. Chiari's description of cerebellar ectopy (1891). *J Neurosurg.* 1991;75:823–826.
14. Chiari H. Über Veränderungen des Kleinhirns, des Pons und der Medulla Oblongata infolge von congenitaler Hydrocephalie des Grosshirns. *Denkschr Kais Akad Wiss Math-Naturw.* 1896;63:71–116.
15. Cleland J. Contribution to the study of spina bifida, encephalocele, and anencephalus. *J Anat Physiol.* 1883;17:257–292.
16. Arnold J. Myelocyste, Transposition von Gewebskeimen und Sympodie. *Zieglers Beitr Pathol Anat.* 1894;16:1–28.
17. Schwalbe E, Gredig M. Ueber Entwickelungsstörungen des Kleinhirns, Hirnstamms und Halsmarks bei Spina bifida (Arnold'sche und Chiari'sche Missbildung). *Beitr Pathol Anat.* 1907;40:132–194.
18. Bertrand G. Anomalies of the craniovertebral junction. In: Youmans J R, ed. *Neurological Surgery.* 2nd ed. Philadelphia: Saunders 1982;3:1482–1508.
19. Oakes W J. Chiari malformations, hydromyelia, syringomyelia. In: Wilkins R H, Rengachary S S, eds. *Neurosurgery.* 2nd ed. New York: McGrawHill 1996;3:3593–3616.
20. Gardner W J. Anomalies of the craniovertebral junction. In: Youmans J R, ed. *Neurological Surgery.* Philadelphia: Saunders 1973;1:628–644.

43

CREUTZFELDT-JAKOB DISEASE

Charles M. Poser and George W. Bruyn

Creutzfeldt–Jakob disease (CJD) is one of the transmissible spongiform encephalopathies (TSEs) characterized clinically by the triad of rapidly devastating dementia, pyramidal and extrapyramidal disease with myoclonus, and triphasic discharges in the electroencephalogram. The pathologic hallmarks are neuronal loss, spongy changes in the gray matter, and an astrocytic response.

It has been argued by a number of authors, most convincingly by Walter Kirschbaum,[1] a student of Alfons Maria Jakob, and by F. Katscher,[2] that the correct eponymous designation should be Jakob–Creutzfeldt disease. There is now a majority view that it was indeed Jakob who first described this disease. Kirschbaum titled his 1968 book *Jakob–Creutzfeldt Disease,* despite the fact that in 1922 the foremost German neuropathologist, Walther Spielmeyer,[3] had given precedence to his erstwhile student Creutzfeldt. The CJD eponym continues to be so widely used that any attempt to redress a slight to the memory of Alfons Jakob seems futile. Consequently, we use CJD in this essay.

Hans-Gerhard Creutzfeldt was born in Harburg, near Hamburg, on 2 June 1885. His father was Dr. Otto Creutzfeldt. He studied medicine in Jena, Rostock, and Kiel, where he received his degree in 1908. He then studied pathology under Professor Morris Simmonds and wrote his thesis on tumors of the pituitary gland. The lure of the sea led him to travel extensively as a young ship's doctor from 1910 to 1912, which resulted in his lifelong interests in tropical diseases, exotic art objects, and linguistics. He studied neuropathology with Ludwig Edinger in Frankfurt-am-Main in 1912, and then spent the next two years with Alois Alzheimer in Breslau. During World War I, he was a German naval medical officer in the North Sea. In 1917 he married Clare Sombart, whose father was the famous sociologist Werner Sombart. In 1919–1920, he worked with Walther Spielmeyer in Munich and with Ernst Siemerling at the University of Kiel. For the next 14 years, he worked in the

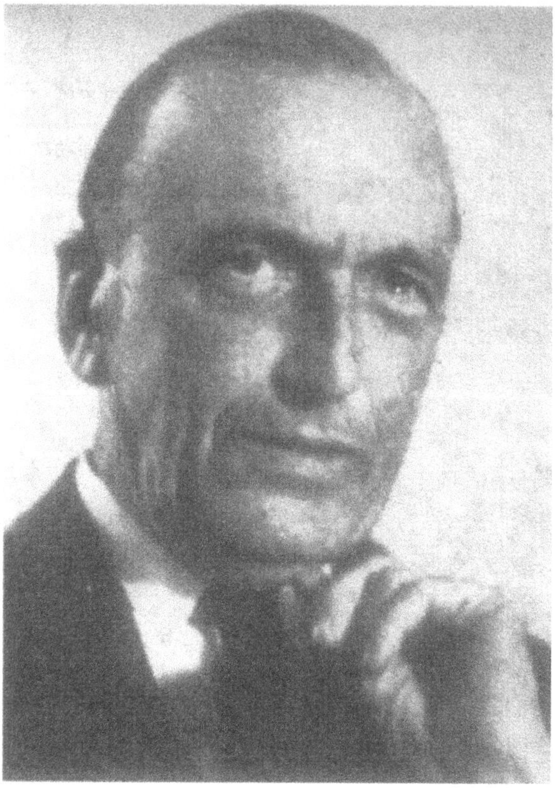

Figure 43–1. Hans-Gerhard Creutzfeldt (1885–1964). Courtesy of the Archives of the Christian-Albrechts University of Kiel.

Department of Psychiatry of the Charité Hospital in Berlin with Karl Bonhoeffer. He returned to Kiel in 1938, was appointed director of neuropsychiatry at the Christian Albrechts University, and served there until 1953. He became the first postwar rector of the university in 1945 and 1946, by appointment of the British military government. He ended his academic career at the Psychiatric Institute of Munich in 1955.

Creutzfeldt was one of the few academics who refused to join the Nazi party. His wife was imprisoned for her anti-Nazi stand and his son Harald defected from the German navy to join the Dutch underground resistance. At war's end, Harald was commissioned in the British army and spent the last 20 years of his life in England. Two of Creutzfeldt's sons became distinguished physicians: Otto became director of the Max-Planck Institute of Neurobiology in Göttingen, and Werner was professor and chairman of the Department of Medicine at the same university.

Hans Creutzfeldt was an original thinker, a modest man, and a devout Christian. As an anatomist and neuropathologist, he regarded neuropathology as the true link between neurology and psychiatry, antedating Harvard's Derek Denny-Brown's dictum that neuropathology was the true basic science of neurology, thus continuing in the Kraepelin–Alzheimer–Spielmeyer tradition of the Deutsche Forschungsanstalt für Psychiatrie in Munich. He died at the age of 80, after a long and agonizing illness, on 30 December 1964. An obituary was published by Laux in 1965.[4]

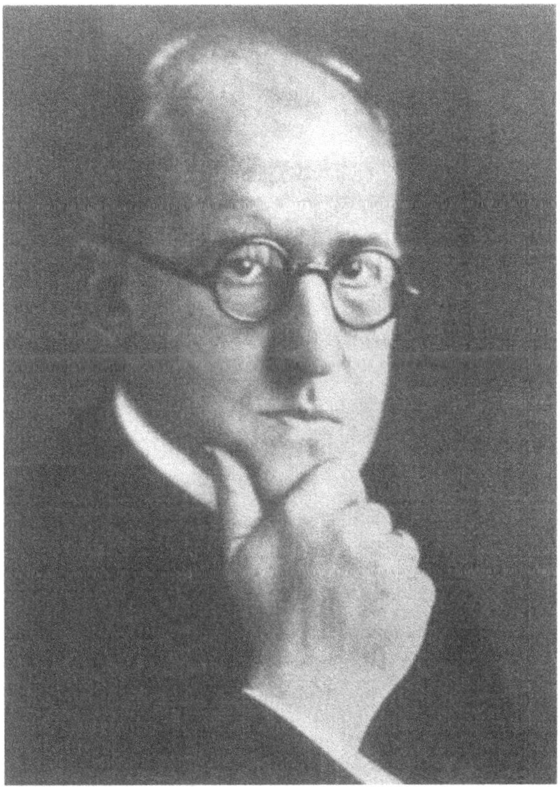

Figure 43–2. Alfons Maria Jakob (1884–1931). Personal collection of Prof. Emer G. W. Bruyn.

Alfons Maria Jakob was born in Aschaffenburg-am-Main on 2 July 1884. He came from a family of shopkeepers. He studied medicine at the universities of Munich, Berlin, and Strassburg. He obtained his degree from the latter in 1909 after writing a thesis on the *Pathogenesis of Pseudobulbar Paralysis.* Even during his internship he volunteered to work as assistant physician in Emil Kraepelin's Psychiatric Clinic and its neuropathology laboratory in Munich, then headed by Alois Alzheimer and Franz Nissl. Neither Kraepelin nor Nissl was known to be lavish with praise, yet they described Jakob as being "diligent, conscientious, clinically talented, scientifically motivated and of humane, amiable and optimistic disposition." On 15 November 1911, Jakob accepted the invitation of Wilhelm Weygandt, director of the Friedrichsberg State Hospital in Hamburg, to work as clinical assistant.

He was to make this institute a center of worldwide fame. In addition to his clinical duties, he spent progressively more time in the pathological–anatomical laboratory run by the prosector Theodor Kaes, who had published a widely acclaimed atlas *cum* textbook *Die Grosshirnrinde des Menschen* in 1907. Jakob succeeded Kaes as prosector in 1913.

For three years, 1915–1918, he served as an army physician at the front in Flanders, Belgium, and spent the rest of his short life at Friedrichsberg. After the war, the laboratory included new sections for serology, genetics, and experimental psychology. Jakob strived to maintain the high quality of the laboratory's scientific output.[5] He also had a large private practice. He was invited to make a lecture tour in the United States in 1924, and another one in South America in 1928. Jakob was the author of five authoritative monographs and nearly 80 scientific papers on varied subjects including pseudobulbar palsy, trauma, yellow fever, leprosy, glial nodule encephalitis (later to be called subacute sclerosing panencephalitis), diffuse and multiple sclerosis, muscular dystrophy, cerebral syphilis, epilepsy, the extrapyramidal diseases, and a two-volume textbook on the normal and pathological anatomy of the brain. Foreign neurologists flocked to his laboratory, many to become famous neuropathologists themselves; one was Kirschbaum, whose monograph eventually enlarged and established the importance of Jakob's contribution. Jakob died on 17 October 1931, only 47 years old.

In 1913, while working at Alzheimer's neuropsychiatric clinic in Breslau (now Wroclaw, Poland), Hans Creutzfeldt studied a case of a "new and unusual type of neurological disease" in a 22-year-old woman who had been seen at the clinic at the age of 16 because of gait ataxia. The patient's mother had died of unknown cause at age 56, and two siblings were mentally defective. She had tremors, spasticity, and pyramidal signs, and she soon became progressively more ataxic and demented. Her later symptoms included nystagmus, rigidity, myoclonus, and mutism. She died in *status epilepticus* 12 months after the onset. The brain revealed moderate cerebral atrophy with a patchy, diffuse neuronal loss, pronounced astroglial hypertrophy, and bilateral degeneration of the corticospinal tracts. Neuronal vacuolation or spongy state was not mentioned. Alzheimer approved the case for publication but, because of the war, it did not appear until 1920,[6] when Creutzfeldt was working in Spielmeyer's laboratory in Munich.

In 1921, Alfons Jakob described four cases at the University of Hamburg, the first three under the name "spastic pseudo-sclerosis, disseminated encephalomyelopathy."[7] He referred to previously published cases he thought similar to these, and particularly the one described by Creutzfeldt.[6] A fourth case was published by Jakob[8] in the same year, which he described as "resembling pseudosclerosis." The fifth case was included in his 1923 book *The Extrapyramidal Diseases.*[9] Jakob had been able to examine Creutzfeldt's slides and had received a preprint of Creutzfeldt's article in Nissl and Alzheimer's 1920 book.[10] He noted that the changes were similar to those of one of his patients. He grouped them together as examples of spastic pseudosclerosis. In turn, Creutzfeldt, commenting on Jakob's first three cases, agreed that they appeared to be identical but objected that "spastic pseudosclerosis" was an oxymoron; he insisted that their cases constituted a completely new entity.[11]

The term "pseudosclerosis" had been introduced in 1883 by Carl Westphal,[12] who had followed two young patients with tremor, thinking they had multiple sclerosis. At autopsy he was unable to find any gross or microscopic lesions. A few years later, Adolf Strümpell was also unable to find any gross lesions of the nervous system.[13] The next year pseudosclerosis became regarded as a variety of Wilson's disease, to which Samuel Alexander Kinnier Wilson vehemently objected. Jakob was aware of this when he published his report, but he still thought there might be a separate form of pseudosclerosis exemplified by his patients and those of Creutzfeldt. He was much impressed by the evidence of corticospinal tract disease that he and Creutzfeldt had found, and for that reason, he designated his subgroup of pseudosclerosis as "spastic."

In retrospect, the most important of Jakob's initial cases was the third, a 42-year-old man with aching legs, vertigo, and abdominal pain, followed by leg weakness, ataxia, diplopia, and progressive mental deterioration. He later developed dysarthria and facial twitching, before dying totally demented and stuporous some nine months after the onset of his illness. Microscopy showed changes that closely resembled Creutzfeldt's case. Neuronal vacuolation or spongiosis was not mentioned. The slides from Creutzfeldt's case were lost during World War II and therefore have never been reviewed. After reexamination of the slides of Jakob's cases, from the Hamburg neuropathological laboratory, Kirschbaum,[1] van Rossum,[14] Masters and Gajdusek,[15] and Richardson[16] all agreed that the diagnosis of CJD was probably correct only in cases 3 and 5. Most importantly, the histology from Jakob's third and fifth cases revealed a diffuse vacuolation of the neuropil involving all areas of the cerebral cortex as well as the molecular layer of the cerebellum. This was eventually recognized as a cardinal feature of CJD and of all the TSEs.

It is most curious that even though Jakob and Creutzfeldt agreed that their cases, including the former's case 3, were identical, the validity of the Creutzfeldt's 1920 case as an instance of CJD is in dispute. According to Manuelidis, Creutzfeldt stated 25 years later that his case was probably not one of CJD.[17] His son, Professor Werner Creutzfeldt, disputes that such a statement was ever made by his father (personal communication, April 1999).

After his first five cases, Jakob examined the brains of two additional patients, which were subjected to further study after he died, and later published by Kirschbaum.[1] The first occurred in a 44-year-old man, Paul Bacher. The patient's maternal grandmother and eight of her siblings had died of unexplained cerebral disease, as eventually did his sister. Paul Bacher's autopsy, and that of the sister, showed the spongiform changes that were thought to be typical of CJD; so did those of two of Paul Bacher's children. These observations established with certainty dominant as well as sporadic transmission. In 1929 Adolf Heidenhain reported three patients in late middle age with cortical blindness in two.[18] Spongy changes were prominent, although Heidenhain thought that his cases differed fundamentally from those with CJD because such changes had been noted by neither Creutzfeldt nor Jakob. Proof that Jakob's later patients were in fact cases of CJD was elegantly provided by Brown and his colleagues, who obtained DNA from an archived slide of the brain of one of the Bacher family cases, sequenced the *PRNP* gene using polymerase chain reaction (PCR) techniques, and found a mutation that we now recognize as being the cause of the disease.[19]

The definitive answer to the nosological question of CJD was to come in stages, culminating in the concept of the prion diseases (or "prionoses," a term that one of us [GWB] prefers), formulated in 1982 by Stanley Prusiner, a neurologist and biochemist in San Francisco, who was awarded the 1997 Nobel Prize for that discovery.[20] It states that there exist infectious proteins which are able to replicate themselves, despite their lack of nucleic acid—a feature that was first pointed out in 1967 by Tikvah

Alper,[21] a British radiation pathologist—by modifying normal "prion proteins" in the neuron causing the cell's eventual death.

This discovery was preceded in 1957 by the description by Carleton Gajdusek and Vincent Zigas of *kuru* in cannibalistic natives of New Guinea.[22] Efforts to transmit the disease to experimental animals including primates failed until William Hadlow, an American veterinary neuropathologist working in England, pointed to the remarkable similarity between the brain lesions of scrapie, a transmissible infectious disease of sheep with an unusually prolonged incubation period, and those of kuru.[23] With his colleagues Clarence Joseph Gibbs Jr. and Michael Alpers, Gajdusek eventually transmitted kuru to chimpanzees in 1966, a feat for which Gajdusek alone received the 1976 Nobel Prize.[24] In a letter to Gajdusek dated 13 September 1957, Igor Klatzo, a neuropathologist, had noted the similarity between kuru and CJD, stating: "The closest condition I can think of is that described by Creutzfeldt and Jakob."[25] Klatzo, Gajdusek, and Zigas more formally stressed the resemblance between kuru and CJD in a 1959 publication.[26] Finally, in 1968, Gibbs et al. induced the disease in chimpanzees by injecting brain tissue from CJD patients.[27] Scrimgeour et al. conjectured that kuru developed following cannibalism of a case of sporadic CJD in a New Guinea native who died in 1900.[28]

In 1971, Kirschbaum stated

> No definite pathogenic relationship is established. However, the concept of slow virus infection should not be dismissed . . . If confirmation is obtained by additional research, some principal pathogenetic questions will be elucidated. It is still worthwhile to remember that from the beginning Jakob considered etiologic relations to chronic *metencephalitis epidemica* . . . Jakob–Creutzfeldt disease is most likely a multiple and not a single disease concept. A nearly identical tissue response may result from hereditary and constitutional liabilities, metabolic–toxic changes and chronic infectious agents.[29]

He had also been prophetic when he suggested that the disease might have different forms. About 15% of cases of CJD are familial. There are two other forms of the disease in addition to the sporadic one. Not only was the disease produced iatrogenically by corneal and dura mater transplantation, scalp needle electrodes, growth hormone, and gonadotrophin obtained from cadaveric pituitary glands, but more recently, in 1996, in Great Britain a different human form of the disease, termed "new variant CJD" (nvCJD), was discovered and attributed (but not proved) to the ingestion of meat from cows with bovine spongiform encephalopathy, a prion disease related to scrapie.[30]

In 1989, before the definition of TSE and the identification of a putative common etiologic agent, Masters had counted no fewer than 84 "types" or variants of CJD.[31] These were based either on the clinical triad of dementia and pyramidal and extrapyramidal symptoms, or on rather loosely interpreted neuropathological features.

Currently CJD is classified as a prion disease, a TSE. There is still much controversy regarding the exclusive role of the prion as the sole etiologic agent of the TSEs. Prions are normal cellular proteins (PrP 27–30) encoded by the gene *PRNP* on the short arm of human chromosome 20. Abnormal PrP (PrPsc) are encoded as a result of a variety of mutations which, in CJD, are at codons 178, 200, and 210. By means of an unknown mechanism, PrPsc are able to replicate and to change normal PrP into its own abnormal configuration leading to cell destruction. While codon 200 mutations are characteristic for familial CJD, they are also found in the other forms of the disease. Close to 20 coding mutations of *PRNP* have been described. Other genetic factors, including zygosity at codon 129, influence the phenotypic manifestations of the disease. Because of analysis of *PRNP* mutations, the Gerstmann–Straussler–Scheinker syndrome (GSSS) and fatal familial insomnia (FFI) are recognized as major CJD variants. In animals the TSEs include scrapie, mink encephalopathy, and bovine spongiform encephalopathy ("mad cow disease").

In 1995, Budka and his colleagues proposed surprisingly imprecise neuropathological diagnostic criteria for the TSEs.[32]

The correct nosological situation of what was once an ill-defined mysterious condition came about as the result of an extraordinary sequence of events. The first clue came in 1959 when William Hadlow noted the similarity between the pathological changes of the brain in kuru and scrapie, with its extremely long incubation period.[23] A search for the cause of scrapie eventually led to the still controversial etiological concept of a nucleic acid–free infectious protein, the prion. Thus a number of superficially disparate diseases of humans and animals, including CJD, were grouped under the term TSE or prion diseases.

Acknowledgments

We are extremely grateful to Professor Emeritus Werner Creutzfeldt, University of Göttingen, Germany, for biographical details about his father, Hans-Gerhard Creutzfeldt, and for constructive criticism of the text.

References

1. Kirschbaum W. *Jakob-Creutzfeldt Disease.* New York: Elsevier, 1968.
2. Katscher F. It's Jakob's disease, not Creutzfeldt's. *Nature.* 1998;393:11.
3. Spielmeyer W. Die histopathologische Forschung in der Psychiatrie. *Klin Wochenschr.* 1922; 1:1817–1819.
4. Laux I. In memoriam Hans-Gerhard Creutzfeldt. *Med Klin.* 1965;60:553–554.
5. Jakob A. Die Entwicklung der gehirnanatomischen Abteilung der Staatskrankenanstalt und psychiatrischen Universitätsklinik Hamburg-Friedrichsberg. *Z Ges Neurol Psychiatr.* 1930; 128:172–178.
6. Creutzfeldt H. Über eine eigenartige herdformige Erkrankung des Zentralnervensystems. *Z Ges Neurol Psychiatr.* 1920;57:1–18.
7. Jakob A. Über eigenartige Erkrankungen des Zentralnervensystems mit bemerkenswerten anatomischen Befunden (spästische Pseudosklerose-Encephalomyelopathie mit disseminierten Degenerationsherden). *Dtsch Z Nervenheilk.* 1921;70:132–146; *Z Ges Neurol Psychiatr.* 1921;64:147–228.
8. Jakob A. Über ein der multiplen Sklerose klinisch nahestehende Erkrankung des Zentralnervensystems (spästische Pseudosklerose) mit bemerkenswerten anatomischen Befunde. *Med Klin.* 1921;13:372–376.
9. Jakob A. *Die Extrapyramidale Erkrankungen.* Berlin: Springer; 1923:218–245.
10. Creutzfeldt H. Über eine eigenartige herdformige Erkrankung des Zentralnervensystems. In: Nissl F, Alzheimer A, eds. *Histologische und histopathologische Arbeiten über die Grosshirnrinde.* Jena: Gustav Fischer; 1921:1–48.

11. Creutzfeldt H. [A review of Jakob's first three cases.[5]] *Z Ges Neurol Psychiatr.* 1921;25: 321–322.
12. Westphal C. Über eine dem Bilde der cerebrospinalen grauen Degeneration. *Arch Psychiat Nervenkrankh.* 1883;4:87–134.
13. Strümpell A. Über die Westphalische Pseudosklerose der Wilsonsche Krankheit. *Dtsch Z Nervenheilk.* 1898;12:115–149.
14. Van Rossum A. Spastic pseudosclerosis (Creutzfeldt-Jakob disease). In: Vinken PJ, Bruyn GW, eds. *Handbook of Clinical Neurology.* Amsterdam: North Holland; 1968;6:726–760.
15. Masters C, Gajdusek D. The spectrum of Creutzfeldt-Jakob disease. In: Smith W, Cavanagh J, eds. *Recent Advances in Neuropathology.* 2nd ed. Edinburgh: Churchill-Livingstone; 1982: 139–165.
16. Richardson E. Introduction to myoclonic dementia. In: Rothenberg D, Hochberg F, eds. *Neurological Classics in Modern Translation.* New York: Hafner; 1977.
17. Manuelidis E. Creutzfeldt-Jakob disease. *J Neuropathol Exp Neurol.* 1985;44:1–17.
18. Heidenhain A. Klinische und anatomische Untersuchungen über eine eigenartige Erkrankung des Zentralnervensystems im Praesenium. *Z Ges Neurol Psychiatr.* 1929;118:49–114.
19. Brown P, Cervenakova B, Boellaard J, et al. Identification of a PRNP gene mutation in Jakob's original Creutzfeldt-Jakob disease family. *Lancet.* 1994;344:130–131.
20. Prusiner S. Novel proteinaceous infectious particles cause scrapie. *Science.* 1982; 216: 136–144.
21. Alper T, Cramp W, Haig D, et al. Does the agent of scrapie replicate without nucleic acid? *Nature.* 1967;214:764–766.
22. Gajdusek D, Zigas V. Degenerative disease of the central nervous system in New Guinea. *N Engl J Med.* 1957;257:974–978.
23. Hadlow W. Scrapie and kuru. *Lancet.* 1959;2:289–290.
24. Gajdusek D, Gibbs C Jr, Alpers M. Experimental transmission of a kuru-like syndrome to chimpanzees. *Nature.* 1966;209:794–796.
25. Klatzo I. Letter to Gajdusek, September 13, 1957. In: Farquhar J, Gajdusek D, eds. *Kuru: Early Letters and Field Notes in the Collection of D. Carleton Gajdusek.* New York: Raven Press; 1981:155.
26. Klatzo I, Gajdusek D, Zigas V. Pathology of kuru. *Lab Invest.* 1959;8:799–847.
27. Gibbs C Jr, Gajdusek D, Asher D, et al. Creutzfeldt-Jakob disease transmission to the chimpanzee. *Science.* 1968;161:388–389.
28. Scrimgeour E, Masters C, Alpers M, et al. A clinico-pathological study of a case of kuru. *J Neurol Sci.* 1983;59:265–275.
29. Kirschbaum W. Jakob-Creutzfeldt disease. In: Minckler J, ed. *Pathology of the Nervous System.* New York: McGraw-Hill; 1971;2:1410–1419.
30. Will R, Ironside J, Zeidler M, et al. A new variant of Creutzfeldt-Jakob disease in the UK. *Lancet.* 1996;347:921–925.
31. Masters C. Creutzfeldt-Jakob disease, its origin. *Alzheimer Dis Assoc Disord.* 1989;3:46–51.
32. Budka H, Aguzzi A, Brown P, et al. Neuropathological diagnostic criteria for Creutzfeldt-Jakob disease and other spongiform encephalopathies (prion disease). *Brain Pathol.* 1995;5: 459–466.

44

CURSCHMANN–STEINERT DISEASE

Richard P. M. Bruyn

Hans Gustav Wilhelm Steinert was born on 10 April 1875 in Dresden. He was the son of a lawyer, Otto Steinert, and his wife, Louise Westen. Virtually nothing is known of his boyhood. He attended the Gymnasium in Dresden from 1884 to 1893, studied medical sciences and philosophy, and subsequently studied medicine in Dresden, Freiburg, Berlin, and Kiel. He graduated in 1898, in the same year defending his thesis, *Über zwei Embryonalkystome des Ovariums und über eine Dermoidzyste des Hodens* [On two embryonal cystic tumors of the ovary and a dermoid cyst of the testis].

From 18 September 1898 to 1 July 1899 he was assistant in Halle. He worked at the outpatient department for nervous diseases in Berlin until 1 January 1900, and from 1 January 1900 to 1 April 1900 he worked at the Leipzig Pathological Institute, then he spent four months as assistant at the outpatient department. From 1 October 1900 to 1 April 1901 Steinert worked in the City Hospital of Dresden. Finally, Heinrich Curschmann invited Steinert to come to Leipzig to work at the University Clinic. With his *Habilitation, Neue Beiträge zur Lehre von der Muskelatrophie bei supranukleären Lähmungen, besonders bei der cerebralen Hemiplegie* [New contributions to the theory of muscle atrophy associated with supranuclear palsy, in particular in the cerebral hemiplegia], Steinert obtained the right to teach *(venia legendi)* at the Leipzig medical faculty. On 10 October 1910 he became extraordinary professor at the medical faculty of the Leipzig University. Shortly thereafter he became ill and sought medical treatment in Davos. He died probably of adrenal carcinoma on 3 November 1911. He was married to an ophthalmologist, Dr. Löwenhain, and they had three children. Because of her Jewish background her position became precarious in 1933. Nothing further is known of her whereabouts or of their children.

Steinert's original description of myotonic dystrophy[1] dealt with six patients who all showed facial weakness, ptosis, atrophy of the sternocleidomastoid and forearm muscles, soft speech, and areflexia. Testicular atrophy was present in four of them, and mild sensory deficit in some. All patients but the sixth were known in Leipzig medical circles, having frequently been examined at medical meetings. They were regarded as curiosities. Three of them had been presented at the Leipzig Medical Society meeting of 1904.

Steinert's first patient in 1899 was a baker who had been without complaints up to the age of 26. His family allegedly was healthy. He developed progressive muscular stiffness with atrophy and weakness, successively spreading from the fingers to the arms, face, tongue, and legs. The examination showed baldness, myopathic face, marked generalized muscle atrophy with weakness, and myotonia of face, tongue, masseter, and forearm muscles. Areflexia was associated with hypesthesia of fingers and toes, the latter having disappeared on reexamination in 1907.

The second patient, aged 44, had myotonia since childhood, as had his father and brother. In addition, baldness, facies myopathica, ptosis, areflexia, testicular atrophy, weakness, and atrophy were noticeable. He died of tuberculosis in 1905. Autopsy revealed muscular "fibrosis," degeneration of spinal dorsal columns, and an unremarkable brain. Patient 3 was 30 years old and came from a family with "Thomsen's disease." He had all the classical symptoms. Patients 4 and 5 were brothers, again exhibiting all the classical features, their ages at manifestation being 24 years. Finally, patient 6 had onset of symptoms when a schoolboy; none of his sisters reached the age of 16 and his father had died of tuberculosis, while his mother died in a psychiatric hospital.

Steinert found previous reports on 26 patients in whom muscular atrophy accompanied myotonia. He stressed the predilection of the disorder for certain muscles, the symmetry, the usual sequence of muscle involvement, and he confirmed the finding of Curschmann that paresis and dystrophy in certain extensor muscles went together with myotonia in their antagonists. Following a discussion of the baldness and testicular atrophy, he outlined the disease as "Thomsen's disease," of which the primary process would be myotonia, subsequently associated with dystrophy, unlike the myotonia due to a myopathy.

Hans Curschmann was born on 14 August 1875 in Berlin, where his father, Professor Heinrich Curschmann, was the director of the Moabit Hospital, a hospital especially built for infectious diseases. Hans Curschmann had one brother and one sister. In 1879 the family moved to Hamburg, where they stayed until Hans was 13. Just like his father, Hans was a talented draftsman and had a passion for painting and sculpture. He loved music and frequently sang in a choir. He studied medicine in Freiburg and Munich, and he graduated in Leipzig in 1900. He was one of Erb's pupils in Heidelberg for four years; subsequently he spent six months with Professor Kraus in Berlin. In 1904, he became assistant of one of his father's pupils, Ernst Romberg, in Tübingen. In 1906 he acquired his *Habilitation* and in the following years he served as chief of the internal medicine department of the Rochus Hospital in Mainz. In 1916 he left for Rostock to become director of the outpatient department of internal medicine. In 1921 he was appointed professor and chairman, positions he held until his retirement in 1941. Curschmann was an inspiring teacher, warm-hearted, direct, a nonaggressive debater, a dedicated consultant, and an optimistic human being.

Figure 44–1. Hans Curschmann (1875–1950). Courtesy of Karl-Sudhoff Institute for History of Medicine and Natural Sciences, Leipzig, Germany.

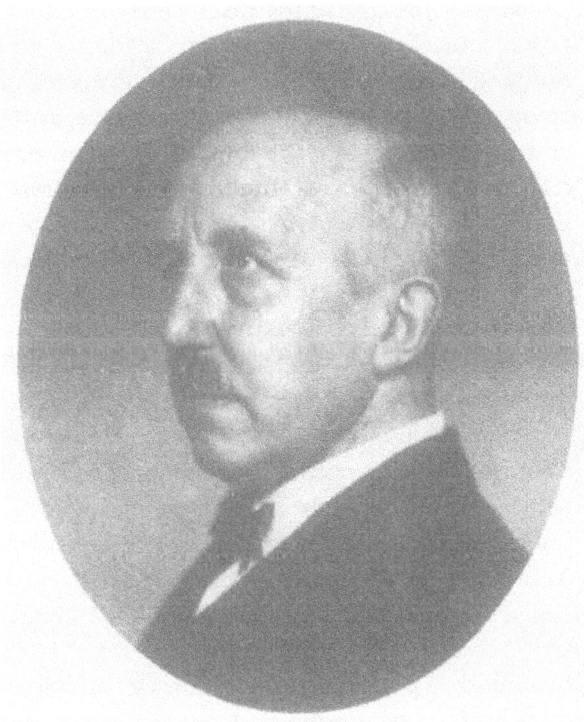

Curschmann's extensive oeuvre contains masterpieces on endocrinology and other subjects, but his real interest, neurology, induced him to write *Lehrbuch der Nervenkrankheiten* (1909) and *Leitfaden der Neurologie* (1913). He followed Erb to chair the Society for German Neurologists (which was founded by Erb, Strümpell, Schultze, and Lichtheim) for ten years. He founded the Northwest German Society for Internal Medicine in 1925; later he became its honorary president.

Curschmann was married to Leni Wendt and they had five children (Otto Heinrich, Grete, Hedwig, Johanna, and Hans Friedrich). One son died of spotted fever in Russia during World War II. Curschmann died of a stroke on 10 March 1950.[2–4]

Curschmann[5] gave Steinert credit for describing myotonic dystrophy as a distinct entity. After 1905 he examined six patients exhibiting the same symptom complex as Steinert's cases. His first case, a 33-year-old baker of low intelligence, complained of stiff hands from the age of 12, and he had difficulty loosening his grip. Only after repeating the same procedure several times did the muscles loosen up. His legs also became stiff, especially after sitting still. Initiation of walking was particularly difficult, but after walking several meters his stiffness faded away. His muscle strength decreased after several years, he became bald, and there was a loss of libido.

On examination, a slim man was found to have thinning of the hair and left-sided testicular atrophy, but otherwise no abnormalities. On neurological examination, atrophy and paresis were found of the facial musculature, showing the facies myopathica, atrophy of the sternocleidomastoid muscles, forearm muscles, and small hand muscle atrophy. Myotonic symptoms were present in the hands and feet.

His second and third cases were the father and an aunt of the first case. The father, a teacher, showed symtoms at the age of 42. Myotonia of legs and hands was followed by dysarthria and baldness. A classical facies myopathica, nasal speech, and atrophic sternocleidomastoids were found, as well as paresis and atrophy of forearm and hand muscles and the muscles of the lower legs. The aunt, a sister of the second case, said to be not very intelligent, showed myotonia at the age of 42. On examination, 14 years later, a typical facies myopathica was present, intact sternocleidomastoids, and atrophy of forearm and lower leg muscles.

The fourth patient, a 36-year-old male, was the youngest of 10 sibs. A brother 21 years older and a sister 10 years older had the same symptom complex, very much like the first three cases. His fifth case is only briefly described in a footnote, and for the sixth patient he refers to an earlier publication (1905).

Curschmann, in the commentary, defined the hand, forearm, sternocleidomastoid, and facial atrophy type as Steinert's disease. He explicitly stated that myotonia became manifest before the atrophy and paresis, and he accentuated the baldness in four of his five male patients, as well as the loss of libido; three had testicular atrophy. Another as yet unidentified sign was the presence of bilateral cataract in his fourth case at the age of 30. Curschmann was the first to draw attention to this nonmuscular sign. He also noticed the tendency for earlier onset in successive generations in the first family, a phenomenon we now call anticipation.

Finally, a paragraph is devoted to symptomatology and pathogenesis. First he mentioned the hereditary nature of the disease. Furthermore, he noticed a peculiar distribution of the paretic and atrophic extensor forearm muscles and the myotonic antagonists. He also observed (as an involuntary myotonic phenomenon) the tendency for identical contralateral movements upon movement of the myotonic muscles. His contribution to the pathogenetic mechanism is minimal, autointoxication and hormonal agents being proposed as causes.

Myotonic dystrophy is an autosomal dominant disorder in which a characteristic pattern of dystrophic muscles is accompanied by myotonia and by specific abnormalities of a variety of other systems.[6] The myotonic dystrophy gene is located on chromosome 19q13.3, and the underlying molecular defect is an unstable trinucleotide repeat sequence CTG in the protein kinase–encoding gene.[7–9] The size of the repeat in patients varies from 50 to several thousands of times versus less than 38 in controls. The matter of anticipation thus seems clearly explained. It is fascinating to note that Curschmann also was aware of this phenomenon, albeit unable to explain it.[5]

Among the early descriptions of myotonic dystrophy were Erb's paper in which he mentioned "genetic heterogeneity" in families suffering from Thomsen's myotonia congenita, including cases with muscle wasting. Johann Hoffmann reported a case with myotonia and wasting of the facial, sternomastoid, and forearm muscles. He also mentioned a brother and sister with facial, sternomastoid, and distal limb wasting, weakness, and myotonia. Other cases were described by Rossolimo, Nonne, and Pässler, and a less convincing case by Dana.[10]

However, it was Steinert who described the clinical picture in minute detail,[1] and it has been settled since then and later by others.[5, 11] Batten and Gibb[1] gave a detailed description in the same year as Steinert's study of the localization of atrophic muscles, but other dystrophic signs remained unmentioned, and their article lacked a post-mortem study. Curschmann essentially did not add to Steinert's observations except for the important occurrence of cataracts. And he honored Steinert as the first one to recognize the characteristic symtom complex as a distinct disease entity.

The clinical syndrome described by Steinert has not lost its immense value. In the future, it may well be that the present eponym will bear another name reflecting modern genetic techniques pinpointing genes and gene products. But until then, Steinert's name will be linked unforgettably to dystrophia myotonica.

Acknowledgments

The help of Jens Blecher and Petra Hesse of the Leipzig University Archives (Director Dr. Gerald Wiemers); Mrs. L. Künstling of the Leipzig University Library "Albertina"; and Dr. Natalja Decker of the Leipzig University Karl-Sudhoff Institute for History of Medicine and Natural Sciences, who provided me with hitherto unpublished biographical data of Hans Steinert as well as the photograph of Hans Curschmann has been invaluable and is very much appreciated.

References

1. Steinert H. Myopathologische Beiträge, I: Ueber das klinische und anatomische Bild des Muskelschwunds der Myotoniker. *Dtsch Z Nervenheilk.* 1909;37:58–104.
2. Nonne M. Hans Curschmann. *Dtsch Z Nervenheilk.* 1950;164:423–426.
3. Deusch G. Hans Curschmann. *Dtsch Med Wochenschr.* 1950;75:686.
4. Meythaler F. Hans Curschmann. *Ärtzliche Forschung.* 1950;4:229–231.
5. Curschmann H. Über familiäre atrophische Myotonie. *Dtsch Z Nervenheilk.* 1912;45:161–202.
6. Harper P S. *Myotonic Dystrophy.* 2nd ed. London: WR Saunders Company; 1989.
7. Aslanidis C G, Jansen G, Amemiya G, et al. Cloning of the essential myotonic dystrophy region and mapping of the putative defect. *Nature (Lond).* 1992;355:548–551.
8. Buxton J, Shelbourne P, Davies J, et al. Detection of an unstable fragment of DNA specific to individuals with myotonic dystrophy. *Nature (Lond).* 1992;355–548.
9. Harley H G, Brook J D, Rundle S A, et al. Expansion of an unstable DNA region and phenotypic variation in myotonic dystrophy. *Nature (Lond).* 1992;355:545–546.
10. Pearce JMS. Early accounts of dystrophia myotonica. *J Neurol Neurosurg Psychiatry.* 1992; 55:920.
11. Batten F E, Gibb H P. Myotonia atrophica. *Brain.* 1909;32:187–205.

45

DOWN'S SYNDROME

Conor Ward

John Langdon Down was born in 1828, in Torpoint in Cornwall. He worked in his father's grocery shop until he was 18 years old. Having first qualified in pharmacy, he entered the London Hospital Medical School at the age of 25. He was a triple gold medalist and immediately after taking his degree he was appointed medical superintendent of the Royal Earlswood Asylum for Idiots in Surrey. Within a year he was successful in the examinations for the membership of the Royal College of Physicians and for the M.D. of London University.[1]

Langdon-Down, as he called himself after 1868, is best remembered for his description of the eponymous syndrome. He was also one of the most distinguished London physicians of his day. He correctly forecast that his case of Prader Willi syndrome would be found to have ovarian hypoplasia.[2] His outlook was liberal. He left his well paid post in Earlswood in 1868, following a dispute with the hospital board concerning his wife's right to work. He then established Normansfield, a highly successful training and educational center for the upper classes. Normansfield remained under the control of the Langdon-Down family for 102 years, responsibility passing first to his medical sons Reginald and Percival and then to Percival's son Norman. Langdon-Down had an extensive private practice and at the time of his death (1896) he was one of London's wealthiest doctors. His granddaughter Stella married the neurologist, Russell Brain.

Langdon-Down supported every liberal cause. He was in favor of the admission of women to all the professions, including the clergy, and of women's right to vote. He was an opponent of slavery. He wrote about the need to provide special learning opportunities for the educationally disabled of all classes.[3] He was a man of deep religious conviction and he employed a full-time chaplain in Normansfield. At the age of 26 he published a pamphlet emphasizing the scriptural account of creation.[4] He was indeed an eminent Victorian.

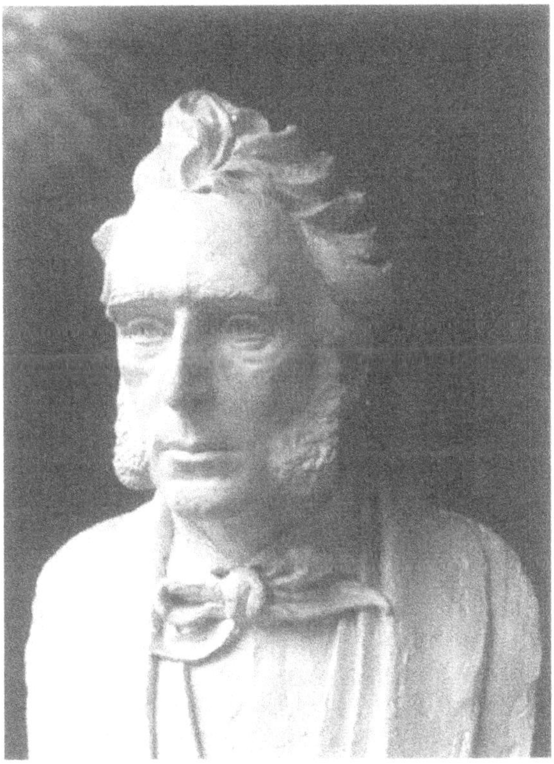

Figure 45–1. John Langdon Down (1828–1896). Bust in the Normansfield Hospital.

Earlswood had been beset by public criticism and by suggestions of neglect. Langdon Down initiated wide-ranging and successful reforms. In 1859 he was appointed to a parallel post as assistant physician to the London Hospital. He began to study the Earlswood patients in depth. He carried out autopsy examinations on those who died and he started a unique photographic survey of his patients. He rapidly established an international reputation.

John Connolly (1794–1866), the reformer of psychiatric hospitals, was official Visitor to Earlswood. Connolly was one of the small remaining group of enthusiasts for phrenology, involving the correlation of the external contours of the skull with specific intellectual and psychological characteristics. In 1862 Langdon Down gave the first indication that he had identified a specific group of patients of special interest. He had examined the palate and tongue of 200 out of 320 residents. Reporting on the tongue he said:

> In 16 cases the tongue presented a sodden appearance and exhibited transverse furrows on its dorsal surface; in all these patients one is able to trace a marked physiological and psychological agreement. So much do they resemble one another that they might readily be taken for members of the same family. Twelve appeared to have very large tongues which in most cases interfered with speech.[5]

In 1865 he began to use Blumenbach's anthropological classification to group the residents as Caucasian, Ethiopian, Malayan, American Indian, and Mongolian.[6]

He reported that there were numerous representatives of the great Caucasian family. Concerning the Mongolian group he wrote:

> It is to this division I wish, in this paper, to draw special attention. A very large number of congenital idiots are typical Mongols. So marked is this that when placed side by side it is difficult to believe that the specimens compared are not children of the same parents. The number of idiots who arrange themselves around the Mongolian type is so great, and they present such a close resemblance to one another in mental power, that I shall describe an idiot member of this racial division, selected from the large number to have fallen under my observation . . .
>
> The face is flat and broad and destitute of prominence. The cheeks are roundish and extended laterally. The eyes are obliquely placed and the internal canthi more than normally distanced from one another. The palpebral fissure is very narrow. The forehead is wrinkled transversely . . . The lips are large and thick with transverse fissures. The tongue is long, thick, and much roughened. The nose is small. The skin has a slight dirty yellowish tinge and is deficient in elasticity, giving the impression of being too large for the body. The boy's aspect is such that it is difficult to realise that he is the child of Europeans, but so frequently are these characteristics presented that there can be no doubt that these ethnic features are the result of degeneration.
>
> The Mongolian type of idiocy occurs in more than 10% of the cases which are presented to me. They are always congenital and never result from accidents after uterine life. They have considerable powers of imitation, even bordering on being mimics. They are humorous and a lively sense of the ridiculous often colours their mimicry. This faculty of imitation may be cultivated to a very great extent, and a practical direction given to the results obtained. They are usually able to speak; the speech is thick and indistinct but may be improved very greatly by a well directed scheme of tongue gymnastics. The co-ordinating faculty is abnormal, but not so defective that it cannot be greatly strengthened. By systematic training considerable manipulative skill may be obtained. The circulation is feeble and however much advance is made intellectually in the summer, some amount of retrogression may be expected in the winter. Their mental and physical capabilities are, in fact, directly as the temperature. The improvement which training effects in them is greatly in excess of what would be predicated if one did not know the characteristics of the type. The life expectancy, however, is far below average and the tendency is to the tuberculosis which I believe to be the hereditary origin of the degeneracy.

Addressing the Obstetric Society in 1876 he referred to the oblique position of the eyes and to the "semi-lunar folds of skin at the inner canthus, which I have been accustomed to describe as epicanthic folds." He referred to "the site of implantation of the ear which was usually placed further back in relation to the head and face than in normal children." No feature was more worthy of attention, he said, than the configuration and position of the external ear.[7]

Mongolism, or Mongolian idiocy, gradually became a descriptive term. Ireland used it in 1877,[8] Tanner and Meadows in 1879,[9] Ashby and Wright in 1882,[10] and Brush in 1891.[11] Tredgold in his major 1903 review entitled "Amentia" devoted a section to Mongolism, but without mentioning Langdon-Down.[12]

There was a diversion in 1876 when Mitchell and Fraser published a detailed report on what they described as Kalmuc idiocy. This was clearly the same condition which Langdon-Down had called Mongolian idiocy. They had overlooked Langdon-

Down's previous description.[13] Shuttleworth used both terms,[14] but Kalmuc idiocy never gained acceptance and in the twentieth century Mongolism was generally used by authors such as Rainsford[15] and Penrose.[16]

A new proposal emerged in 1961. A group of the world's leading geneticists wrote to the *Lancet* pointing out that the term Mongolism was offensive and embarrassing to overseas research workers. They listed four alternatives—Langdon Down anomaly, Down's syndrome or anomaly, congenital acromicria, or trisomy 21 anomaly.[17] The first of these was clearly inappropriate. When Langdon Down described the condition in 1866 his family name was Down. He changed it to Langdon-Down two years later when he went into private practice in Welbeck Street in London. Congenital acromicria might be seen as too restrictive.

Jerome Lejeune, who discovered the extra chromosome 21, was one of the signatories and indeed there was a case for linking his own name to a new descriptive term.[18] Many, however, favor a convention that eponyms should be conferred posthumously only.[19] If accepted, his name could perhaps have been linked with that of Edouard Seguin, a distinguished French doctor working in the United States. Seguin suspected that there was something different about a group whom he called "furfuraceous cretins," but he said that "the incomplete studies did not permit of the group being accurately classified and it was better to leave things as they were." Seguin had described a nine-year-old girl, small for her age, gay in temperament, with short fingers, described as "unfinished," and a rounded head. He considered her to have the special form of cretinism, which he described as "furfuraceous."[20] The distinction between Mongolism and cretinism continued to be debated for almost a century. Seguin suspected that there was something different about the "furfuraceous" patients, but if he had seen them as being specifically different from cretins rather than special type of cretin, his publication would have appeared a few months ahead of Langdon Down's and, by convention, would have taken precedence in the naming of the condition.

There were clearly differences of opinion among the signatories of the joint letter on nomenclature. One of them, Cedric Carter from Great Ormond Street Hospital, made a preemptive strike and immediately published a paper using the eponym Down's syndrome.[21] There were two objections which prompted the editor to intervene.[22,23] He pronounced his judgment in a brief notice: Down's syndrome was, he said, an appropriate alternative to Mongolian idiocy until the chromosome abnormality in the disorder had been fully elucidated and a new significant term could be coined.[24] Benda, another of the joint signatories, wrote in 1962 that he had always used the term acromicria.[25] He lauded Fraser and Mitchell, describing their rival 1876 Kalmuc idiocy paper as most important[13] and describing Seguin as more scientific than Down. He gathered no support. There was no further discussion and Down's syndrome came to be universally used. Another alternative, not considered, was Downs' syndrome. Reginald Langdon-Down, the eldest surviving son of the family, described the single palmar crease and reported on the body proportions in Down's syndrome in 1909. His contribution, however, was probably not of sufficient weight to justify linking his name with that of his father.[26]

The *Index Medicus* changed from Down's syndrome to Down syndrome in 1992, although in that year 125 authors used the apostrophe against 101 who referred to Down syndrome. Since then opinion has remained fairly evenly balanced between these alternatives. No authoritative body has pronounced on the matter and many authors will continue to use the term Down's syndrome on the basis of its historical validity. This usage was given the approval of the World Health Organization in 1966 and the decision has never been reversed.[27]

References

1. Ward O C. *John Langdon-Down: A Caring Pioneer.* London: Royal Society of Medicine Press; 1998:19.
2. Ward O C. Langdon-Down's 1864 case of Prader Willi syndrome. *J R Soc Med.* 1997;90: 694–696.
3. Langdon-Down JLH. *On the Education and Training of the Feeble in Mind.* London: Lewis; 1876.
4. Down, JLH. *Nature's balance. A prize essay on the wisdom and beneficience of the Creator as displayed in the compensation between the animal and vegetable kingdoms.* London: Crockfords; 1853.
5. Down JLH. On the condition of the mouth in infancy. *Lancet.* 1862;1:65–68.
6. Down JLH. Observations on an Ethnic Classification of Idiots. *London Hospital Reports.* 1866;3:259–262.
7. Down JLH. The obstetric aspects of idiocy. In: *Transactions of the Obstetric Society 1876.* London: Churchill; 1887:210–217. Reprinted in: *Mental Affections of Childhood and Youth.*
8. Ireland W W. *On Idiocy and Imbecility.* London: Churchill; 1877:55.
9. Tanner T H, Meadows A. *Diseases of Infancy and Children.* London: Renshaw; 1879:213–217.
10. Ashby H, Wright G A. *The Diseases of Children, Medical and Surgical.* London: Longmans Green; 1882:461–464.
11. Brush E. Idiocy. In: Keating JM, ed. *Cyclopedia of the Diseases of Children.* London: J Pentland Young; 1889–1891:1027.
12. Tredgold A F. Amentia. *Practitioner.* 1903;2:354–382.
13. Mitchell A, Fraser R. Kalmuc idiocy. *J Ment Sci.* 1876;22:169–179.
14. Shuttleworth G E. Clinical lecture on idiocy and imbecility. *Br Med J.* 1886;1:183–184.
15. Rainsford A A. Review of the admission of the imbeciles of the Mongolian type during the last 20 years. *J Ment Sci.* 1917;44:238–241.
16. Penrose L S. Mongolism. *Br Med Bull.* 1961;17:184–189.
17. Allen G, Benda C J, Böök G A, Carter C O, et al. Letter. *Lancet.* 1961;2:935.
18. Lejeune J, Gautier M, Turpin R. Étude des chromosomes somatiques de neuf enfants mongoliens. *C R Acad Sci.* 1959;248:1721–1722.
19. Warkany J. *Congenital Malformations.* Chicago: Year Book Publishers; 1971:47.
20. Seguin E. *Idiocy and Its Treatment by the Physiological Method.* New York: Wood; 1866:381.
21. Carter C O. Risk of parents who have had one child with Down's syndrome (Mongolism) having another child similarly affected. *Lancet.* 1961;2:785–788.
22. Spalding JMK. Letter. *Lancet.* 1961;2:935.
23. Papworth M H. Letter. *Lancet.* 1961;2:935.
24. *Lancet.* Editorial comment. 1961;2:935.
25. Benda C E. Letter. *Lancet.* 1962;1:163.
26. Langdon-Down R L. Report. *Br Med J.* 1909;2:665.
27. Howard-Jones N. On the diagnostic term Down's syndrome. *Med Hist.* 1979;22:102–104.

46

DUCHENNE'S DYSTROPHY

Peter Hudgson

The use of eponyms in human biology tends to confuse nosologic clarity. The same cannot be said of Duchenne muscular dystrophy (DMD) which was a clear-cut pathological and genetic entity, well before the introduction of recombinant DNA technology. In light of this, the words of Lord Walton in his foreword to the Emerys' classic study[1] of the history of the disease—that DMD remains "an apposite term"—elicits some sympathy. Nevertheless, the historical evidence that DMD may be a rather less than completely "apposite" eponym is accumulating steadily and we owe the Emerys a considerable debt of gratitude for their unique contribution.[2,3]

Guillaume Benjamin Amand Duchenne "de Boulogne" chose his *post-nom* to distinguish himself from Duchesne (de Paris), who was an esteemed physician in the local salons at the time. He was born of maritime stock in Boulogne-sur-mer (or Boulogne, as it is known elsewhere in Europe) on 17 September 1806, and was blessed with a provincial accent which probably cost him dear in Paris in his earlier years.[4] In spite of this, he had clearly inherited his father Jean's courage and determination. The latter was awarded the Légion d'Honneur by Napoleon for his distinguished contribution as a sea captain fighting against the English in the Napoleonic Wars.

He underwent his then traditional medical training in Paris, graduating with his thesis *Essai sur le Brûlure* [Treatise on burn] in 1831, after what was regarded as "an undistinguished career,"[1] with the firm intention of becoming a family practitioner. However, his return to Boulogne was blighted by the death in 1833 of his young wife with puerperal sepsis, some two weeks after giving birth to their son Emile. He was subsequently estranged from his son through the malevolent agency of his mother-in-law—a classic example of life imitating art! He returned to Paris in 1842, at the age of 36. He started a private practice and never had a hospital or university appointment.

Gradually he became recognized for his clinical insights and skill. He used to visit several hospitals in Paris, accompanied by his electrical equipment (*avec sa pile et sa bobine;* i.e., his electric battery and his spool), to examine various interesting patients.[4] He communicated his knowledge of neurological diseases to staff members and students while trying to increase his knowledge of nervous diseases. Charcot and Trousseau, with whom he became friendly, spread his fame. Gradually Duchenne turned from the clinic to pathological investigation. Next to applying electricity, he also used the new technique of photography, notably in his book on the study of facial muscles and human expression, which was referred to by Charles Darwin.[5,6] He described locomotor ataxia (1858–1859), which Ernst Horn and Moritz Romberg had published on previously[7] (see Chapters 26 and 48). Duchenne died from cerebral hemorrhage on 15 September 1875. The medical journals of Paris only briefly mentioned his death. However, Charcot considered him one of his most important teachers and he is now considered one of the founders of modern electrodiagnostics and electrotherapy.[8]

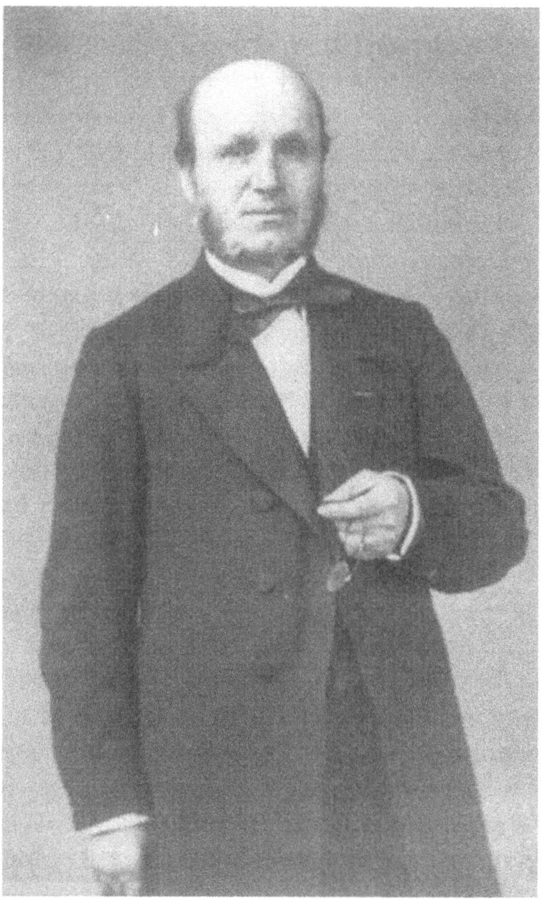

Figure 46–1. Guillaume Benjamin Amand Duchenne (1806–1875). Courtesy of Medizinhistorisches Institut, Zurich, Switzerland.

Duchenne developed electrical therapy of muscles and later applied it as a diagnostic tool. He distinguished two types of muscle disorders: (1) degenerated muscles that did not respond to stimulation or proportionately to the number of residual muscle fibers; and (2) muscles that reacted to stimulation as they had recently been denervated. He published his experience and knowledge of muscles and muscle diseases in several papers, and in *De l'électrisation localisée de son application à la pathologie et à la thérapeutique*[9] and *La physiologie des mouvements.*[10]

His interest in the electrical stimulation of weak, paralyzed muscles led to his seminal study of what we now call DMD.[11]

> La découverte de la paralysie pseudo-hypertrophique remonte au commencement de l'année 1858 . . . Ayant recueilli, en trois années, quelques faits absolument semblables, et dont je ne connaissais pas d'analogues dans la science, je me suis cru fondé à considérer cette affection musculaire comme une espèce morbide non encore décrite et propre à l'enfance.[12]

[The discovery of pseudohypertrophic muscular paralysis goes back to the beginning of the year 1858 . . . Having collected, in 3 years, several similar cases, for which I knew nothing analogous in science, I believed myself justified in regarding this muscular affection as a disease entity not previously described and peculiar to childhood.][13]

Duchenne had published the clinical characteristics in the second edition of his *Electrisation localisée* (1861), but he had since observed new cases. Similar observations had been made in Germany and France, influencing his ideas about the condition. He summarized his first case as follows:

> Paralysie pseudo-hypertrophique; début dans la première enfance, par la faiblesse des membres inférieurs; grossissement considérable, à l'âge 7 ans, des muscles moteurs des membres inférieurs et des extenseurs de la colonne vertébro-lombaire; généralisation progressive de la paralysie et abolition complète de tous les mouvements, à 13 ans et demi; intelligence obtuse; mort phthisique, à 15 ans.[12]

[Pseudohypertrophic paralysis; beginning in infancy with weakness of the lower extremities; considerable enlargement of the muscles of the lower extremities and the extensors of the lumbar vertebral column to the age of 7 years; progressive generalization of the paralysis and complete abolition of all movements at 13½ years; intelligence dull; pulmonary death at 15 years].[13]

Duchenne had noticed the weakness in the legs and trunk, leading to lordosis when the child was standing or walking. He also described the lateral swinging of the trunk while walking. He had an instrument constructed in order to be able to perform biopsies. A previously used instrument, *Mideldorff's harpoon,* appeared unsuitable for this purpose.

> The histological punch should be introduced perpendicular to the direction of the muscle. Its hook should grasp the muscle transversely even at the risk of not bringing anything back.

ARCHIVES GÉNÉRALES
DE MÉDECINE

JANVIER 1868.

MÉMOIRES ORIGINAUX

RECHERCHES SUR LA PARALYSIE MUSCULAIRE PSEUDO-HYPERTROPHIQUE OU PARALYSIE MYO-SCLÉROSIQUE,

Par le Dr DUCHENNE (de Boulogne).

INTRODUCTION (1).

A. *Définition et dénomination de la maladie.* — La maladie que je vais décrire est caractérisée principalement 1° par un affaiblissement des mouvements, siégeant généralement, au début, dans les muscles moteurs des membres inférieurs et dans les spinaux lombaires, s'étendant progressivement aux membres supérieurs, dans une période ultime, et s'aggravant en même temps jusqu'à l'abolition des mouvements, 2° par l'augmentation du volume soit (ordinairement) de quelques-uns des muscles paralysés, soit (exceptionnellement) de presque tous les muscles paralysés, 3° par l'hyperplasie du tissu connectif interstitiel des muscles paralysés, avec production abondante ou de tissu fibreux, ou de vésicules adipeuses dans une période plus avancée.

Je propose d'appeler cette maladie *paralysie musculaire pseudo-hypertrophique*, d'après ses principaux signes cliniques objectifs, ou *paralysie myo-sclérosique*, d'après ses caractères anatomiques périphériques. Ces dénominations seront justifiées ultérieurement par l'étude de la symptomatologie, et de l'anatomie pathologique

(1) Les figures qui se rapportent aux observations IV et XII paraîtront, dans le numéro prochain, aux articles Symptomatologie et Anatomie pathologiques.

Figure 46–2. Title page of Duchenne's paper on muscular dystophy.[12]

In the first case to which he applied the method, which he called *living pathological anatomy*, he found:

> Hyperplasia of the interstitial connective tissue, with proliferation of more or less abundant fibrous tissue . . . [it is] associated with a slight or moderate number of fatty vesicles. According to the observations in Germany, it is replaced by a considerable quantity of adipose tissue.[13]

Duchenne emphasized the absence of fever and sensory disturbance. He had also noted that the functions of the bladder and intestine remained normal.*

Whether or not the perpetuation of the unshared eponym can be justified remains to be seen, as the Emerys have made a powerful case for wider recognition of the pioneering contribution the English physician Edward Meryon made some 13 years earlier.[1] Edward Meryon was born of Huguenot ancestry in Rye in 1807. He was registered as a medical student on 1 October 1829 at the University of London (now University College, London) and had a distinguished undergraduate career, gaining many "glittering prizes." There followed a period of several years in which he married, raised five children, gradually established himself as a physician, and proceeded to the M.B. (London) in 1841 (University College, London did not offer a degree in medicine until 1839). He was awarded the M.D. in 1844 and was elected Fellow of the Royal College of Physicians in 1859. He also became a Fellow of the Royal Medical and Chirurgical Society (later the Royal Society of Medicine) and spent two sessions as a lecturer in comparative anatomy at St. Thomas' Hospital during this period. It seems likely that he developed his interest in diseases of the nervous system and skeletal muscle at the same time (his first publication, "On Fatty Degeneration of the Voluntary Muscles," appeared in 1851).

In Meryon's original paper presented to the Royal Medico-Chirurgical Society on 9 December 1951, he described three families, P, H, and T, all of whom were tainted with the genetic defect now known to be responsible for X-linked primary muscle cell disease. The affected children in families P and H had clinical courses consistent with Duchenne's disease, whereas the later onset and relatively mild course of the affected boys in family T were much more in keeping with Becker muscular dystrophy. In the discussion following his presentation which was reported in *Lancet*,[14] Meryon made it clear that he believed the condition to be a primary disorder of skeletal muscle, not the spinal cord, a vital point he reiterated in the more detailed account published in the Society's *Transactions* the following year.[15] (Duchenne in 1868 mistakenly claimed that Meryon had confused his cases with progressive muscular atrophy, an error corrected by Meryon himself[16] and by Gowers.)[17,18]

In the latter publication, Meryon's description of the postmortem histopathology of DMD was infinitely superior to that of later authors, for instance, Erb.[19] This writer has had the privilege of seeing Professor Emery's color reproductions of Meryon's *camera lucida* drawings of "granular degeneration of the voluntary muscles." Meryon (1852) emphasized the early disappearance of the transverse striae

* For further reading of Duchenne's work see G.B.A. Duchenne, *Selections from the Clinical Works of Dr. Duchenne (de Boulogne)*. Translated, edited, and condensed by G. V. Poore. London: Sydenham Society, 1883, pp. 173–191.

together with the ultimate replacement of the internal structure of the fibers with "granular material" and fat droplets.[14]

Meryon also noted that "the sarcolemma or tissue of the elementary fibre was broken down and destroyed," a process now known to be fundamental to the inception of the disease process in DMD *in utero* because of the abnormal cytoskeletal protein in the sarcolemma, the phenotypic expression of the genetic abnormality in this disease. (The concept of "preclinical" disease in the affected male child has been well recognized since the 1960s.)[20,21] Certainly neuropathological studies on the early sarcolemmal abnormalities in DMD have preoccupied many authorities since the mid-1980s and certainly antedated the identification of dystrophin.[22]

Meryon recognized the selective affection of male issue in the eight sibships he analyzed in detail, but he mistakenly concluded *all* males in a tainted family would be affected.[15,16] Mendelian genetics were unknown until the turn of the century. It is likely that he also probably (unknowingly) identified manifesting carriers in one of the families he studied, describing "a very uncommon development of the gastrocnemii muscles" in (female) members of the mother's family.[16] This has proved to be the single most useful clinical pointer to carrier status in young women from families carrying the gene.

The Emerys, in analyzing the possible reasons for previous neglect of Meryon's seminal contribution, concluded that his brief publications were simply not read by others working in the field.[1] In sharp contrast, Duchenne's encyclopedic description of the clinicopathological features of DMD in a French journal no longer extant attracted a great deal of attention,[12] although it was clear that he was aware of Meryon's work (see below). His reasons for refusing to acknowledge priority remain obscure, and he may have misunderstood (perhaps because of the translation) how Meryon had characterized the disease. In addition, his judgment in this respect may well have been skewed by his prolonged and severe unhappiness (which was presumably a consequence of his early domestic travails).

There can be no argument about Duchenne's comprehensive description of the clinical features of the disease that bears his name. Certainly it was much more detailed than Meryon's earlier account, although it was refined to a certain extent by later writers, notably Gowers,[17,18] and reviewed relatively recently by Brody and Wilkins.[13] Further, Duchenne's development of the muscle biopsy punch (*emporte-pièce histologique*) enabled him to study the antemortem histopathology of DMD. Not surprisingly, he was struck by the proliferation of fibrous connective tissue, which he thought might be fundamental to the pathogenesis of the disease. He also noted the accumulation of fat with the passage of time and the loss of the transverse striae described previously by Meryon. However, he was not particularly concerned about the state of the sarcolemma and most certainly did not record the active necrobiotic changes characteristic of the earlier stages of Duchenne muscular dystrophy.[20] This is scarcely surprising, since he was investigating boys with well-established clinical disease. Duchenne's pathological observations led him to coin the term *"paralysie pseudo-hypertrophique"* to account for the striking enlargement of calf and other muscles in clinical cases. We know now that this feature is due to genuine hypertrophy of surviving muscle fibers, particularly in the earlier stages of the disease.

Other descriptions of the affliction had been published before Duchenne. Wilhelm Griesinger (1817–1868) professor of psychiatry in Berlin (predecessor of Carl Westphal), well known for his bon mot "*Geisteskrankheiten sind Nervenkrankheiten*" (mental diseases are brain diseases), described muscular dystrophy with pseudohypertrophy in 1865.[23] The condition has been called "Duchenne–Griesinger disease" for some time. Probably Pierre Paul Broca (1824–1880) described the condition as well (1851).[24]

One has to decide issues like this on their historical merits alone and it is hard to escape the conclusion that Meryon deserves priority in this case if eponyms are to be in any way meaningful (the Emerys' subtitle for their monograph was "*Duchenne Muscular Dystrophy or Meryon's Disease?*" Nevertheless, it would be a major (if not revolutionary) semantic somersault to overturn a century-old tradition and one that would be bound to generate more than a few ripples among our friends and colleagues in neuroscience on the other side of the *pas de Calais.*

Acknowledgments

I am deeply indebted to David Gardner-Medwin and several colleagues for their generous help in providing reference material. I thank Alan and Marcia Emery and their tireless researches into the historical background of this model of genetically determined muscle disease. Irene Lea typed the manuscript with her customary skill and diligence.

References

1. Emery AEH, Emery MLH. *The history of a genetic disease: Duchenne Muscular Dystrophy or Meryon's Disease?* London: Royal Society of Medicine Press; 1995.
2. Emery AEH. Duchenne muscular dystrophy—Meryon's disease. *Neuromusc Dis.* 1993; 3:263–266.
3. Emery MLH, Emery AEH. Edward Meryon (1807–1880): his life and Huguenot background. *J Med Biogr.* 1998;6:1–10.
4. Adams R D. Amand Duchenne (1806–1875). In: Haymaker W, Schiller F, eds. *Founders of Neurology.* 2nd ed. Springfield, Ill: Charles C Thomas; 1970:430–434.
5. Duchenne G-B. *Mécanisme de la physionomie humaine.* Paris: Renouard; 1862.
6. Cuthbertson R A. The highly original Dr. Duchenne. In: Duchenne de Boulogne G B; Cuthbertson R A, ed-trans. *The mechanism of human facial expression.* Cambridge: Cambridge University Press; 1990:225–241.
7. Duchenne de Boulogne GBA. De l'ataxie locomotrice progressive. *Arch Gén Méd.* 1858; 12:641–652; 1859;13:36–62, 158–181, 417–451.
8. Hirsch A *Biographisches Lexikon der hervorragenden Aerzte aller Zeiten und Völker.* Wien: Urban & Schwarzenberg; 1885.
9. Duchenne GBA. *De l'électrisation localisée et de son application à la pathologie et à la thérapeutique.* Paris: Baillière; 1855.
10. Duchenne GBA. *La physiologie des mouvements, démontrée à l'aide de l'expérimentation éléctrique et de l'observation clinique.* Paris: Baillière; 1867.
11. Duchenne GBA (de Boulogne). De la paralysie atrophique graisseuse de l'enfance. *Arch Gén Méd.* 1864;2:28–50; 184–209; 441–455.
12. Duchenne GBA. Recherches sur la paralysie musculaire pseudo-hypertrophique, ou paralysie myosclérosique. *Arch Gén Méd.* 1868;11:5–25, 179–209, 305–321, 421–443, 552–588.

13. Brody I A, Wilkins R H. Duchenne's muscular dystrophy. *Arch Neurol.* 1968;19:628–636.
14. Meryon E. On fatty degeneration of the voluntary muscles. *Lancet.* 1851;2:588–589.
15. Meryon E. On granular and fatty degeneration of the voluntary muscles. *Medico-Chir Trans.* 1852;35:73–84.
16. Meryon E. *Practical and Pathological Researches on the Various Forms of Paralysis.* London: Churchill; 1864:200–215.
17. Gowers W R. *Pseudo-hypertrophic Muscular Paralysis: A Clinical Lecture.* London: Churchill; 1879.
18. Gowers W R. *A Manual of Diseases of the Nervous System.* London: Churchill; 1888;2:836–842.
19. Erb W. Über die juvenilen Form der progressiven Muskelatrophie und ihre Beziehung zur sogenannten Pseudohypertrophie der Muskeln. *Dtsch Arch Klin Med.* 1884;34:467–519.
20. Pearson C M. Muscular dystrophy: review and recent observations. *Am J Med.* 1963; 35:632–645.
21. Hudgson P, Pearce G W, Walton J N. Preclinical muscular dystrophy: histopathological changes observed on muscle biopsy. *Brain.* 1967;90:565–576.
22. Hoffman E P, Brown R H, Kunkel L M. Dystrophin: the protein product of the Duchenne muscular dystrophy locus. *Cell.* 1987;51:919.
23. Griesinger W. Ueber Muskelhypertrophie. *Arch Heilkd.* 1865;6:1–13.
24. Schiller F. *Paul Broca: Founder of French Anthropology, Explorer of the Brain.* New York: Oxford University Press; 1992:94.

47

VON ECONOMO'S ENCEPHALITIS

Nicolaas J. M. Arts

In the winter of 1916–1917, Europe was seized by a strange epidemic. In some patients the disease started abruptly, in others insidiously, like influenza. After the initial phase, the patients developed cranial nerve palsies, motor disorders, behavioral changes, and variable lethargy. Some patients were only mildly affected, others were stuporous. An English physician who had witnessed the epidemic in Glasgow wrote afterwards:

> There is nothing in the history of medicine to compare with the phantasmagoria of disorder manifested in the course of this strange malady . . . Into the maze of contradictory phenomena it seemed almost impossible to read anything like a rationalized order of events which might be termed a disease entity.[1]

The epidemic spread to Asia, Australia, and the Americas within a few years, thus becoming a veritable pandemic. After ten years it disappeared as mysteriously as it had come, leaving millions dead and an untold number of patients in nursing homes, suffering from postencephalitic syndromes.

More than anyone else, it was Constantin Von Economo, a baron of Greek–Macedonian descent, who managed to find order in this maze of contradictory phenomena. He was an adventurous man, who loved flying, but who remained firmly on the ground when conducting scientific work. His methodical study of the first cases in Vienna enabled him to publish an accurate and comprehensive description of the disease, after having examined only seven patients with autopsy in two brains.

Constantin Alexander Von Economo was born on 21 August 1876 in Braila, Romania, not far from the Black Sea.[2–5] His ancestors were bishops in the Greek Orthodox Church—"Economo" means "elder of the parish." Von Economo was a cosmopolitan from birth. Born in Romania, of Greek parents, and educated by a French governess, he was raised in Trieste and spent his summers in the Salzkammergut, near Salzburg. He spoke Greek with his father, German with his mother, French with his sister Sophia and his older brother Dmitri, and Italian with his brother Leo. At school he was a very bright pupil. His interest in the brain and human behavior was aroused when, as a youth, he read *L'Uomo Delinquente* [The criminal] and *L'Uomo di Genio* [The man of genius] by the then famous Italian criminologist Cesare Lombroso. At 17, Von Economo was sent to Vienna to continue his studies at the Vienna Technical School, because his father had decided that he was to become an engineer. The story goes that Von Economo was fond of art, nature, and women, but most of all he loved books; as a student he skimped on his meals to be able to buy them. Engineering was definitely not his vocation and after a few years he was allowed to switch to medicine. He entered Vienna Medical School in 1895.

In 1899 he published his first scientific paper, "The Development of the Hypophysis in Birds," in which he gave the original description of the *pars infundibularis.* After qualifying as a doctor in 1901, he embarked on an open-ended "postgraduate course" at Europe's most celebrated neurological and psychiatric centers: a year at the Paris hospitals, a few months at the hospitals in Nancy and Strassburg, 18 months at Kraepelins clinic in Munich, a few months in Berlin, and several months in Trieste; but eventually he returned to Vienna.

In 1907, a new passion seized him: flying. He went to France to take flying lessons. After a year, he returned to Vienna with his pilot certificate and his own plane, the first in Austria. Before going to the clinic in the morning, he flew for two or three hours, and after finishing work at five in the evening, he immediately returned to the airfield. Eventually he had his own hangar, with several planes. In World War I, Von Economo organized the Austrian air force and volunteered as a battle pilot. His parents begged him to end his military career, but it was only after his younger brother had been killed on a battlefield in Italy in 1916 that Von Economo gave in and returned to his old post as assistant in the Psychiatric–Neurological Clinic of the University of Vienna.

In January 1917 Von Economo saw seven patients with many bizarre symptoms, but also with one common characteristic: a persistent, intractable stupor. He remembered a story his mother had told him about an epidemic witnessed in northern Italy in the 1890s, of a strange disease called *nona.* This disease appeared "in the form of a lethargy with delirium, and it developed a malignant character." Within three months after the outbreak of the Vienna epidemic, Von Economo published his first paper on "Encephalitis Lethargica."[6]

In 1918, both the war and the epidemic ended, at least in Vienna. For some time Von Economo's life became quiet and peaceful. He worked from 9 A.M. to 2 P.M. at the Psychiatric–Neurological Clinic. The remaining part of the afternoon he usually spent in his library, reading Dante, Shakespeare, Russian novels, religious classics, and books on Einstein's theory of relativity.

In 1919 Von Economo married Princess Karoline von Schönburg-Hartenstein. At the university he was given the position of an extraordinary professor, but without a salary; never in his entire career did Von Economo receive any money for his medical and scientific work.

In the same year, new epidemics of encephalitis lethargica occurred in Vienna and in many other cities all over the world; it had now become a pandemic. From

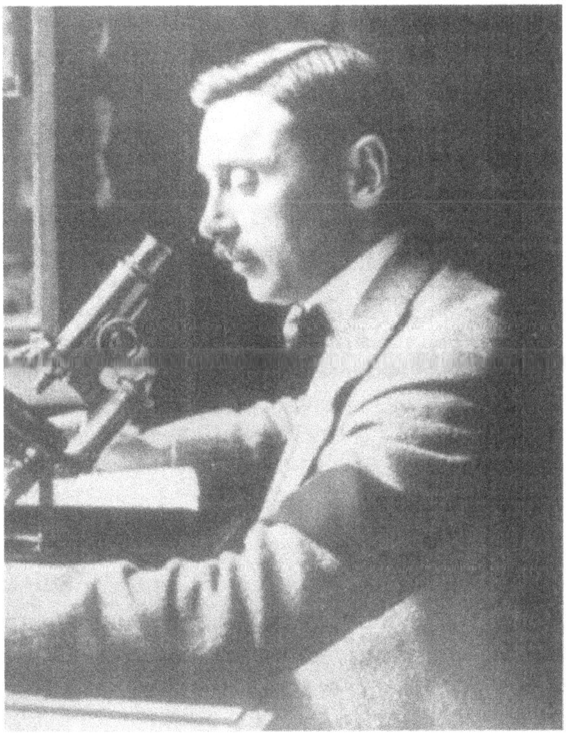

Figure 47–1. Constantin Alexander von Economo (1876–1931). From Ref. 4, permission of Thieme Verlag, Stuttgart, Germany.

everywhere, doctors turned to Von Economo as the preeminent authority on encephalitis lethargica, now also called "Von Economo's disease" or "Von Economo's encephalitis." The great number of patients enabled him to refine his knowledge of the disease and eventually he published 27 papers on it. Meanwhile he continued his high-society life, visiting salons, galleries, and operahouses with his wife. Full professorships were offered to him in Athens, Frankfurt, Munich, and Zurich, but he always declined. He preferred the freedom of an unsalaried extraordinary professorship as well as life among Viennese aristocratic circles. Though he visited his laboratory at the hospital no more than once or twice a week, he worked very hard. At home—a castle near Schneeberg—he worked tirelessly on a project begun in 1912 and which after 13 years resulted in *Die Cytoarchitektonik der Grosshirnrinde des erwachsenen Menschen,* a monumental atlas with an accompanying 810-page text on the microscopic anatomy of the human cerebral cortex.[7]

Sleep was another focus of interest for Von Economo.[8] He was the first to suggest the existence of a cerebral "sleep center," actively responsible for all physiological and behavioral changes that occurred during the transition from wakefulness to sleep. He correctly located it in an area adjacent to the hypothalamus.

In June 1931 Von Economo admitted, for the first time that his wife could recall, that he was tired. In the following months his condition deteriorated. A severe attack of angina pectoris was followed by coronary artery obstructions and cerebral embolism. He had to cut short his attendance at the first International Congress of

Neurology, in Berne, August 1931, where his vote was the only opposition to the separation of neurology and psychiatry. After a month of progressive illness, Von Economo died in his sleep on 21 October 1931, at the age of 55.

Von Economo's original description of encephalitis lethargica was published in the *Wiener klinische Wochenschrift* of 10 May 1917:

> Since Christmas, we have had the opportunity to observe a series of cases at the psychiatric clinic that do not fit any of our usual diagnoses. Nevertheless, they show a similarity in type of onset and symptomatology that forces one to group them into one clinical picture. We are dealing with a kind of sleeping sickness, so to speak, having an unusually prolonged course. The first symptoms are usually acute, with headaches and malaise. Then a state of somnolence appears, often associated with active delirium, from which the patient can be awakened easily. He is able to give appropriate answers and to comprehend the situation. He can follow commands correctly and is able to walk and stand, but if left by himself, relapses in the somnolent state.[6]

In five out of the seven cases the disease had started acutely, while in the other two there was an insidious onset. In the mildest cases, the sleepiness persisted only briefly, in other cases there was a delirious somnolence that lasted for weeks or even months, sometimes leading to stupor, coma, and death. In some cases there were signs of meningeal irritation and fever.

Usually these symptoms were followed by oculomotor palsies, palsies elsewhere, dystonia, spasms, increased reflexes, and pathological Babinski reflexes. A peculiar form of rigidity and cerebellar ataxia with tremor were also frequently observed—often unilaterally, like the pyramidal signs.

In his first report, Von Economo already tried to determine the cause of the new disease. Toxins and chemical agents were ruled out, as were bacteria and several viruses, such as influenza and poliomyelitis. Nevertheless, everything suggested some form of encephalitis. When two of the patients died rapidly, Von Economo was able to study their brains:

> The microscopic findings, which are identical in both cases, prove indisputably that we are dealing with a single inflammatory process. There is a tremendous infiltration by small cells of the vessels in the gray matter around the third ventricle, the area of the ocular nuclei, around the aqueduct of Sylvius and the floor of the fourth ventricle. This infiltration at first is limited to the vascular sheaths. It extends caudally into the medulla oblongata. The vessels of the spinal cord are less affected . . . We found the same alterations in the cerebrum, quite pronounced in certain areas. The blood vessels of the cortex were surrounded by a mantle of lymphocytes and plasma cells. Here too, we found the peculiar nests of polymorphonuclear leukocytes, as well as much more distinct neuronophagia than in other parts of the nervous system . . . The greater part of the cerebral cortex appears to be free of severe inflammatory lesions. The cerebral white matter remains, for the most part, free of the disease process. Only close to the cortex are the vessels of the white matter also infiltrated at times.[6]

In the spinal cord, the inflammation with lymphocytic infiltration did not show any clear predilection for nerve cells, which differentiated the new disease from poliomyelitis, the only established neurotropic virus at that time. Though there was severe hyperemia of the cerebral cortex and the spinal cord, bleeding generally did not occur—a fact Von Economo emphasized because influenzal encephalitis generally has a hemorrhagic character:

> Therefore, [he concluded,] we have the histological picture of a polioencephalitis cerebri, pontis et medullae oblongatae, with a slight poliomyelitis of a perivascular, inflammatory and diffusely infiltrative but not hemorrhagic and only slightly neuronophagic character.
>
> We therefore think that this encephalitis of somewhat epidemic occurrence, with the peculiar symptom of somnolence, and with characteristic anatomic-histologic findings, is a specific disease sui generis and must be caused by a specific, living virus. We also think that the remarkable paucity of the general symptoms of "Grippe" [flu] and the severity of the cerebral symptoms indicate a special affinity for the central nervous tissue, similar but not identical to the virus of poliomyelitis.[6]

Between 1917 and 1927, Von Economo continued to investigate all aspects of encephalitis lethargica; the results were described in 27 papers and a comprehensive monograph.[9] Eventually he discerned three types of encephalitis lethargica:

1. The somnolent–ophthalmoplegic form, with a prodrome of fever, malaise, chills, and nasal catarrh, followed by somnolence, delirium, meningism, ophthalmoplegia, and oculogyric crises; this form often ended in stupor, coma, and death.
2. The hyperkinetic form, with a flulike prodrome, followed by motor unrest and behavioral symptoms. Myoclonic twitching, tics, chorea, and athetosis were frequently seen, as were other forms of hyperactivity, such as continuous jerking, rolling, whistling, and fidgeting. Anxiety, delirium with visual hallucinations, hypomania, and violent outbursts were the usual mental symptoms. The psychomotor unrest was worse at night and led to "sleep inversion"—sleeplessness at night and hypersomnia during the day.
3. The amyotatic–akinetic form, with the same prodrome, succeeded by rigidity, bradykinesia, retropulsion or propulsion, and sometimes tremors; depression and mutism were the most frequent mental symptoms.

Other manifestations, described by other authors, were obsessive–compulsive behaviour, compulsive palilaliac shouting (Benedek's klazomania), sexual aberrations, and schizophrenialike psychoses.[10,11]

In his original paper, Von Economo spoke of an encephalitis "of a somewhat epidemic occurrence." This would prove to be an understatement: between 1916 and 1927, worldwide, an estimated 5 million people fell victim to the disease. Some 30%–35% did not survive the acute phase, an equal percentage recovered completely, and the remainder were left with postencephalitic symptoms.

These postencephalitic symptoms were as strange and baffling as the original disease.[10,12,13] They could appear many years—sometimes even ten years or more—after an apparent recovery, and often they bore no obvious relation to the symptoms experienced during the initial attack, either in character or severity. In some patients these postencephalitic symptoms were fatal, resulting in death within five to ten years after onset. Generally, the same neuropsychiatric symptoms as in the acute phase could be seen, but the relative incidence had changed.

One of the most characteristic postencephalitic syndromes was postencephalitic parkinsonism, resembling a chronic, late-onset variant of Von Economos amyotatic–akinetic form of encephalitis lethargica. More than 85% of the patients with postencephalitic symptoms developed this parkinsonian syndrome.

During the 1920s interest in encephalitis lethargica was intense, but with the sudden disappearance of the pandemic in 1927 medical and scientific interest in the disease vanished almost as quickly; Sacks spoke of a "medical catatonia which had followed the initial excitement and enthusiasm."[12] From the 1920s extending until late in the 1970s, thousands of patients with postencephalitic syndromes were living in nursing homes, scattered all over the world, slowly fading away, forgotten by science and society.

The outlook for many survivors with postencephalitic parkinsonism changed when levodopa became available in the late 1960s. At Beth Abraham Hospital in New York, Sacks treated several postencephalitic patients with the new drug and the results were often spectacular; veritable "awakenings" occurred.[11,12] Thanks to levodopa, these patients were liberated not only from lethargy, catatonia, and parkinsonism, but also from the varied crises and tics, the impulsional disorders, and the other neuropsychiatric syndromes from which they had suffered. Unfortunately, in several patients these spectacular benefits were only temporary or were followed by disagreeable side-effects.

In the 1970s, Sacks had hoped for an "awakening" of the medical community, too, but nothing of the sort happened and the last opportunity to help the survivors of the pandemic and to make observations as revealing as those of Von Economo was lost.

Perhaps this awakening will occur in the near future. Scientists are starting to realize that encephalitis lethargica and the postencephalitic syndromes often resemble unexplained neuropsychiatric disorders, such as dystonia, tardive dyskinesia, mania, schizophrenia, obsessive–compulsive disorders, and Tourette's syndrome.[13,14] Although the last survivors have died, a reexamination of the old records and a study of the numerous papers published in the 1920s might still provide many insights. Von Economo might have foreseen this when he wrote:

> Encephalitis lethargica demonstrates to us the possibility of an organic basis for those apparently functional symptoms whose true cause may be found in the particular chemical affinity of the agent of encephalitis lethargica for quite definite gray masses at the base of the brain . . . Every psychiatrist who wishes to probe into the phenomena of disturbed motility and changes of character, the psychological mechanisms of mental inaccessibility, of the neuroses, etc., must be thoroughly acquainted with the experience gathered from encephalitis lethargica.[9]

Rare cases resembling Von Economo's disease continue to be reported,[15–17] but no further epidemics have occurred since 1927. The cause of the pandemic has never been determined, although most experts agree with Von Economo that a virus is the most likely candidate.[18,19] Scientific studies have recently been performed on old tissue specimens from encephalitis patients, but without any unequivocal results. Casals et al.[19] concluded that after 80 years our knowledge of the cause of encephalitis lethargica has scarcely gone beyond Von Economo's summary in the conclusion of his initial paper.

References

1. McKenzie I. Discussion of epidemic encephalitis: epidemiological considerations. *Br Med J.* 1927;1:532–534.
2. *Constantin Freiherr von Economo. Sein Leben und Wirken. Erzählt von seiner Frau und von Prof. J. Von Wagner-Jauregg.* Wien: Mayer; 1932.
3. Seitelberger F. Das wissenschaftliche Werk Constantin von Economos. *Wien Klin Wochenschr.* 1966;78:729–731.
4. Stransky E. Constantin von Economo. In: Kolle K, (ed). *Grosse Nervenaerzte.* Stuttgart: Thieme; 1970;2:180–185.
5. Bendiner E. Economo: the daring young man's flight from the clouds to the brain. *Hosp Pract.* 1991;26:133–142.
6. Economo C von. Encephalitis lethargica. *Wien Klin Wochenschr.* 1917;30:581–585. Translation in: Wilkins R H, Brody I A. *Neurological Classics.* Park Ridge, Ill: American Association of Neurological Science; 1973, 1997. Slightly modified in this chapter.
7. Economo C von, Koskinas GN. *Die Cytoarchitektonik der Grosshirnrinde des erwachsenen Menschen.* Wien: Springer; 1925. Abridged English translation 1929.
8. Economo C von. Sleep as a problem of localization. *J Nerv Ment Dis.* 1930;71:249–259.
9. Economo C von. *Die Encephalitis lethargica; ihre Nachkrankheiten und ihre Behandlung.* Berlin: Urban & Schwarzenberg; 1929. In English: Newman K O, trans. *Encephalitis Lethargica: Its Sequelae and Treatment.* London: Oxford University Press; 1931.
10. Yahr M D. Encephalitis lethargica. In: Vinken P J, Bruyn G W, Klawans H G, eds. *Handbook of Clinical Neurology, 34.* Amsterdam: Elsevier; 1978.
11. Sacks O W. *Awakenings.* London: Duckworth; 1973, 1990.
12. Sacks O W. Postencephalitic syndromes. In: Stern G M, ed. *Parkinson's Disease.* London: Chapman & Hall; 1990.
13. Ward C D. Encephalitis lethargica and the development of neuropsychiatry. *Psych Clin N Am.* 1986;9:215–224.
14. Cheyette S R, Cummings J L. Encephalitis lethargica: lessons for contemporary neuropsychiatry. *J Neuropsych Clin Neurosci.* 1995;7:125–134.
15. Rail D, Scholtz C, Swash M. Post-encephalitic parkinsonism: current experience. *J Neurol Neurosurg Psychiatry.* 1981;44:670–676.
16. Howard R, Lees A. Encephalitis lethargica. *Brain.* 1987;110:19–33.
17. Blunt S B, Lane RJM, Turjanski N, Perkin G D. Clinical features and management of two cases of encephalitis lethargica. *Mov Dis.* 1997;12:354–359.
18. Dourmashkin R R. What caused the 1918–30 epidemic of encephalitis lethargica? *J R Soc Med.* 1997;90:515–560.
19. Casals J, Elizan T S, Yahr M D. Postencephalitic parkinsonism: a review. *J Neural Transm.* 1998;105:645–676.

48

FRIEDREICH'S ATAXIA

Peter J. Koehler

Friedreich's ataxia is an autosomal-recessive disease with a prevalence of between 1 and 2 per 100,000, characterized by symptoms and signs including progressive ataxia, absent tendon reflexes in the legs, distal impairment of position and vibration sense, Babinski reflexes, and dysarthria. Other signs may be present, such as pes cavus, scoliosis, diabetes mellitus, and cardiomyopathy. In most cases it starts between the age of 8 and 15, the patients becoming wheelchair bound after approximately 14 years. During the nineteenth century it was gradually distinguished from other types of ataxia. Nikolaus Friedreich played a major role in defining the disease.

The medical faculty of Würzburg (Germany) employed members of the Friedreich family for several decades in the nineteenth century. Nikolaus Anton (1761–1836), professor of surgery (1796–1824), described peripheral facial nerve paralysis in 1798, some 23 years before Charles Bell.[1,2] His son Johannes Baptist Friedreich (1796–1862) became extraordinary professor of surgery at the age of 24 and ordinary professor 10 years later. According to his list of publications, he was interested in the nervous system: *Handbuch der allgemeinen Pathologie der psychischen Krankheiten* [Handbook of general pathology of psychic diseases] (1830) and *System der gerichtlichen Psychologie* [System of forensic psychology] (1835). He adhered to the somatic school of psychiatry.

Nikolaus Friedreich, the son of Johannes Baptist, was born in Würzburg in 1825.[3–5] He began studying medicine in his native city in 1844 and went to Heidelberg for six months in 1847. Nikolaus graduated in 1850 and became first assistant of the blind physician Karl Friedrich Marcus (1802–1862). He wrote his thesis, *Beiträge zur Lehre von den Geschwülsten innerhalb der Schedelhöhle* [Contributions to the study of tumors inside the skull] in 1853. Although Friedreich had studied under Rudolf Albert Kölliker (1817–1905), who held the chair of anatomy from 1849, he was influenced above all by Rudolf Virchow (1821–1902), who came to Würzburg in 1849, and whom he succeeded to the chair of pathological anatomy in Würzburg in 1856, when

Figure 48–1. Nikolaus Freidreich (1825–1882). Courtesy of Medizinhistorisches Institut, Zurich, Switzerland.

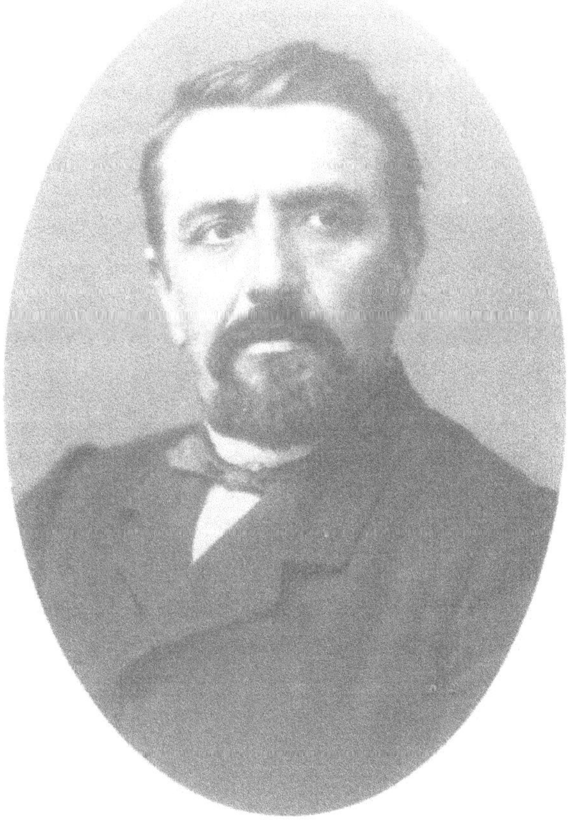

Virchow moved to Berlin (see Chapter 54). Only two years later, Friedreich was appointed chief of the medical clinic in Heidelberg, where he took the chair of pathology and therapy, remaining there for the rest of his life. Virchow mentioned his characteristics at that time:

> Ich muss dagegen besonders hervorheben, dass er seine Assistentenstellung von vornherein mit einem Eifer, einem Scharfsinn und einer Selbständigkeit ausbeutete, welche des höchsten Ruhmes würdig sind.[6]

[I have to emphasize, on the other hand, that he exploited his position as registrar from the start with such enthusiasm, cleverness, and independence that he deserves the highest fame.] Adolf Kussmaul (1822–1902) described him as a person with a noble expressive bronzed face with beautiful dark eyes, dignified but friendly behavior, tactful reserve in conversation, delicacy in his comments, good humor, and sharp wit.[5] On the other hand, Friedreich raised suspicions quite early, because his father had made many enemies in academic circles by his offensive tongue and the son was still regarded by many with reserve.

He published papers on several subjects, including abdominal typhus; corpora amylacea; leukaemia; ear, nose, and throat diseases; and cardiac and blood vessel diseases. His main interest was diseases of the nervous system. One of the early works in this field was his study on progressive muscular atrophy, which he dedicated to his teacher Virchow.[7] Friedreich, however, erroneously considered all muscular dystrophy of myogenic origin. His most important contribution to neurology was the study of hereditary spinal ataxia, which will be discussed shortly. In addition to the eponymic Friedreich's ataxia, his name also became associated with paramyoclonus multiplex.[8] His strength was his industriousness in collecting clinical material and in sorting and correlating clinical and pathological–anatomical observations. A sound judgment of physiological and pathological subjects is reflected in all his publications. He took detailed patients' histories and performed examinations with great precision. As such, he was an exemplary teacher and had a very extensive practice. According to Kussmaul, there was not a greater expert in physical examination than Friedreich:

> Niemand kam ihm gleich in der Kunst des Percutirens, man konnte keine besseren Percussionshämmer oder Plessimeter finden als Freidreich's Finger. Auch an dem korpulentesten Individuum lockte er die Töne weithin vernehmlich hervor.[5]

[Nobody could equal his art of percussion; one could find no better percussion hammer or plessimeter than Freidreich's finger. Even in the most obese person could he arouse clearly perceptible sounds.] He taught many well-known physicians, including Kussmaul, Friedrich Schultze (1848–1934), and Wilhelm Erb (see Chapter 32), who succeeded him to the chair of pathology and therapy in Heidelberg in 1882. Friedreich dedicated most of his time to medicine, the only diversion coming from his family life. Finally, an incurable aneurysm of the thoracic aorta was diagnosed. He survived another three years until he died on 6 July 1882.

Friedreich began his observations on ataxia in the 1850s and discussed the patients with his colleagues, including Kussmaul and Virchow. Gradually he became aware that these patients were not suffering from ordinary locomotor ataxia as described in 1858–1859 by Guillaume Benjamin Amand Duchenne (1806–1875; see Chapter 46),[9] but from a variant. Although Duchenne was not the first to describe this condition, also known as tabes dorsalis (see Chapter 26), he presented a classic account resulting in the eponym "Duchenne's disease." Friedreich presented the first data at a meeting in Speyer, Germany, in 1861. Subsequently, he published several papers on the hereditary type of ataxia between 1863 and 1877.[10,11] In the introduction to the first paper, he expressed his expectation that he would delineate a characteristic type of spinal degeneration within the group of tabes dorsalis. In the 1863 papers, he described six patients in two families.[12] He added three other patients in the 1876–1877 papers, resulting in nine patients from three families.

In these papers, he also presented a follow-up of patients from the earlier papers. One of these patients, the 49-year old Charlotte Lotsch, who had had symptoms since the age of 18, had been admitted to the hospital in 1862 and again in the year of the publication, 1876. She had become unable to walk. On examination,

> Die Sprache ist in viel erheblicheren Grade gestört, als bei ihrer Entlassung aus der Klinik vor 13 Jahren. Pat. articulirt so schlecht, dass man die Worte oft kaum versteht . . . An die Pupillen keine Veränderungen.[11]

[Speech is disturbed in a more considerable degree than at dismissal from the clinic 13 years ago. The patient articulates so badly, that one often hardly understands the words . . . No abnormalities of the pupils.]

The eye movements were disturbed, with saccadic horizontal pursuit movements interrupted by sudden upward movements, "wie es in den Bewegungen der Extremitäten als Störung der Coordination, als locomotorischen Ataxie hervortritt [as occurs in the movements of the extremities like disturbed coordination, or locomotor ataxia].

Nystagmus was present. The head could not be kept still and made balancing movements. There was marked kyphoscoliosis, which had much worsened since the examination in 1862.

> Im höchsten Grade aber ist die locomotorische Coordination an den oberen Extremitäten beeinträchtigt, viel mehr, als beim ersten Aufenthalt der Kranken in der Klinik . . . das Schreiben ist nahezu unmöglich geworden; das Ergreifen eines vorgehaltenen Gegenstandes, das Führen des Löffels zum Munde . . . geschieht unter mannigfaltigen, von der richtige Linie abweichenden und dem Zwecke durchaus nicht entsprechenden Nebenbewegungen. Augenschluss bedingt keine Steigerung der atactischen Symptome.

[The locomotor coordination of the upper limbs is restricted to the highest degree, much more than at the first stay in the clinic . . . writing has become almost impossible; directing the spoon to the mouth . . . happens with multiple additional movements deviating from the right line and from the target. Closing the eyes does not increase the ataxic symptoms.]

The legs were almost completely paralyzed, the feet in equinovarus contracture. The sensitivity of the legs was diminished.

> Stärkere Reizungen der Fusssohlenhaut erzeugen noch ziemlich lebhafte Reflexe; dagegen fehlen die Erb'schen Sehnenreflexe vollständig.

[Stronger stimuli at the sole of the foot generate rather brisk reflexes; yet the tendon reflexes of Erb are completely lacking.] Obviously, Friedreich referred to the knee tendon reflex described by Erb (and Westphal) a year earlier. He commented that there had been pure locomotor ataxia of the four limbs, with normal sensitivity and without nystagmus 13 years previously.[11]

The disease could be distinguished from tabes dorsalis because of the hereditary occurrence, the early age of onset, the long duration, the fact that seven of the nine patients were female, and the absence of sensory loss, at least in the early stages of the disease.[13] He found that the lower part of the spinal cord was involved at the beginning of the disease; later it spread to involve the medulla oblongata. The disease started with ataxia, initially present only in the legs, later in the arms. Dysarthria was found later, sometimes accompanied by nystagmus and scoliosis. Sensory loss in the legs was only observed after many years, whereas loss of deep sensation was present in only one patient, in such a way that walking in darkness or with the eyes closed was more difficult.

Autopsy on four patients demonstrated degeneration of the dorsal spinal columns, particularly in the lower part. Upon microscopic examination, nerve atrophy and demyelination were noticed as well as replacement by fine fibrillary tissue. The lateral columns were also involved, and degeneration of cells in Clarke's column as well as in the hypoglossal nuclei was found. Interestingly, Friedreich concluded the article by mentioning a remarkable fatty degeneration of the cardiac muscle in three cases, which he associated with the increasing tendency of the patients to collapse.[11,13]

His belief that he had discovered a new disease was not endorsed by the medical world at first. Several colleagues considered it a variant of tabes dorsalis. Charcot's pupil Bourneville in Paris believed it was multiple sclerosis, as he thought nystagmus and dysarthria did not belong to the syndrome of locomotor ataxia. The lack of sensory and visual disturbances was unusual as well.[14] It is obvious that many physicians tried to fit the syndrome into one of the existing diagnoses, including tabes dorsalis or multiple sclerosis.[12] Friedreich replied to Bourneville in his 1876–1877 papers, pointing to the pathologic–anatomic findings in the dorsal colums of the spinal cord.[11]

In a chapter on tabes dorsalis, Wilhelm Erb mentioned "Friedreich's type of tabes" in 1878.[15] William Gowers wrote on hereditary ataxy, or Friedreich's disease, in 1880,[16] and again in the first volume of his well-known *Manual* (1886), stating that in approximately 65 cases distributed in 19 families, "the family tendency of the disease . . . shown by the affection . . . of brothers and sisters,"[17] had been recorded at that moment, including 57 cases reviewed by a certain Dr. Everett Smith (1885; he observed 6 cases and presented a review of 51 including 6 cases of Friedreich.[18] One year later, Bury summarized data of 100 published cases.[19]

In the meantime, Brousse of Montpellier dedicated a thesis to the "maladie de Friedreich" (1882).[20] The approval of Friedreich's findings, however, had to await Charcot's work two years later. In his 1876 paper, Friedreich had already expressed his wish that Charcot should find similar cases among his patients. Indeed, Charcot demonstrated a young patient suffering from a hereditary type of ataxia, not fitting the diagnosis of tabes or multiple sclerosis, in 1884.[12,21]

During the past few decades, the knowledge of hereditary ataxia has increased considerably. Several genes have been found to code for autosomal-dominant cerebellar ataxia (ADCA) and a few for autosomal-recessive ataxias. The responsible gene for Friedreichs ataxia was mapped to chromosome 9 in 1988. It was recently discovered that the frataxin gene codes for a 210 amino acid protein of unknown function, the mutation being an unstable expansion of a GAA repeat in the first intron.[22] Whereas expansion of trinucleotide repeats has been found in several neurological disorders, it was the first time to be noticed in an autosomal-recessive disorder. Most patients suffering from Friedreich's ataxia are homozygous for the GAA expansion. The clinical features are related to the number of GAA repeats and atypical cases; for example, Friedreich's ataxia with retained reflexes and late-onset Friedreich's ataxia have been shown to carry fewer repeats than typical patients.[23]

References

1. Bird T D. Nicolaus A. Friedreich's description of peripheral facial nerve paralysis in 1798. *J Neurol Neurosurg Psychiatry*. 1979;42:56–58.

2. Friedreich N A. De paralysis musculorum faciei rheumatica. *J Erfindungen (Gotha).* 1798; 8:no 25. Quoted in: *Ann Med (Edinb).* 1800;5:214–222.
3. Richter R B. Nikolaus Friedreich (1825–1882). In: Haymaker W, Schiller F, eds. *The Founders of Neurology.* 2nd ed. Springfield, Ill: Charles C Thomas; 1970:439–441.
4. Hirsch A, *Biographisches Lexikon der hervorragenden Aerzte aller Zeiten und Völker.* Wien: Urban & Schwarzenberg; 1885.
5. Kussmaul A. Nikolaus Friedreich. Erinnerungen. *Dtsch Arch Klin Med.* 1882;32:191–208.
6. Virchow R. Zur Erinnerung an Nicolaus Friedreich. *Virchow's Arch Pathol Anat.* 1882; 90:213–220.
7. Friedreich N. *Ueber progressive Muskelatrophie, ueber wahre und falsche Muskelhypertrophie.* Berlin: Hirschwald; 1873.
8. Friedreich N. Paramyoclonus multiplex. *Arch pathol Anat (Berl).* 1881;86:421–430.
9. Duchenne de Boulogne GBA. De l'ataxie locomotrice progressive. *Arch Gén Méd.* 1858; 12:641–652; 1859;13:36–62, 158–181, 417–451.
10. Friedreich N. Ueber degenerative Atrophie der spinalen Hinterstränge. *Virchows Arch Pathol Anat.* 1863;26:391–419, 433–459; 1863;27:1–26.
11. Friedreich N. Ueber Ataxia mit besonderer Berücksichtigung der hereditären Formen. *Virchow's Arch Pathol Anat.* 1876;68:145–245; 1877;70:140–152.
12. Keppel Hesselink J M. A discussion from the previous century: multiple sclerosis or tabes dorsalis; or Friedreich's disease? *Ned Tijdschr Geneeskd.* 1986;130:2353–2356.
13. Tyrer J H. Friedreich's ataxia. In: Vinken P J, Bruyn G W, DeJong JMBV, eds. *Handbook of Clinical Neurology, vol 21: System Disorders and Atrophies,* pt 1. Amsterdam: North-Holland Publishing Company; 1975:359–364.
14. Bourneville M. Nouvelle étude sur quelques points de la sclérose en plaques disséminées. In: Bourneville M, Guérard L, eds. *De la sclérose en plaques.* Paris: Delahaye; 1869.
15. Erb W. *Handbuch der Krankheiten des Nervensystems, I.* Leipzig: Vogel; 1878.
16. Gowers W R. A family affected with locomotor ataxy. *Clin Soc Trans.* 1880;14:27–36.
17. Gowers W R. *A Manual of Diseases of the Nervous System, 1. Diseases of the Spinal Cord and Nerves.* London: Churchill; 1886:349–356.
18. Smith W E. Hereditary or degenerative ataxia. Six cases in one family. Death of one case, and autopsy. *Boston Med Surg J.* 1885;113:361–368.
19. Bury J S. A contribution to the symptomatology of Friedreich's disease. *Brain.* 1886; 9:145–177.
20. Lapresle J. La dystasie aréflexie héréditaire de Roussy-Lévy. *Rev Neurol.* 1982;12:967–978.
21. Goetz C G. *Charcot the Clinician: The Tuesday Lessons.* New York: Raven Press; 1987:141–163.
22. Campuzano V, Montermini L, Molto M D, et al. Friedreich's ataxia: autosomal recessive disease caused by an intronic GAA triplet repeat expansion. *Science.* 1996;271:1423–1427.
23. Brice A. Unstable mutations and neurodegenerative disorders. *J Neurol.* 1998;245:505–510.

49

HORTON'S SYNDROME

John M. S. Pearce

Bayard T. Horton was a prominent figure in the development of scientific investigation in the United States. Much of received medical wisdom until the 1930s had been based on uncritical and often untested opinions, founded on empirical methods and passed from chief to student. Among others, the Mayo and Harvard groups in the United States and Sir Thomas Lewis and Sir George Pickering in England were to challenge accepted dogma by devising and implementing physiological and pharmacological tests and by applying scientific methods to clinical phenomena. This was the foundation of a new era of critical and inquiring clinical investigation, in which Horton was to play a significant role.

Bayard Taylor Horton was born in Gate City, Virginia, on 6 December 1895. He attended the University of Virginia and received the degree of M.D. in 1922. In 1917 he served in the U.S. Navy. Returning to civilian life he was appointed an intern at the University of Virginia Hospital, later becoming professor of biology and physician at Emory and Henry College at Emory, Virginia.

Horton moved to Rochester, Minnesota, on 1 July 1925, as a fellow in medicine of the Mayo Foundation. The early basic training he received in the Section of Pathologic Anatomy was under the direction of H. E. Robertson and J. W. Kernohan, for a period of 18 months; during that time he helped to perform more than 1000 postmortem examinations. The scientific training he received under Leonard G. Rowntree and George E. Brown laid the foundation for his future work at the Mayo Clinic. Horton received the M.Sc. in Medicine from the University of Minnesota in 1928. He was appointed to the staff of the Mayo Clinic in July 1929 and became instructor in medicine in the Mayo Foundation Graduate School, University of Minnesota.

Horton carried out studies on hypertension, cold allergy, duodenal diverticula, uremia, and, in particular, diseases of the blood vessels. Vascular investigations remained a prime interest and became the bedrock of much of his future work. By

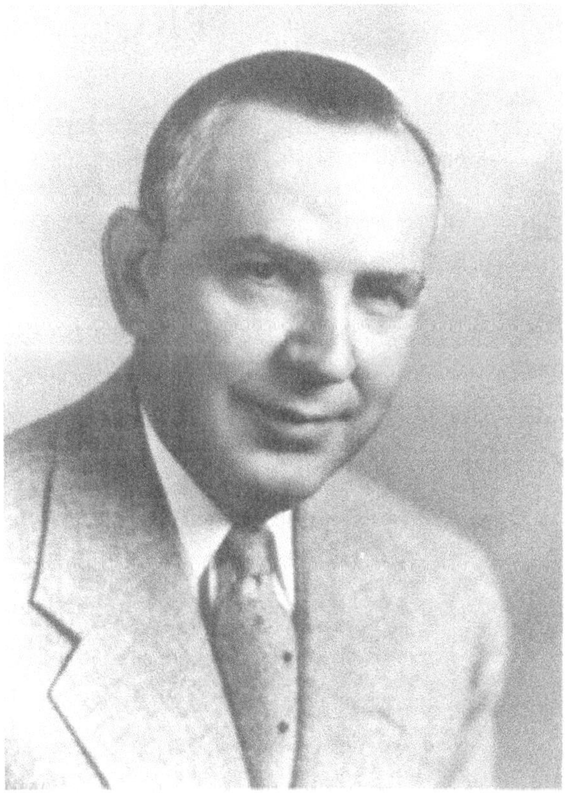

Figure 49–1. Bayard T. Horton (1895–1980). By permission of Mayo Historical Suite, Mayo Foundation, Rochester, Minnesota.

1927 he was widely known for his studies on hypersensitivity to cold, an abnormal condition in some persons which he showed could cause involuntary drowning.

Many celebrated physicians are known for their work on one illness, but Horton became internationally known for his descriptions of two diseases: histaminic cephalgia (Horton's headache) and temporal arteritis. Horton wrote his celebrated paper on the syndrome of cluster headache in 1939 (Fig. 49–2).[1] In 1941 he decided to change its name to histaminic cephalgia.[2,3] Wilfred Harris in 1926 had named the same condition "migrainous neuralgia" and "ciliary neuralgia," a nomenclature that was adhered to in Britain for many years after World War II. In 1952 Kunkle et al. used "cluster headache" after an analysis of 30 patients.[4]

Giant cell arteritis was also described by Horton with Magath and Brown in 1932 in a 55-year-old woman and in a 68-year-old man. They presented the features of "fever, weakness, anorexia, loss of weight, anemia, mild leukocytosis, and painful, tender areas over the scalp and along the temporal vessels."[5] In a later paper: "The physician should be aware of headache in the senior citizen. Sudden loss of vision in one eye in an elderly person with headache and high sedimentation rate should indicate: the patient most likely has temporal arteritis."[6] Horton also clearly described intermittent claudication of the jaw and the microscopical granulomatous necrosis of the arteritis. Jonathan Hutchinson (1828–1913) has the prior claim in describing

PROCEEDINGS

OF THE

STAFF MEETINGS OF THE MAYO CLINIC

Published Weekly for the Information of the Members of the Staff and the Fellows of The Mayo Foundation for Medical Education and Research

Vol. 14 Rochester, Minnesota, Wednesday, April 26, 1939 No. 17

CONTENTS

A NEW SYNDROME OF VASCULAR HEADACHE: RESULTS OF TREATMENT WITH HISTAMINE: PRELIMINARY REPORT*

B. T. Horton, M. D., Division of Medicine, A. R. MacLean, M. D., Section on Neurology, and W. McK. Craig, M. D., Section on Neurosurgery: In the last eighteen months we have observed and treated eighty-four patients with a specific type of headache which has not been described adequately in the literature. We believe that our observations warrant the establishment of this type of headache as a distinct clinical entity, classical in its symptomatology and unique in its response to histamine. Our patients were disabled by the disorder and suffered from bouts of pain from two to twenty times a week. They had found no relief from the usual methods of treatment. Diagnoses of their condition ran the gamut of the nomenclature for headaches, from "psychoneurosis" to "organic" lesions. Their pain was so severe that several of them had to be constantly watched for fear of suicide. Most of them were willing to submit to any operation which might bring relief.

THE CLINICAL PICTURE

The majority of the patients were in the fourth and fifth decades of life. They could relate the onset of the headache to no definite cause. Although several of the patients gave a history of classical migraine earlier

Figure 49–2. Horton's celebrated 1939 paper on the syndrome of cluster headache.[1] By permission of Mayo Historical Suite, Mayo Foundation, Rochester, Minnesota.

"an old man . . . the father of a well remembered beadle at the London Hospital College 30 years ago . . . I was asked to see him because he had 'red streaks on his head' which were painful and prevented his wearing his hat. The 'red streaks' proved to be his temporal arteries which . . . were inflamed and swollen."[7] But Horton's exposition of this malady could fairly be considered a more original contribution than his work on cluster headache.

Horton's interests and experiments were diverse.[8] He continued his basic research studies with Sheard, Williams, and Grace Roth, studying skin temperatures of the limbs under various environmental and physiological conditions. He made extensive studies on congenital and acquired arteriovenous fistula, and in 1932 he was the first to demonstrate arteriovenous fistula by means of arteriography in the living subject. With E. J. Baldes he developed a photographic method of recording bruits by which aneurysm and arteriovenous fistula could, he believed, be accurately differentiated. In 1938 Horton gave the Alpha Omega Alpha Address on short circuits in the circulation of the blood, at the University of Virginia.

Horton with G. A. Peters and L. S. Blumenthal, in 1945, published on the use of dihydroergotamine in the treatment of migraine. In 1948, with Robert Ryan and J. L. Reynolds, he described the first control studies on the use of Cafergot in the treatment of headache. He carried out research with Henry P. Wagener over a period of 11 years on the long-continued intravenous administration of histamine in cases of lesions of the optic nerve, retina, and choroid. Some of these patients apparently regained normal vision. His clinical investigations were recorded in 184 publications.

Preferment led to appointment as assistant professor in 1933 and associate professor in 1937. By 1940 he had become head of a section of clinical investigation, later known as "Dr. Horton's Laboratory." The University of Virginia in 1957 elected him to membership in Phi Beta Kappa for "distinguished achievement in field of medical research." He retired from the Mayo Clinic on 1 January 1958.

Bayard Horton was married to Jane Heyl, of Charlottesville, on 14 June 1922. They had three children. After a long retirement, he died on 6 July 1980 in Sun City, Arizona. These are verbatim excerpts from his 1939 paper:

> In the last eighteen months we have observed and treated eighty four patients with a specific type of headache which has not been described adequately in the literature. We believe that our observations warrant the establishment of this type of headache as a distinct clinical entity, classical in its symptomatology and unique in its response to histamine. Our patients were disabled by the disorder and suffered from bouts of pain from two to twenty times a week . . . Their pain was so severe that several of them had to be constantly watched for fear of suicide. Most of them were willing to submit to any operation which might bring relief.

The Clinical Picture

> The majority of the patients were in the fourth and fifth decades of life. They could relate the onset of the headache to no definite cause. Although several of the

patients gave a history of classical migraine earlier in life, the majority denied periodic headaches in their earlier years. There were no familial or hereditary characteristics.

The pain of which the patients complained was limited to one side of the head. It was a constant, excruciating, burning, boring type of pain which involved the eye, the temple, the neck, and often the face. It had none of the tic-like qualities of trigeminal neuralgia, and there were no trigger zones. There was frequently marked tenderness on pressure over the branches of the external carotid and common carotid arteries.

The bouts of pain appeared and disappeared very quickly. The onset and cessation frequently could be measured in minutes. The duration of the headache varied from fifteen minutes to several hours. In most cases the headache occurred with clock-like regularity particularly at night, the patients awakening with pain night after night and week after week at a certain hour. Although night pain was characteristic, pain during the waking hours was common. Remissions and exacerbations in many cases occurred spontaneously. As a general rule, however, the patient had had frequent attacks of pain for at least a year without a remission before admission to the Clinic.

Coincident with the onset of the pain, our patients invariably described the onset of phenomena of vasodilatation on the same side of the head as the pain. These consisted of swelling of the temporal vessels, engorgement of the soft tissues of the eye, injection of the conjunctiva, plugging of the nose, profuse watering of the eye and nose and flushing of the side of the face. At least some of these phenomena were present in each case. Scotoma and also intestinal upsets were not associated with the headache, although occasionally nausea was associated. The relationship of alcoholic beverages to exacerbations of pain in some cases was evident . . . The relationship between the menstrual cycle and bouts of pain of the women patients was not as striking as that observed in migraine . . . Salicylates, however, had no effect on the rhythmic recurrence of the bouts of headache.

Many patients obtained some relief by making strong pressure over the eye and temporal vessels. A few discovered that digital compression of the common carotid artery on the side of the pain gave relief. During the bout of pain, a reclining position was intolerable . . . Many of the patients slept propped up by pillows or in chairs; on awakening with their pain paced the floor holding their temples.

Tests Employed

We were able to produce the typical syndrome of headache described in twenty-five cases by the subcutaneous injection of 0.3 to 0.5 mg. of histamine. In twenty of these cases we were able completely to control an attack induced by histamine by the intravenous administration of epinephrine and other vasoconstricting agents. Spontaneous attacks were controlled in a similar manner . . . Associated with the pain following the injection of histamine, the phenomena of vasodilatation, noted in the spontaneous attacks were reproduced. Patients were unable to differentiate between induced and spontaneous attacks . . . That the pathogenesis of the pain lies in this phenomena (sic) of abnormal vasodilatation, appears evident when we consider that spontaneous attacks were induced with histamine and alcohol, both of which are vasodilating substances, and that relief was obtained by administration of vasoconstricting substances.

Method and Results of Treatment

> The method of treatment used consisted in giving subcutaneously 0.05 milligram of histamine twice each day for two consecutive days . . . [increasing until] by the fifth day 0.1 mg. twice a day is well tolerated. The injection of 0.1 mg. twice a day is continued for two to three weeks . . . A careful follow-up study has revealed: Sixty-five patients obtained definite permanent relief for periods of from two weeks to eighteen months . . . Several of these patients have suffered from a recurrence of their symptoms, but these recurrences promptly responded to another course of treatment with histamine. In cases treated recently we have been giving 0.1 mg. of histamine subcutaneously at weekly intervals whenever possible in an attempt to prolong the period of freedom from attack. Ten patients received no benefit from the two weeks' course of histamine and nine patients have not been heard from since dismissal from our care.[1]

In a 1952 paper however, although still calling the syndrome "histaminic cephalgia," Horton advocated intravenous dihydroergotamine (1 cc), which

> will frequently abort an attack in 1–5 minutes, if it is administered at the onset of the attack. The breathing of 100% oxygen will alleviate an attack to a marked extent especially if the attack is mild . . . A rectal suppository which contains 2 mg. Of ergotamine tartrate and 100 mg caffeine [Cafergot], if used at bedtime, frequently prevents nocturnal attacks.[9]

He also later recommended corticotrophin intravenously.

At the time, judging from his paper, Horton and his co-workers appear to have been wholly unaware of previous publications; it seems he had not seen Wilfred Harris's detailed clinical descriptions of "periodic migrainous neuralgia."[10,11] "Ciliary neuralgia" described by Harris in the same text is clearly the same condition except for its location in the eye. Harris reported cases in either sex:

> Attacks invariably on one side of the head only, though in the majority the pain may attack either side, but even then severe neuralgia is limited to one side . . . neuralgia continues for several hours yet occasional attacks are much shorter lasting only from ten minutes to an hour and may recur within twenty-four hours . . . In other cases migrainous neuralgia may occur daily at about the same time and last for several hours for a period of a few weeks only in the year, and may recur annually at about the same time.[10(p303)]

Furthermore, several earlier accounts of variant forms (by Eulenburg, Bing, Sluder, and Vail) also seem to have escaped Horton's attention. Raymond Hierons suggested in 1955 that Thomas Willis's account (1672) may have been the first record of this malady.[12] His patient was a lady who began to suffer from headaches "each afternoon at about 4 o'clock"; this continued daily for some five weeks.[13]

However, the following account, recognized by Isler[14] the first description known to date of episodic cluster headache, was the work of Gerard van Swieten (1700–1772), a student of the famous Herman Boerhaave in Leiden. In 1745, van Swieten published in Latin a renowned textbook that contains this history:

> A healthy, robust man of middle age was, each day, at the same hour troubled by pain above the orbit of the left eye, where the nerve leaves through the bony frontal

> opening; after a short time the left eye began to redden and tears to flow; then he felt as if his eye was protruding from its orbit with so much pain that he became mad. After a few hours all this evil ceased and nothing in the eye appeared at all changed . . .
>
> The patient reminded me, whilst I sat with him, that in the medial canthus of the eye he felt a large pulsation: I applied the apex of my little finger to the artery, which goes around the medial canthus of the eye, then with the other hand explored the carpal pulse; and thus I manifestly perceived how the artery in the canthus of the eye was pulsing more rapidly, and strongly than it naturally does.[15]

Perhaps earlier still Nicolaas Tulp (1593–1674), a Dutch physician, had observed the same syndrome. He tells of an Isaak van Halmaal, who,

> in the beginning of the summer season, was inflicted with a very severe headache, occurring and disappearing daily on fixed hours, with such intensity, that he often assured me that he could not bear the pain any more or he would succumb shortly. For rarely it lasted longer than two hours. And the rest of the day there was no fever, nor indisposition of the urine, nor any infirmity of the pulse. But this recurring pain lasted until the fourteenth day.[16]

In 1747 Joannes Christoph Ulricus Oppermann published his little acknowledged Dissertatio Medica Inauguralis, entitled *Hemicrania Horologica* which so far is the first known account of the cluster headache variant "chronic paroxysmal hemicrania" (CPH). Horton's description of "pain—they often occur every two hours, day and night" suggests that he may have observed cases that would now be classified as CPH.

Benjamin Hutchinson's "neuralgia spasmodica" was probably trigeminal neuralgia. Romberg in his *Manual* gave a convincing description of cluster headache, for which he coined the term "ciliary neuralgia," with "the pupil contracted . . . the eye generally weeps and becomes red. These symptoms occur in paroxysms of a uniform or irregular character, and isolated or combined with facial neuralgia and hemicrania."[17] But he stressed "excited by rays of light and visual effort—not a characteristic feature in current thinking.

Horton and his colleagues deserve full credit for the excellence and detail of their clinical description, but not for originality. They described precipitation not only by histamine but also by alcohol; this should have suggested a vulnerability to vasodilators in general rather than a specific histamine reaction. It is likely that gastric hyperacidity during an attack was no more than a nonspecific effect of stress, though an association with peptic ulcer is well known. Finally, desensitization after histamine injections was not shown, by controlled experiments, to be due to a desensitizing effect; antihistamine drugs proved unreliable in Horton's syndrome. The more characteristic response to vasoconstrictor noradrenergic ergotamine α-agonist, ergotamine (Symonds)[18] and the 5-HT agonist sumatriptan (Humphrey)[19] were recognized later, though ergot was widely used in migraine in Horton's time.

Horton has no just claim for originality of the description of cluster headache. His notion of histamine sensitivity—as the cause—was proved to be wrong not long after his paper achieved widespread recognition. However, he did provide an excellent, detailed, and admirable description of a condition little known and seldom recognized at the time. That was an important contribution, though to this day misdiagnosis in primary care practice sadly remains a commonplace error.

Acknowledgments

I am greatly indebted to Jack P. Whisnant, M. D., and Andrew G. Engel, M. D., of the Mayo Clinic for providing invaluable biographical information from the *Rochester Post-Bulletin,* 30 September 1957, and the portrait, reproduced by kind permission of Mayo Historical Suite, Mayo Foundation, Rochester, Minnesota.

References

1. Horton B T, MacLean A R, Craig W M. A new syndrome of vascular headache: results of treatment with histamine. *Proc Staff Meet Mayo Clin.* 1939;14:257–260.
2. Horton B T. The use of histamine in specific types of headaches. *JAMA.* 1941;116:377–383.
3. Horton B T. Histaminic cephalgia: differential diagnosis and treatment. *Proc Mayo Clin.* 1956;31:325–330.
4. Kunkle E C, Pfeiffer J B, Wilhoit W M, Hamrick L W. Recurrent brief headache in cluster pattern. *Trans Am Neurol Assoc.* 1952;77:240–243.
5. Horton B T, Magath T B, Brown G E. An undescribed form of arteritis of the temporal arteries. *Proc Staff Meet Mayo Clin.* 1932;7:700–701.
6. Horton B T. Headache and intermittent claudication of the jaw in temporal arteritis. *Headache.* 1962;2:29–40.
7. Hutchinson J. Diseases of the arteries. *Arch Surg.* 1890;1:323–333.
8. Capobianco D J, Swanson J W. Neurologic contributions of Byard T. Horton. *Mayo Clin Proc.* 1998;73:912–915.
9. Horton B T. Histaminic cephalgia. *Lancet.* 1952;72:92–98.
10. Harris W. *Neuritis and Neuralgia.* London: Oxford University Press; 1926:293–314.
11. Harris W. *The Facial Neuralgias.* London: Oxford University Press; 1937:70–76.
12. Hierons R. Willis's contributions to clinical medicine and neurology. *J Neurol Sci.* 1967;4:1–7.
13. Willis T. *Two Discourses concerning the soul of brutes (De anima brutorum). Part 1. 1672.* Cited by Spillane J D in: *The Doctrine of the Nerves.* New York: Oxford University Press; 1981:58–61.
14. Isler H. Episodic cluster headache from a textbook of 1745: van Swieten's classic description. *Cephalalgia.* 1993;13:172–174.
15. Van Swieten G. *Commentaria in Hermanni Boerhaave Aphorismos de cognoscendis et curandis morbis.* Lugduni Batavorum [Leiden]: Apud Johannem et Hermanum Verbeek; 1745;ii,34:533.
16. Koehler P J. Headache in Tulp's "Observationes Medicae" (1641). *Cephalalgia.* 1993;13: 318–320.
17. Romberg, M H; Sieveking E H, trans. *A Manual of Nervous Diseases of Man.* London: Sydenham Society, 1853;1:56.
18. Symonds C P. A particular variety of headache. *Brain.* 1956;79:217–232.
19. Feniuk W, Humphrey PPA. The development of a highly selective 5-HT-1 receptor agonist, sumatriptan, for the treatment of migraine. *Drug Dev Res.* 1992;26:235–240.

50

HUNTINGTON'S CHOREA

George W. Bruyn and Richard P. M. Bruyn

Huntington's hereditary progressive chorea is characterized by choreatic, often stereotyped, movements (less abrupt and coarser than those in Sydenham's chorea), which in the course of time acquire dystonic features, and by dementia, paranoid hypochondriac psychosis, and loss of weight. The neuropathological matrix consists of progressive depletion of the small to medium spiny interneurons of the neostriatium, particularly of the caudate nucleus, and also of the other gray matter, such as cortex, thalamus, and hypothalamus.

The disease usually becomes manifest between the ages 30 and 50; it is caused by a point mutation in gene *IT15* (from "interesting transcript"). The gene normally contains a CAG repeat near the 5′ end; if there are more than 36 CAG repeats, Huntington's chorea will manifest. The number of repeats is unstable. The *IT15* gene is requisite for normal embryonal development; it encodes a ±300 KD protein, called "*huntingtin,*" of unknown function and expressed in both neural and nonneural tissues. The protein contains a long polyglutamine stretch in the patients ranging from 36 to 120. Why certain cerebral grisea bear the brunt of *huntingtin*'s noxious effect is as yet unelucidated, but *huntingtin* seems to bind to cerebral "*huntingtin*-associated proteins" and interacts with glyceraldehyde-3-phosphate dehydrogenase, essential for glycolysis, which might explain the cachexia.

George Huntington and George Sumner Huntington, anatomist, have been frequently confused in reports on the early history of the disease. They were cousins five times removed.[1,2]

George Huntington was born in East Hampton, New York, 9 April 1850, son of George Lee Huntington, who was born in that town in 1811 and practiced medicine there all his life, having obtained his medical degree at New York University, and Mary Hoogland, whose typically Dutch name reflects her Knickerbocker family roots. George's paternal grandfather Abel was born in Norwich, Connecticut, in 1777 and settled in East Hampton in 1797 as a general practitioner. By that date, the eponymous disease was already firmly established among the population. East Hampton, a drowsy, secluded village between the ocean and the woods, is about 100 miles east of the town of Huntington on Long Island.

George Huntington, as a boy, played the flute, sang in the choir, and spent many hours in hunting. He attended the East Hampton Clinton Academy and the College of Physicians and Surgeons of Columbia University, graduating early 1871 (with a thesis on "Opium"), then returning to his birthplace to assist his father. Later that year, he made notes of the choreic cases they saw together, for a lecture on Sydenham's chorea. His father's penciled remarks figure in the margin of the original draft of his paper. Only in the last pages did George draw attention to the hereditary type that now bears his name, regarding it as a particular type of Sydenham's chorea. Unlike the authors preceding him on this subject, he presented an accurate picture of the features and transmission of the affliction.

Late in 1871, he moved to Pomeroy, Ohio, to establish a practice in that booming coal-mining and industrial town, on the advice of a cousin married to a clergyman there. George remained a country doctor. He never scriptorially broached another medical subject, did no research, and did not acquire a faculty appointment.

George, clearly a modest man, devoted to practice and aware of his limitations, exhibited the restless pioneer spirit. In 1874 he married Miss Mary Elisabeth Hackard, whose father was Judge Martin Hackard, and, as the practice there did not flourish, returned to East Hampton. The development of a severe asthma within a few months forced him to leave for La Grangeville, in Dutchess County, New York—Washington Irving territory—where he practiced medicine until 1901. He was member of the Medical Society of New York (1880) and became honorary member of the Brooklyn Society of Neurology in 1898. He served as president of the Dutchess County Medical Society. There, a son was born, Charles Gardiner, to be followed by the birth of another son, Edwin Horton, and three daughters, Catherine, Elizabeth, and Eleanore. Because of his health, the family moved to Asheville, North Carolina, where he practiced until 1903. As his health improved, the family finally settled in Hopewell Junction (Dutchess County) where he set up his practice. At home, he played the piano and the flute and usually went hunting with his setters.

His children persuaded him to retire in 1915. He went to live with his son Edwin at Cairo, in the Catskills (New York). He succumbed there to pneumonia on 3 March 1916. He was survived by his wife, who also died in her son's house, in 1921 at the age of 71.

Not much more is known about him. Even less is known about his progeny, no further historical or genealogical research having been carried out. His son Charles graduated in chemistry and ultimately obtained a high position in the Chicago Nortwestern Banknote & Engraving Company; his son Edwin became a medical practitioner in Cairo, where he hospitably housed his parents. Some further details about George Huntington can be found in early sources[3, 4] and in a recent one.[5]

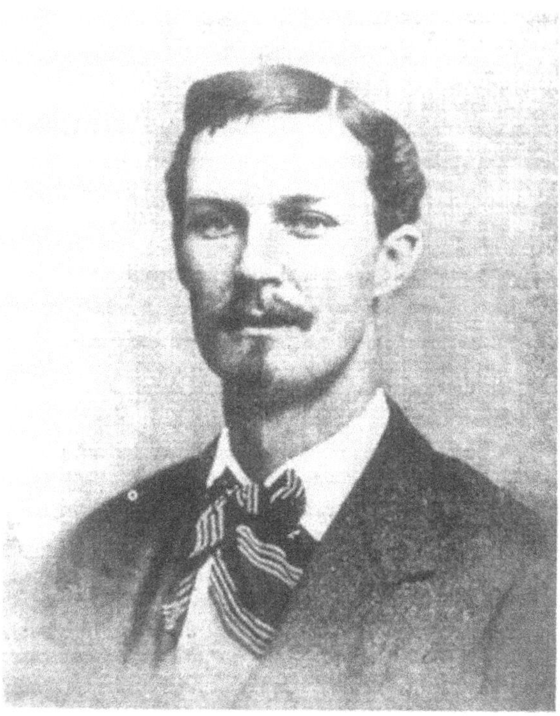

Figure 50–1. George Huntington (1850–1921). Courtesy of the late Dr. Russell W. DeJong.

Huntington read his (now historical) essay on 15 February 1872, to the Meigs and Mason Academy of Medicine—probably a local medical society with monthly meetings, of which the records have been lost. In the essay, he ends by observing

> And now I wish to draw your attention more particularly to a form of the disease which exists, so far as I know, almost exclusively on the east end of Long Island

and goes on to elaborate on its hereditary nature, its tendency to insanity and suicide, and its manifestation as a grave disease only in adult life. He points out that "it never skips a generation to manifest itself again in another; once having yielded its claims, it never regains them," and that

> in my grandfather's and father's experience which conjointly cover a period of 78 years, nervous excitement in a marked degree almost invariably attends upon every disease the patient may suffer from.

He emphasized the impairment of mind, the tendency to suicide and uninhibited erotic behavior, and closed by saying

> I have drawn your attention to this form of chorea, gentlemen, not that I consider it of any great practical importance to you, but merely as a medical curiosity, and as such it may have been of interest.

Apparently the lecture was so well received that he submitted the text—on a "medical curiosity" prevalent 500 miles to the east—to the editors of the *Medical and Surgical Reporter of Philadelphia,* nearer to the malady's focus. They published it within weeks of receipt.[6] The fact that this essay from an obscure and very young country practitioner published in a parochial journal was taken up in abstract form by Virchow and Hirsch's *Jahresbericht* (1872) decisively contributed to a rapid and widespread recognition.[7] The eponym "Huntington's chorea" was soon coined by Huber.[8]

Huntington referred to "his" chorea only twice,[9,10] mentioning in a paper read to the New York Neurological Society on 7 December 1909 that he had seen practically no other cases since 1871, and, as stipulated by de Jong,[11] that he

> without the facts and observations handed down to him by his grandfather and father, never could have formulated a picture of the salient characteristics of the disease so true and so complete.

Huntington closed by observing that

> over fifty years ago, in riding with my father on his professional rounds, I saw my first case of 'that disorder' which was the way the natives always referred to that dreadful disease . . . It made a most enduring impression upon my boyish mind, an impression which was the very first impulse in my choosing chorea as my virgin contribution to medical lore.

Since the mid-1980s, this eponym, having enjoyed wide recognition for a century, is being replaced by the expression "Huntington's disease." The new term has lost information with respect to the most conspicuous symptom of the disorder, without imparting new or essential information, or really implying that there are more symptoms than chorea. Moreover, the new term does not cure the inexactitude of the old, as running true to Stiegler's law of eponymy, George Huntington was not by far the first physician to describe the malady.[12,13]

Indeed, George's father, George Lee Huntington, and his grandfather, Abel Huntington, both medical practitioners at East Hampton, were familiar with hereditary progressive chorea. George Lee, in fact, read and corrected the text of his son's essay. Accordingly, while still disregarding the six or seven princeps observations antedating those of George's 1872 paper, the term "Huntingtons' chorea" would qualify as more appropriate.

Interest in this relatively rare disease remained tepid for nearly a century. Then, in the late 1960s, two developments concurred: the silent revolution of molecular biology following the Watson–Crick DNA helix discovery, and the founding in Montreal 1967 of the Research Group of Huntington's Chorea. An avalanche of reports started to build up.[14] Soon the gene was located at chromosome 4.p16.3,[15] it was identified,[16] the gene's product was determined,[17] and a predictive test was developed, while the various clinical types and ages at manifestation were correlated with the abnormal protein's structure.[18,19] The cytohistological effects of this protein on neurons are in the stage of clarification, and the promise of prophylactic genetic engineering appears within reach.

Soon the venerable and traditional eponym, already changing, will be swapped—for something like "*IT15* disease"—and the last vestiges of the past events will be buried under the dust of time. Perhaps rightly so: the eponym rests upon a single publication in a modest practitioner's entire life. There are, however, at least three eponyms in neurology which rendered enduring recognition to men who never published a word on their eponym's topic. No valid arguments, therefore, exist to discontinue the charming, resonating use of "Huntington's chorea" at the bedside or in professional script.

References

1. Van der Weiden RMF. George Huntington and George Sumner Huntington: a tale of two doctors. *Hist Phil Life Sci.* 1989;11:297–304.
2. Van der Weiden RMF. George Huntington and George Summer Huntington. In: Cerens E F, Tricot J P, eds. *Proceedings of the 32nd International Congress of the History of Medicine.* Bruxelles: Société Belgique de L'Histoire de la Médecine, 1991;615–620.
3. Winfield J M. A biographical sketch of George Huntington. *Neurographs (Brooklyn).* 1908; 1:89–95.
4. Stevenson CS. A biography of George Huntington. *Bull Hist Med.* 1934;2:53–76.
5. Durbach N, Hayden M R. George Huntington, the man behind the syndrome. *J Med Genet* 1993;30:406–409.
6. Huntington G. On chorea. *Med Surg Reporter Philad.* 1872;26:317–321.
7. Kuszmaul A, Nothnagel H. Krankheiten des Nervensystems. In: Virchow R, Hirsch A, eds. *Jahresbericht über die Leistungen und Fortschrine der ges amlen Medizin Berlin, A. Hirschwald* 1872;7:32.
8. Huber E. Chorea hereditaria der Erwachsenen (Huntingtonscher Chorea). *Virchow's Arch Pathol Anat.* 1887;108:267–285.
9. Huntington G. Huntington's chorea. *Brooklyn Med J.* 1895;9:173.
10. Huntington G. Recollections of Huntington's chorea as I saw it at East Hampton, Long Island, during my boyhood. *J Nerv Ment Dis.* 1910;37:255–257.
11. De Jong RN. The history of Huntington's chorea in the United States. In: Barbeau A, Chase T N, Paulson G W, eds. *Advances in Neurology.* New York: Raven Press; 1973;1:19–27.
12. Bruyn G W. Huntington's chorea. In: Vinken P J, Bruyn G W, eds. *Handbook of Clinical Neurology.* Amsterdam: North-Holland, Publishing Company; 1968;6:298–302.
13. Bruyn G W, Went L N. Huntington's chorea. In: Vinken P J, Bruyn G W, eds. *Handbook of Clinical Neurology.* Amsterdam: Elsevier; 1986;49:267.
14. Bruyn G W, Baro F, Myrianthopoulos NC. *A Centennial Bibliography of Huntington's Chorea 1872–1972.* The Hague: Nijhoff; 1974:3–14.
15. Gusella J F, Wexler N S, Conneally P M. A polymorphic DNA marker genetically linked to Huntington's disease. *Nature.* 1983;306:234–238.
16. Huntington's Disease Collaborative Research Group. A novel gene containing a trinucleotide repeat that is expanded and unstable on Huntington's disease chromosomes. *Cell.* 1993;72:971–978.
17. Strong T, Tagle D, Valdes J. Widespread expression of human and rat Huntington's disease gene in brain and nonneural tissues. *Nat Gen.* 1993;5:259–265.
18. Snell R, MacMillan J, Cheadle J. Relationship between trinucleotide expansion and phenotype variation in Huntington's disease. *Nat Gen.* 1993;4:393–397.
19. Andrew S, Goldberg P, Franz M. Correlation between the onset age of Huntington's disease and length of the trinucleotide repeat in IT 15. *Hum Mol Genet.* 1993;2:1547–1549.

51

PARKINSON'S DISEASE

Frank Clifford Rose

This condition is probably the eponymous disease most widely recognized by the general lay public. In spite of this, few know the details of Parkinson's life.

He was born in April 1755 in Hoxton (to the northeast of the City of London), an area which in the late eighteenth century was more salubrious than now. Baptized and married in St. Leonards Church, he was buried in its churchyard as were his father, grandfather, and great-grandfather, all four generations practicing as surgeon–apothecaries for a continuous period of 80 years.[1] There is no portrait of Parkinson, but his friend, Dr. Mantell, wrote

> Mr Parkinson was rather below middle stature, with an energetic intellect, and pleasing expression of countenance, and of mild and courteous manners; readily imparting information, either on his favourite science, or on professional subjects.

Having been apprenticed to his father, he was one of the earliest medical students to enter the London Hospital Medical College, where he studied for a period of six months. He married Mary Dale in St. Leonards Church in 1781, and they had six children, four of whom survived infancy. Eight years later (1784–1785) he attended a course of surgical lectures given by John Hunter (1728–1793), the "Father of British Surgery," where his knowledge of shorthand was invaluable; a transcription of his verbatim account of the lectures is preserved in the library of the Royal College of Surgeons. He was elected a Fellow of the Medical Society of London (founded 1773) in 1787 and gave his first paper to that society on "Some Account of the Effects of Lightening".[2]

In 1814, Parkinson wrote a letter to the editor of the *London Medical Repository*[3] concerning two cases of hydrophobia he had observed some 26 years earlier in conjunction with Sir William Blizard (1743–1835). Parkinson gave his notes on these cases to Dr. Andrew Marshall and they appeared unabridged in Dr. Marshall's posthumously published *The Morbid Anatomy of the Brain.*[4]

A politically active supporter of parliamentary and electoral reform, he was an early member of radical societies and wrote several political tracts during the years 1793–1795, after the French Revolution and during the opening stages of the Napoleonic Wars between England and France. These writings were under the pseudonym "Old Hubert," but his publishers were repeatedly prosecuted for seditious libel. When called to give evidence before the Privy Council, Parkinson admitted being the author of such tracts as *Revolution Without Bloodshed; or, Reformation Preferable to Revolt,*[5] *Pearls Cast Before Swine,*[6] and *An Address to the Hon Edmund Burke: From the Swinish Multitude.*[7]

In 1807, Samuel Whitbread, both member of Parliament and son of the brewer, introduced a bill in the House of Commons "for providing and encouraging industry amongst the labouring classes of the country and the relief and regulation of the criminal and necessitous poor." Among other measures, it sought to establish parochial schools throughout the country, providing free education for pauper children for a period of two years. Parkinson was one of a number of authors, including Reverend Thomas Robert Malthus (1766–1834, author of *An Essay on the Principle of Population,* 1798), who criticized the bill. An account of the work and aims of the school is given in his tract *Remarks on Mr Whitbread's Plan for the Education of the Poor.*[8] One pragmatic criticism of Whitbread's provisions was that the parents of children in employment would be unlikely to forgo their income for the sake of their education. When Parkinson gave evidence before the Privy Council, in the so-called Pop-Gun Plot to assassinate George III, he acquired some public notoriety.

Even before his famous essay, he published several medical works, two of which were on domestic medicine: *Medical Admonitions to Families*[9] and *The Villager's Friend & Physician.*[10] Other works were *Dangerous Sports,*[11] stories for children warning against dangerous games; *The Hospital Pupil,*[12] which consisted of letters from Parkinson to a father whose son wanted to be a doctor, outlining the necessary qualities and recommending a suitable course of study; *The Chemical Pocket-Book;*[13] and *Observation on the Nature & Cure of Gout,*[14] which gave a detailed account of personal experience of the disease which he had had for 15 years.

Later in life, Parkinson became famous for his research into fossils and as a student of orycytology (paleontology), he amassed one of the largest collections of fossils in Britain. Between the years 1804 and 1811 he published the three quarto volumes entitled *Organic Remains of a Former World,*[15] a comprehensive study of paleobotany and paleozoology trying to link paleontology to the study of strata. A founding member of the Geological Society of London (established 1807), he published several contributions in its *Transactions.*[16]

For more than 25 years Parkinson was a regular medical attendant to Holly House, Hoxton, a private madhouse of 118 beds, and in 1810 was a medical witness at the trial of a man found guilty of confining his aunt who, it was alleged, was of sound mind. Parkinson was severely reprimanded for having certified the woman as insane only on the report of her relatives and not as a result of his own observations.

Because of this criticism, he defended himself by publishing *Observations on the Act for Regulating Madhouses.*[17] He was also active in promoting vaccination, which had been recently introduced by Edward Jenner (1749–1823).

James Parkinson died on 21 December 1824 in Hoxton, two days after the sudden onset of aphasia and right hemiplegia.

After accumulating a wealth of clinical experience during more than 32 years of practice, he published his seminal work, *An Essay on the Shaking Palsy,*[18] at the age of 62. In this medical classic, he reported six cases of what he termed "a tedious and most distressing malady." The essay was well reviewed by several medical and literary periodicals and his clinical description became gradually accepted during the nineteenth century, both in Britain and on the Continent. Charcot established the eponymous term "*la Maladie de Parkinson*" but ironically its anglicized form was accepted only later, possibly because Parkinson was not a pillar of the medical establishment. His clinical accuracy in describing the disease remains unbeaten. *The Essay* was published as an octavo volume of 66 pages of text, divided into five chapters, with a four-page preface. The chapters bear the following summary headings:

Chap. I Definition—History—Illustrative cases
Chap. II Pathognomonic symptoms examined—Tremor Coactus—Scelotyrbe Festinans
Chap. III Shaking Palsy distinguished from other diseases with which it may be confounded
Chap. IV Proximate cause—Remote causes—Illustrative cases
Chap. V Considerations respecting the means of cure

In the preface, Parkinson tendered "some conciliatory explanation" for publishing the *Essay,* in the hope that "the offering of the following pages to the attention of the medical public, will not be severely censured." Shaking palsy, he emphasizes,

> is of a nature highly afflictive. Notwithstanding which, it has not yet obtained a place in the classification of nosologists; some have regarded its characteristic symptoms as distinct and different diseases, and others have given its name to diseases differing essentially from it; whilst the unhappy sufferer has considered it as an evil, from the domination of which he had no prospect of escape.[18]

As the disease is of long duration, continued observation of the same cases over several years was required in order to establish the precise course of the symptoms at each stage. Parkinson had this opportunity. By making these observations of the disease in its different stages, Parkinson hoped that he

> had been led to a probable conjecture as to the nature of the malady, and that analogy had suggested such means as might be productive of relief, and perhaps even of cure, if employed before the disease had been too long established.[18]

In the final two chapters of the *Essay,* Parkinson tentatively identified as the proximate cause of the disease a lesion of the cervical portion of the spinal cord, extending to the medulla oblongata, and suggested blistering and withdrawal of

AN

ESSAY

ON THE

SHAKING PALSY.

BY

JAMES PARKINSON,

MEMBER OF THE ROYAL COLLEGE OF SURGEONS.

LONDON:

PRINTED BY WHITTINGHAM AND ROWLAND,

Goswell Street,

FOR SHERWOOD, NEELY, AND JONES,

PATERNOSTER ROW.

1817.

Figure 51–1. Title page of Parkinson's An Essay on the Shaking Palsy.

blood from the upper part of the neck. In the rationale for his diagnosis and therapy, Parkinson acknowledges

> that mere conjecture takes the place of experiment; and that analogy [is] the substitute for anatomical examination, the only sure foundation for pathological knowledge.[18]

In Chapter II, Parkinson remarks that

> certain affections, the tremulous agitations, and the almost invincible propensity to run, when wishing only to walk, each of which has been considered by nosologists as distinct diseases, appear to be pathognomonic symptoms of this malady.[18]

He also outlined some earlier ideas concerning the other major symptom of the shaking palsy: the "propensity to bend the trunk forwards, and to pass from a walking to a running pace."[18]

In Chapter III, Parkinson presents the evidence for the shaking palsy being distinct nosologically from other diseases involving tremor:

> If the trembling limb be supported, and none of its muscles be called into action, the trembling will cease. In the real Shaking Palsy the reverse of this takes place, the agitation continues in full force whilst the limb is at rest and unemployed; and even if sometimes diminished by calling the muscles into employment.[18]

Tremors which are liable to be confused with the shaking palsy include those due to alcohol abuse, tea and coffee abuse, and old age.

Chapter IV considers the causes of the disease, but Parkinson is careful to state that he has never performed a postmortem on a case. He argues that since the senses and the intellect remain unimpaired, "the morbid state does not extend to the encephalon."[18]

Parkinson's essay acknowledges the writings of Juncker, who distinguished tremors, either "Active—sudden affections of the mind, terror, anger or, Passive—dependant on debilitating causes such as advanced age, palsy etc." He credits Franciscus dele Boë (see Chapter 8) for showing the difference between rest (tremor coactus) and action tremor in 1680. François Boissier de Sauvages de Lacroix (1706–1767) had described the festinant gait, which "I think cannot be more fitly named than hastening or hurrying Scelotyrbe (scelotyrbem festinantem, seu festiniam)," as did Hieronymus David Gaubius (1705–1780) some ten years earlier. Sauvages also observed that "the tremulous parts leap, and as it were vibrate, even when supported: whilst every other tremor, he observes, ceases, when the voluntary exertion for moving the limb stops . . . but returns when we will the limb to move." Parkinson also referred to Gerard van Swieten (1700–1772), who had described resting tremor (1749). In none of these pre-Parkinson records, however, is there a distinctive clinical picture.

Parkinson's description of paralysis agitans as constituting a distinct disease quite separate from other forms of tremor was remarkable, but it was only gradually recognized. All of his six cases had involuntary tremor of the limbs, varying only in degree and distribution; five of these had the "propensity to bend the trunk forwards, and to pass from a walking to a running pace."[18] Although each of these symptoms had previously been observed, they had not been considered as distinct clinical entities.

Parkinson's originality lay in his recognition that the two components were pathognomic of a single malady, which he termed "shaking palsy, paralysis agitans."

Several years elapsed before the teachers of medicine in the London medical schools began to take notice of Parkinson's identification of the shaking palsy as a clinical entity. It took 40 years or more until the syndrome was recorded in standard works. Robert Bentley Todd in his clinic lectures:

> The patient begins to stoop, he finds he cannot hold himself erect, and in some instances his gait is apt to pass into that which is known as symptomatic of the disease termed "paralysis agitans."[22]

Armand Trousseau[23] (1801–1867) made two important additions to Parkinson's account. He recognized both rigidity and mental impairment in his lectures on clinical medicine. He explained the festinant gait:

> As his center of gravity is thus displaced, he is obliged to run after himself, as it were, so that he keeps trotting and hopping on.

Trousseau also described the progressive slowing of repeated hand opening, the first clear account of bradykinesia. Although Parkinson had said "the senses and intellect being uninjured," Trousseau commented:

> The intellect . . . gets weakened at last; the patient loses his memory and his friends notice soon that his mind is not as clear: precocious caducity sets in.

Jean-Martin Charcot (1825–1893) left a masterly account of paralysis agitans. In a lecture given at the Salpêtrière in Paris, he first differentiated disseminated sclerosis from paralysis agitans.[19] He described a group of cases in which "tremor is only shown when an intentive movement is made," and contrasted it with another group in which "tremor is a constant symptom . . . it rarely departs except during sleep." Of paralysis agitans, Charcot remarked

> Its history, however, does not reach far back. The first regular description of it only dates from 1817; it is due to Dr Parkinson, who published it in a little work entitled *Essay on the Shaking Palsy.*

This Charcot referred to Russell Reynolds's *System of Medicine* (specifically, an article by W. R. Sanders, Vol. II, p. 184),[20] containing the first complete and extensive consideration of paralysis agitans to be found in any English textbook.[19]

> But in all these descriptions, and our own does not at all escape this reproach, there is complete confusion between paralysis agitans and disseminated sclerosis. The line of demarcation between the two diseases was for the first time indicated by myself, if I mistake not, in the thesis of M Ordenstein (*Sur la paralysie agitante et la sclérose en plaques généralisée.* Thèse de Paris, 1868).[21]

It was Charcot who described so aptly a peculiar characteristic of the tremor of the hands where the thumb moves over the fingers, "as when a pencil or paper ball is rolled between them . . . [or] in crumbling a piece of bread."[19] He believed that he had also contributed to the clinical picture of this disease in recognizing the presence of rigidity:

> We shall now point out a characteristic [he said], which, we believe, was overlooked by Parkinson as well as by most of his successors: we allude to the rigidity to be found, at a certain stage of the disease, in the muscles of the extremities of the body and, for the most part, in those of the neck also . . . Generally, the flexor muscles are the first, as they are always the most intensely affected . . . Thus on account of the rigidity of the anterior muscles of the neck, the head, as Parkinson remarked, is greatly bent forward and, as one might say, fixed in that position: for the patient cannot, without much effort, raise it up, or turn it to the right or left. The body is also slightly inclined forward when the patient is standing.[19]

In a note to the second edition of the lectures, Charcot introduced the eponymous name for paralysis agitans, when in describing an illustrative case, he said "A man aged fifty years was attacked by PARKINSON'S DISEASE." This case was of special interest because it was diagnosed as paralysis agitans in the absence of tremor, all the symptoms and signs being present, including rigidity.

Thus, Charcot felt, as all clinical neurologists must, that the disorder justly deserves its eponymous title of Parkinson's disease, and many later writers concur, for example, Rowntree (1912),[24] McMenemy (1955),[25] and Gardner-Thorpe (1987).[26]

References

1 Rose, F C. *James Parkinson: His Life and Times by A D Morris.* Boston: Birkenhauser; 1989.
2. Parkinson, J. Some account of the Effects of Lightening. *Memoirs of the Medical Society of London.* 1789;2:193, 493–503.
3. Parkinson, J. To the Editors of the London Medical Repository. *London Medical Repository.* 1814;1:289–292.
4. Marshall, A. *The Morbid Anatomy of the Brain.* London: Longman, Hurst, Rees & Orme; 1815.
5. Parkinson, J. *Revolutions Without Bloodshed; or, Reformation Preferable to Revolt.* London; 1794.
6. Parkinson, J. *Pearls Cast Before Swine . . . Scraped Together by Old Hubert.* London: DI Eaton; 1793(?).
7. Parkinson, J. *Address to the Hon. Edmund Burke: From the Swinish Multitude. By Old Hubert.* London: J Ridgeway; 1793.
8. Parkinson, J. *Remarks on Mr Whitbread's Plan for the Education of the Poor.* London: HD Symonds; 1807.
9. Parkinson, J. *Medical Admonitions to Families, Respecting the Preservation of Health & The Treatment of the Sick.* London: HD Symonds; 1801.
10. Parkinson, J. *The Villager's Friend & Physician.* 2nd ed. London: C Whittingham; 1804.
11. Parkinson, J. *Dangerous Sports. A Tale Addressed to Children.* London: HD Symonds; 1808.
12. Parkinson, J. *The Hospital Pupil; or, an Essay Intended to Facilitate the Study of Medicine & Surgery. In Four Letters.* London: HD Symonds; 1800.
13. Parkinson, J. *The Chemical Pocket-Book; or, Memoranda Chemica; Arranged in a Compendia of Chemistry.* London; 1800.
14. Parkinson, J. *Observations on the Nature & Cure of Gout; on Nodes of the joints & on the Influence of Certain Articles of Diet in Gout, Rheumatism & Gravel.* London: HD Symonds; 1805.
15. Parkinson, J. *Organic Remains of a Former World.* London: J Robson; 1804–1811.

16. Parkinson, J. Observations on some of the strata in the neighbourhood of London and on the fossil remains contained in them. *Trans Geol Soc.* 1811;1:324.
17. Parkinson, J. *Observations on the Act for Regulating Madhouses.* London; 1811.
18. Parkinson, J. *An Essay on the Shaking Palsy.* London: Sherwood, Neely and Jones; 1817.
19. Charcot, J M; Sigerson G, trans. On paralysis agitans. In: *Lectures on the Diseases of the Nervous System.* London: New Sydenham Society; 1877:129–156.
20. Reynolds, J Russell. *A System of Medicine.* London; 1866–1879.
21. Ordenstein, L. *Sur la Paralysie Agitante et la Sclérose en Généralisées.* Paris: Mortimer; 1867.
22. Todd, R B. *Certain Diseases of the Brain and Other Affections of the Nervous System.* Philadelphia: Lindsay and Blakiston; 1854.
23. Trousseau A; Bazire P V, trans. Lecture XV: Senile trembling and Paralysis Agitans. In: *Lectures on Clinical Medicine delivered at the Hotel-Dieu, Paris.* London: New Sydenham Society, 1868:441–450.
24. Rowntree L G. James Parkinson. *Bull Johns Hopkins Hosp.* 1912;23:33–45.
25. McMenemy W H. James Parkinson 1755–1824: a biographical essay. In: Critchley M, ed. *James Parkinson 1755–1824.* London: Macmillan; 1955:1–44.
26. Gardner-Thorpe C. *James Parkinson 1755–1824.* Exeter: Wheaton & Co Ltd; 1987.

52

PICK'S DISEASE

Nicolaas J. M. Arts

The history of Pick's disease is complex and confusing.[1–4] Over a period of 14 years, Arnold Pick published a series of four papers in which he pointed out that within the large group of the senile demented, there are patients with unusually severe aphasia and apraxia due to circumscribed atrophy of the cortex.[5–8] Being convinced that these patients were suffering from senile dementia, Pick did not even envisage the possibility that he was describing a new disease entity. However, when Alzheimer studied the brains of two demented patients with circumscribed cortical atrophy, he found very characteristic histological abnormalities: argentophile inclusions and swollen neurons.[9] From 1925 on, the name "Pick's disease" was applied both to cases with the microscopic abnormalities described by Alzheimer and to cases with the macroscopic atrophy described by Pick. This led to decades-long confusion, because the former group of cases is considerably smaller and forms a subgroup of the latter—which even includes cases of Alzheimer's disease. These diagnostic problems have only recently been clarified.

Arnold Pick was born of German-Jewish parents on 20 July 1851 in Gross-Meseritsch, near Iglau in Moravia, then a province of the Austro-Hungarian Empire.[10–14] He attended the Gymnasium of Iglau and studied medicine in Vienna. While still a student, he became assistant to the neuropsychiatrist Theodor Meynert (1833–1892), whose influence on him was considerable. In 1874 Pick went to Berlin, to work as a trainee with Carl Westphal (1833–1890) at the Charité. From 1875 to 1877 he was a resident in the asylum of Wehnen and from 1877 to 1880 he worked in the Prague state asylum. He received his teaching qualification as a lecturer in neurology and psychiatry from the University of Prague in 1878. In the Prague asylum he met Otto Kahler (1849–1893), and a lifelong friendship began. Together they published a series of classical papers on oculomotor palsies, ataxia, cortical localization, syringomyelia, and other affections of the spinal cord.

In 1880 Pick was appointed assistant director of the new psychiatric institute in Dobrzan, and two years later he became its director. In 1886, at the early age of 35 years, he was promoted to full professor and soon took over the chair of the Neuropsychiatry Department in Prague. He remained in this post for the next 35 years.

Pick's pupil Otto Sittig (1886–1943) relates that Pick did not have an easy time as director of the department in Prague.[10,11] Although Bohemia, of which Prague was the capital, belonged to the Austro-Hungarian Empire, Czechs were predominant and they were engaged in a struggle for independence. Alongside the German university and hospitals, there was a Czech university and Czech hospitals. The German institutions faced many problems, especially because the hospitals and asylums belonged to the province of Bohemia, whereas the universities were controlled by Vienna. The housing of the German neuropsychiatry department was rented from the state asylum and Pick never had complete authority over it. Formerly a monastery, it was a very old building, overcrowded and ill-adapted to the maintenance of even the most primitive hygiene. Essential facilities such as a psychological laboratory were absent. Personal relationships often suffered from the political difficulties; Pick had to face much small-mindedness, resentment, and hostility, according to Sittig.

Pick was a highly cultivated man; his best friends were from outside the medical school and included the physicist and philosopher Ernst Mach and the psychologist Christian von Ehrenfels. He was an ardent lover of music, especially Beethoven, and collected books in many languages; they were piled from floor to ceiling in his home. He is described as a noble-minded, excessively modest, but fearless man, "the essence of calm serenity."[12]

Pick retired in 1921, but he never stopped working, although his last years were marred by illness. He lost his sight because of cataracts, and one of his eyes had to be enucleated. A renal stone was removed in 1924, unfortunately followed by many complications. On 4 April of the same year, at the age of 73, Pick died of urinary sepsis following an operation for bladder calculus.

Pick made many important contributions to neurology,[11] and the breadth of his publications is remarkable, ranging from microscopic studies of the spinal cord to analyses of visual hallucinations and hysterical psychosis. The majority of his more than 350 papers deal with what are now called neuropsychology and behavioral neurology. Because of the above-mentioned logistic and political difficulties, he was never able to carry out any large-scale scientific projects. He therefore had to confine himself to single case studies, the results of which could eventually be synthesized into more general conclusions. Pick was among the first to give reliable descriptions of visual hallucinations, micrographia, palilalia, and reduplicating paramnesia. He wrote seminal papers on apraxia and on the visual system of rabbits.

According to Sittig, Pick had a very characteristic scientific approach that is evident even in his first paper: a very detailed patient history with autobiographical accounts and comments by the patients, with emphasis on psychological data, meticulous note of the pertinent literature, and a very cautious interpretation of the facts.

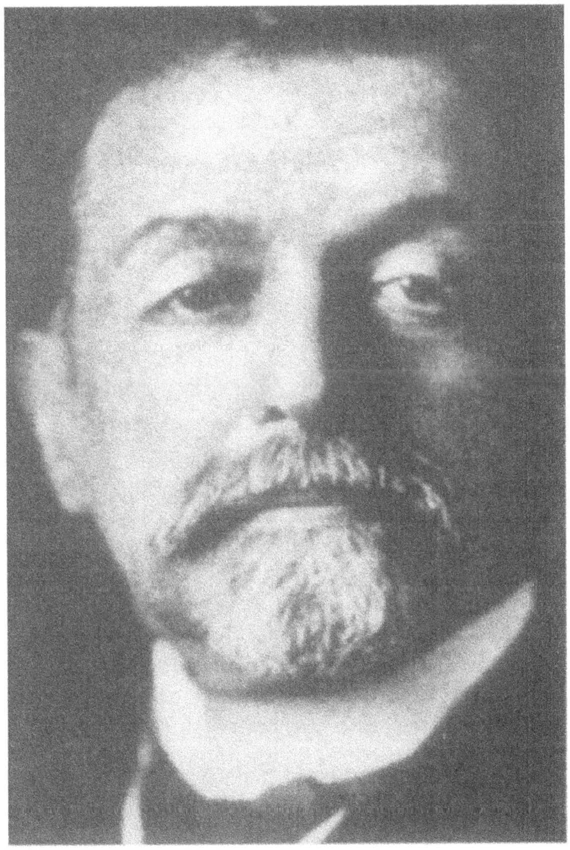

Figure 52–1. Arnold Pick (1851–1924). Courtesy of the Center of Scientific Information, Third Medical Faculty, Prague.

Pick's psychological approach is also apparent in his publications on language pathology, which are undoubtedly his major contribution to neuroscience. In his work on "agrammatism"[15]—a term he introduced—he provided a psychological foundation for aphasiology. He argued that a sentence is not simply an additive summation of words, but a psychological unity. The agrammatical speech disturbances, the disorders of sentence construction, should be considered the core problem of aphasiology. Modern linguists have built a comprehensive theory about syntactical structures in language expression, erected on the foundations laid by Pick.[16]

Carl Wernicke (1848–1905)[17] initially influenced Pick's views on language. Pick was the first to place Wernicke's ideas on a sound pathoanatomical basis, but later he became influenced by John Hughlings Jackson (1835–1911), whose ideas shine through in his work on agrammatism. Jackson and Pick held each other in high esteem and it is not difficult to see their similarities. Both were scientists, not teachers; both were theoreticians, but disliked empty speculation; and both recorded their findings in terse prose, without consideration for the prospective reader, and therefore wrote papers that were often difficult to understand.

Pick corresponded extensively with Dejerine, Marie, Head, and especially Jackson, to whom he dedicated his monograph on agrammatism. This book came to the attention of Henry Head, who was spurred to study Jackson's writings on aphasia. In this way, Pick was instrumental in bringing about the revival of interest in Jackson's work, not only on the Continent but also in England.[18]

Between 1892 and 1906, Pick wrote four papers on patients with aphasia and apraxia due to circumscribed atrophy of cortical areas,[5–8] mostly in the temporal lobe (only the last case had frontal lobe atrophy). In his introduction to the first paper, he clearly stated what he wanted to accomplish:

> While it is certain now that the early stages of general paresis of the insane are characterised by focal symptoms and forms of aphasia which rarely seem to result from a complicating [i.e., an additional] gross focal lesion, nobody has ever considered the possibility that the same could occur with the atrophy underlying simple, uncomplicated senile dementia. The current view is rather that, apart from the so-called "amnestic" variety, all aphasias accompanying senile dementia result from complicating [additional] gross focal lesions. Wernicke . . . once stated that general paresis is the only form of mental disorder which in due course can lead to cortical and subcortical focal symptoms, and therefore occupies a midway position between mental illness and organic brain disease. This paper intends to show that the same does apply to senile dementia, or to the cerebral atrophy that underlies it, thereby providing a further contribution to the attempts to link neuropathology and psychiatry more closely, as a result of which psychiatry will be more accessible to medical understanding.[5]

In other words, he wanted to prove that focal symptoms can result not only of gross focal lesions—such as infarctions and hemorrhages—but also from a more or less circumscribed atrophy; and that they can appear not only in general paresis (dementia paralytica), but also in simple forms of senile dementia, without any complicating gross lesions.

In the 1901, 1904, and 1906 papers, Pick returned to this point.[6–8] Again, he took a stand against Wernicke. In five additional cases he showed that contrary to what Wernicke believed, simple atrophy of a circumscribed cortical area *can* cause loss of function of this area, and *can* cause focal symptoms such as aphasia and apraxia. This vital point apart, Pick had nothing to prove. It is unlikely that the thought of having described a new disease entity ever crossed his mind, because he was convinced that these patients were suffering from senile dementia.

The history of Pick's disease took a different—and in all respects decisive—turn when Alzheimer, in his 1911 paper "on peculiar cases of illness in old age,"[9] described two cases of "a group of senile diseases to which Pick devoted particularly detailed studies, the cases with circumscribed atrophy." Unlike Pick, Alzheimer studied the brains of his patients microscopically, and he discovered abnormalities never seen before: achromatic neuronal ballooning and intraneuronal argentophilic inclusion bodies, later called "Pick cells" and "Pick bodies." These findings remained unnoticed for almost 14 years.

In 1922, the Dutch neurologist Gans wrote a paper on a case of frontal lobe atrophy in which he suggested the eponymic term "Pick's atrophy."[19] He showed that the atrophic areas did not correspond to the areas of arterial supply, and that a vascular cause was therefore unlikely. In a later paper he stressed that a hereditary disposition was involved.

Alzheimer's important observations were rediscovered around 1925. Onari and Spatz were the first to make an attempt to define the local cerebral atrophies—now called "Pick's atrophy" or "Pick's disease"—as a disease entity.[20] In a seminal contribution they gave a more precise description of the atrophy and showed that it was not linked to vascular or inflammatory pathology. They also found that the atrophy always appeared in a phylogenetically young area, while the projection areas generally remain unaffected. In all their patients the microscopic abnormalities were most prominent in the superficial cortical layers, a finding that was to be confirmed by nearly all subsequent investigators.

Carl Schneider was the first to elaborate the symptomatology of Pick's disease.[21,22] He distinguished three stages, the first of which was characterized by a compulsive lack of restraint. Some patients were irritable at first, but soon became indifferent. The second stage was characterized by a progressive dementia, with disturbances of thinking and judgment, while imprinting and memory remained intact for a remarkably long time. Focal symptoms appeared at this stage: a gradual loss of initiative in frontal atrophies and progressive aphasia in temporal atrophies. The third stage showed a complete apathy and mutism, as a result of which it was extremely difficult to determine what the patient was still able to do. In the end, the patient was reduced to an almost complete vegetative existence, with flexion contractures of one or more extremities.

From the 1930s to the 1980s there was no universally accepted definition of Pick's disease. Disagreement, misunderstanding, and confusion reigned supreme.[2] The French tended to diagnose Pick's disease without recourse to any histological examination, while the Genevan school recognized three forms of Pick's disease (without the specific histological abnormalities; with only one of these abnormalities; with both abnormalities) and several subtypes.[23] Many German neurologists used histological criteria but maintained nevertheless that Alzheimer's disease and Pick's disease could be differentiated on the basis of clinical criteria, whereas American neurologists generally believed that this was impossible. Moreover, even in the clinical diagnosis of Pick's disease, French, Swiss, Swedish, and American authors all used different criteria.[2]

In the 1980s, neuropsychiatrists from Lund, Sweden, and Manchester, England, discussed the predominantly frontal or frontotemporal gray matter degenerations associated with behavior that differed from that of typical Alzheimer patients. In April 1994, after several conferences, they published a consensus, on "Clinical and Neuropathological Criteria for Frontotemporal Dementia,"[24] which was revised in 1998.[25] This paper clarified the position of Pick's disease within the frontotemporal dementias: the nature and distribution of neuropathological changes is similar in all these dementias, except that in Pick's disease achromatic swollen neurons (Pick cells) and silver staining inclusions containing immunoreactive tau and ubiquitin (Pick bodies) are present, and the white matter gliosis is more intense. Kertesz et al.[26] introduced the term "Pick complex" to cover the whole family of frontotemporal dementias. In other words, the histological abnormalities first described by Alzheimer define the modern concept of "Pick's disease," while the macroscopic atrophy first described by Pick is now practically covered by the designation "Pick complex." However, the current debate about conceptual distinctions among frontotemporal degeneration, Pick's disease, and corticobasal degeneration testifies that the controversies surrounding frontotemporal dementias have not yet been settled.[27]

References

1. Mansvelt J. *Pick's Disease; A Syndrome of Lobar Cerebral Atrophy, Its Clinico-Anatomical and Histopathological Types.* Enschede; 1954. Thesis (University of Utrecht).
2. Pasquier F, Petit H. Frontotemporal dementia: its rediscovery. *Eur Neurol.* 1997;38:1–6.
3. Kertesz A. Pick's disease and Pick complex: introductory nosology. In: Kertesz A, Munoz D G, eds. *Pick's Disease and Pick Complex.* New York: Wiley-Liss; 1998.
4. Arts NJM, ed. Das schwindende Hirn: *Alois Alzheimer und die Anfänge der Demenzforschung.* Nijmegen: Sylvius; 2000.
5. Pick A. Über die Beziehungen der senilen Hirnatrophie zur Aphasie. *Prag Med Wochenschr.* 1892;17:165–167. Reprinted in: Arts.[4] Present author's translation. A slightly abbreviated and not completely reliable translation in: *Hist Psychiatry.* 1994;5:542–547.
6. Pick A. Senile Hirnatrophie als Grundlage von Herderscheinungen. *Wien Klin Wochenschr.* 1901;14:403–404. Reprinted in: Arts.[4] Translation in: *Hist Psychiatry.* 1995;6:533–537.
7. Pick A. Zur Symptomatologie der linksseitigen Schläfenlappenatrophie. *Monatschr Psychiat Neurol.* 1904;16:378–388. Reprinted in: Arts.[4] Translation in: *Hist Psychiatry.* 1997;8:149–159.
8. Pick A. Über einen weiterer Symptomenkomplex im Rahmen der Dementia senilis, bedingt durch umschriebene starkere Hirnatrophie. *Monatschr Psychiatr Neurol.* 1906;19:97–108. Reprinted in: Arts.[4] Translation will appear in: *Hist Psychiatry.*
9. Alzheimer A. Über eigenartige Krankheitsfälle des Späteren Alters. *Z Ges Neurol Psychiatr.* 1911;4:356–385. Reprinted in: Arts.[4] Translation in: *Hist Psychiatry.* 1991;2:71–102.
10. Sittig O. Professor MUDr. Arnold Pick †. *Jahrb Psychiatr.* 1924;44:i–x.
11. Sittig O. Professor Arnold Pick †. *Arch Psychiatr.* 1924;72:1–20. With a nearly complete bibliography of Pick's works.
12. Brown M R. Arnold Pick. In: Haymaker W, Schiller F, eds. *The Founders of Neurology.* 2nd ed. Springfield, Ill: Charles C Thomas; 1970:358–362.
13. Kertesz A, Kalvach P. Arnold Pick and German neuropsychiatry in Prague. *Arch Neurol.* 1996;53:935–938.
14. Kertesz A. Arnold Pick: a historical introduction. In: Kertesz A, Munoz D G, eds. *Pick's Disease and Pick Complex.* New York: Wiley-Liss; 1998.
15. Pick A. *Die agrammatischen Sprachstörungen.* Berlin: Springer; 1913.
16. Goodglass H. Agrammatism in aphasiology. *Clin Neurosci.* 1997;4:51–56.
17. Wernicke C. *Der aphasische Symptomencomplex: Eine psychologische Studie auf anatomischer Basis.* Breslau: Cohn & Weigert; 1874.
18. Wallesch C W. Hughlings Jackson and European neurology. In: Kennard C, Swash M, eds. *Hierarchies in Neurology: A Reappraisal of a Jacksonian Concept.* London: Springer; 1989.
19. Gans A. Betrachtungen über Art und Ausbreitung des krankhaften Prozesses in einem Fall von Pickscher Atrophie des Stirnhirns. *Z Ges Neurol Psychiatr.* 1922;80:10–28.
20. Onari K, Spatz H. Anatomische Beiträge zur Lehre von der Pickschen umschriebenen Grosshirnrindenatrophie (Picksche Krankheit). *Z Ges Neurol Psychiatr.* 1926;101:470–511.

21. Schneider C. Über Picksche Krankheit. *Monatschr Psychiatr Neurol.* 1927;65:230–275.
22. Schneider C. Weitere Beiträge zur Lehre von der Pickschen Krankheit. *Z Ges Neurol Psychiatr.* 1929;120:340–384.
23. Tissot R, Constantinidis J, Richard J. Pick's disease. In: Vinken P J, Bruyn G W, Klawans H L, eds. *Handbook of Clinical Neurology.* Amsterdam: Elsevier; 1985;46:233–246.
24. The Lund and Manchester Groups. Clinical and neuropathological criteria for frontotemporal dementia. *J Neurol Neurosurg Psychiatry.* 1994;57:416–418.
25. Neary D, Snowden J S, Gustafson L, et al. Frontotemporal lobar degeneration: a consensus on clinical diagnostic criteria. *Neurology.* 1998;51:1546–1554.
26. Kertesz A, Hudson L, Mackenzie IRA, Munoz D G. The pathology and nosology of primary progressive aphasia. *Neurology.* 1994;44:2065–2072.
27. Neary D, Kertesz A, Hachinski V. Frontotemporal degeneration, Pick disease, and corticobasal degeneration. *Arch Neurol.* 1997;54:1195–1196.

53

SYDENHAM'S CHOREA

Howard I. Kushner and David Cortes

Sydenham's chorea is a movement disorder characterized by facial/oral grimaces, fine, fast, uncoordinated movements often resulting from attempted voluntary actions, hypotonia, and obsessive–compulsive symptoms.[1] In the majority of cases the onset of Sydenham's chorea is diagnosed between the ages of 5 and 15, with females three times more likely than males to contract it. Most recover in two to three months, but recurrence takes place in about one-third of all cases.[2,3] The movements and behaviors that characterize this disorder are believed to result from an antibody cross-reaction to basal ganglia epitopes as a sequel to a Group A β-hemolytic streptococcus (GABHS) infection.[1,4]

During his lifetime Thomas Sydenham was known as the "English Hippocrates" because of his rejection of Galenic (scholastic) medicine in favor of careful observation of patients' signs and symptoms and differential diagnoses of seemingly similar conditions.[5,6] Born 10 September 1624 in Dorset, England, Sydenham entered Oxford University in 1642 but left that same year to serve in Cromwell's army.[6,7] He returned to Oxford in 1646, completed a Bachelor of Medicine in 1648, and was then made a fellow at All Souls College.[5,7] In 1655 Sydenham resigned his fellowship, married Mary Geffrey, with whom he later had ten children, and by some accounts moved to London. He ran unsuccessfully for Parliament in 1659 and in 1663 obtained a license to practice medicine from the Royal College of Physicians.[7]

Sydenham's best-known work was *Methodus Curandi Febres, propriis observationibus superstructa,* published in 1666. While that first edition dealt primarily with fevers and smallpox, a 1668 second edition included additional material on the plague.[8] A third edition entitled *Observationes medicae circa morborum acutorum historiam et curationem* was published in 1676,[9] the same year he received his Doctor of Medicine degree from Cambridge.[8,9]

Figure 53–1. Thomas Sydenham (1624–1689). Courtesy of the National Library of Medicine, Bethesda, Maryland.

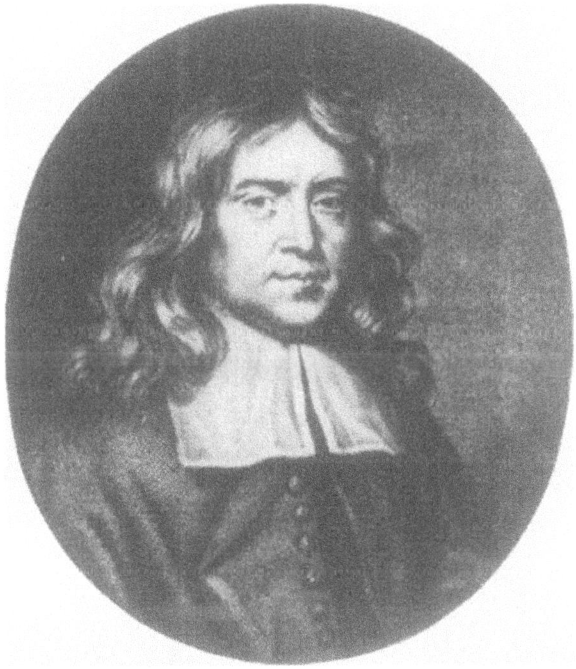

Before his death on 29 December 1689, Sydenham published *Epistola Responsoria* (1680), *Dissertatio Epistolaris* (1682), *Tractus de Podagra et Hydrope* (1683), a treatise on gout (from which he suffered), *Opera Universa* (1685), and his last book, in which he addressed convulsive movements, *Schedula Monitoria* (1686).[10] Among his acquaintances were John Locke, who reviewed *Schedula Monitoria* for *Bibliothèque Universelle,*[7] Robert Boyle, and Daniel Malthus, grandfather of Thomas Robert Malthus.[11] He was known for concocting a popular tincture, called "Sydenham's laudanum," from opium, saffron, cloves, and cinnamon.[6] An advocate of such therapeutics as bloodletting and purging, Sydenham also endorsed the curative powers of fevers, and he encouraged physicians to more carefully monitor patients' responses to treatment.[5]

The main subject of *Schedula Monitoria* was not the chorea that bears Sydenham's name, but a febrile outbreak that reached epidemic proportions during 1685. In describing the symptoms and treatment of this fever, Sydenham noted that an induced sweat during the onset of fever could result in an inordinate pulse accompanied by jerking of the limbs and, shortly thereafter, death.[10] He claimed that the best treatment for convulsing patients was bleeding and purging. To demonstrate to the reader that such therapeutics were appropriate for such convulsions, Sydenham recounted his cure of five patients suffering from St. Vitus dance.

The description in *Schedula Monitoria* collapsed different movement disorders into the term "St. Vitus dance," so named by Paracelsus after the chapel in Dresselhausen, Swabia, where late fourteenth- and early fifteenth-century German sufferers of convulsivelike behaviors made pilgrimages in search of relief (Fig. 53–2).[12,13]

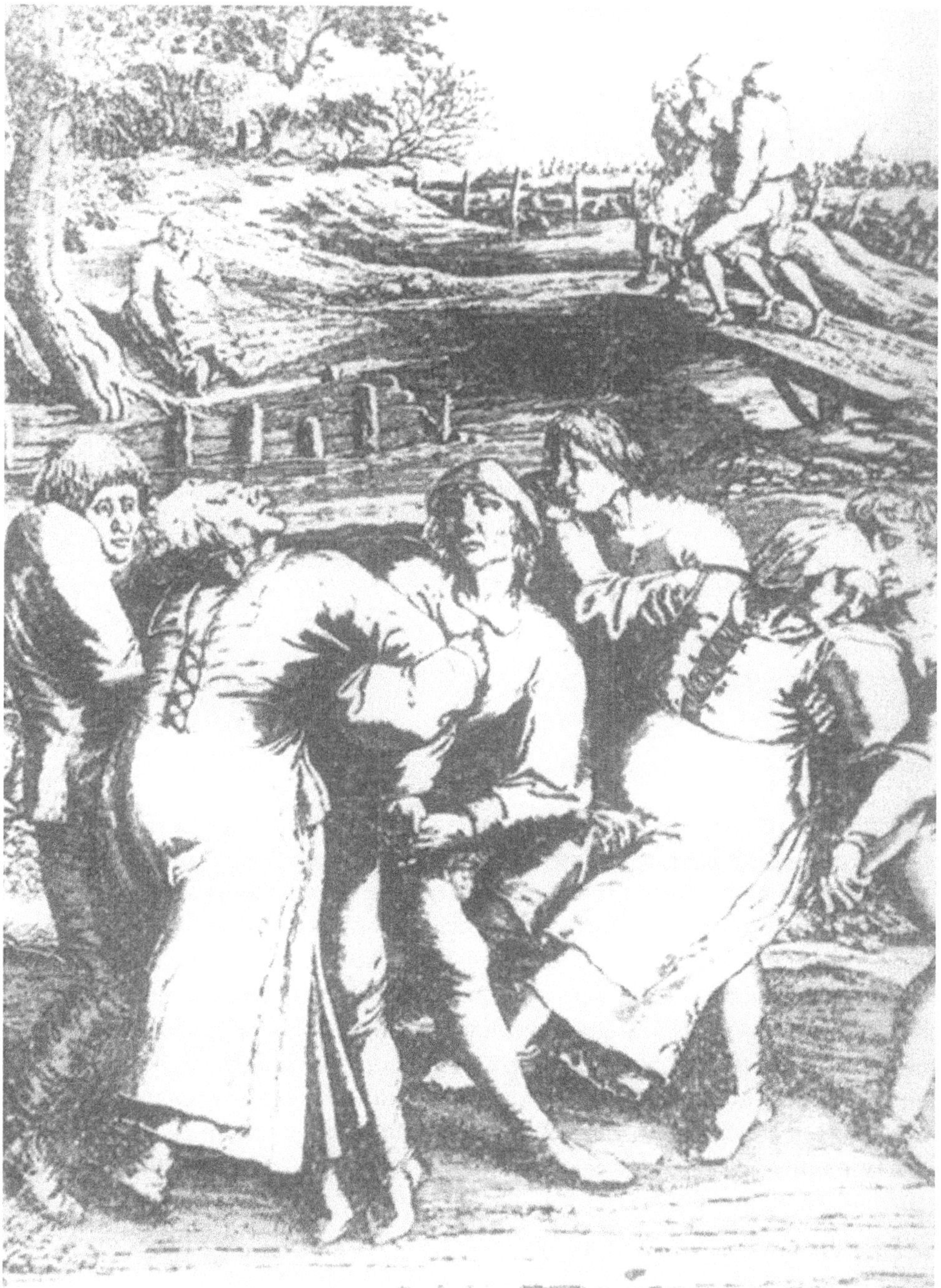

Figure 53–2. St. Vitus Dance. This is one of three engravings published by Hendrik Hondius (1642). (Hondius' title: "How the pilgrims have to dance on St. Jansday, out of Brussels to Meulebeeck"). All three engravings were inspired by Pieter Bruegel's original engraving (1564) from the collection at the Albertina, Vienna (copy, ascribed to Pieter II as well as to Jan Bruegel). Permission of Mercatorfonds, Antwerpen, publisher of Marijnissen RH. *Bruegel. Het volledige oeuvre* [Bruegel. The complete oeuvre]. Antwerpen, Mercatorfonds, 1988, p.388.

According to Sydenham, this particular convulsion affected children starting at ten years of age, and it was characterized

> by a halting, or rather an unsteady movement of one of the legs, which the patient drags. Then it is seen in the hand of the same side. The patient cannot keep it a moment in its place, whether he lay it upon his breast or any other part of his body. Do what he may, it will be jerked elsewhere convulsively. If any vessel filled with drink be put into his hand, before it reaches his mouth he will exhibit a thousand gesticulations like a mountebank. He holds the cup out straight, as if to move it to his mouth, but has his hand carried elsewhere by sudden jerks. Then, perhaps, he contrives to bring it to his mouth. If so, he will drink the liquid off at a gulp; just as if he were trying to amuse the spectators by his antics.[10]

Sydenham attributed this convulsion to "some humour falling on the nerves," and he noted that even after repeated treatments of bleeding and purging the symptoms often returned.[10(p199)]

Written in English and translated into Latin by Gilbert Havers of Trinity College, Cambridge, *Schedula Monitoria* went through three editions by the year of Sydenham's death; a series of related works by other authors soon followed.[4,7,10,11] In 1850 *Schedula Monitoria* appeared in a two-volume English translation of Dr. G. A. Greenhill's early 1840s Latin edition of Sydenham's works. This translation became the primary English reference for what would become known as Sydenham's chorea.[9,10]

By the end of the nineteenth century the label "Sydenham's chorea" became used for the most common manifestation of choreic movement disorders. However, throughout the nineteenth century the term "chorea" was used by physicians to describe a variety of highly variable movement disorders that included random chorea, tics, dystonia, and myoclonus, as well as "variable choreas," or "convulsive tics," labeled *"maladie des tics convulsifs avec coprolalie"* by Georges Gilles de la Tourette.[14] Although several nineteenth-century physicians reported symptomatic differences that justified separating each form of chorea as a distinct disorder, they were reluctant to do so because they assumed that a variety of movements could result from a single underlying cause.[15,16]

A number of late eighteenth- and early nineteenth-century European physicians reported a connection between rheumatic fever and choreic movement disorders. As early as 1802 the *Syllabus, or Outlines of Lectures on the Practice of Medicine,* published by London's Guy's Hospital, concluded that rheumatism was "one of the existing causes of chorea."[17(pp10–11)] French physicians reached parallel conclusions. In 1810, for instance, E. M. Bouteille remarked on the coincidence of rheumatism and St. Vitus dance, which he renamed "chorea."[18] Citing numerous published clinical reports from England, Richard Bright wrote that the "combination of . . . spasmodic disease with rheumatism has long been recognized."[17(p10)] By the middle of the nineteenth century the French physician J. P. Botrel (1850), drawing on the work of English doctors, argued that chorea was one of a number of possible manifestations of rheumatism.[18] That same year the French Academy of Medicine published and awarded a prize to Germain Sée of the Hôpital des Enfants for his *De la Chorée,* which concluded that "in most cases . . . chorea results from a rheumatic predisposition."[19(p390)] Sée also listed more than 30 published accounts of rheumatic chorea in Britain and France between 1810 and 1845.[19] Thus by 1862, Armand Trousseau confidently stated that "of all the predisposing pathological states [of choreas], rheumatism is assuredly the most marked and the least questionable."[18(p831)]

Tied to this view was the logical conclusion that variations in movement symptoms were different manifestations of a common underlying condition. Thus in 1825, Jean Itard had rejected separating the involuntary walking, running, tic, and cursing behaviors from the quasi-purposeful movements displayed in typical choreas that he had encountered in his practice.[20] Similarly, Bright (1838) insisted that rheumatic fevers could cause an array of different disorders, depending on which organs of the body had been diseased.[17] Elaborating this view in 1850, Sée categorized choreas into a variety of "pathological states." No matter what the particular pathological manifestation was, Sée found that clinical evidence demonstrated the ultimate connection between diverse choreas and rheumatism.[19] The clearest statement that a predisposing rheumatic cause undercut the need for separate choreic categories was made in 1851 by Sandras of the Faculty of Medicine of Paris.[21]

But lacking any firm understanding of infections in the brain, nineteenth-century practitioners diagnosed choreas by their symptoms. Thus Trousseau's influential two-volume *Clinique Médicale de l'Hôtel-Dieu de Paris* (republished in 11 editions in France, Britain, America, and Germany from 1861 to 1913) distinguished the symptoms described by Sydenham from other involuntary motor movements and vocalizations.[18] Even though Trousseau believed that choreas ought to be differentiated by symptom complexes, he insisted, nevertheless, that the "hereditary predisposition" of all choreas was "unquestionable."[18(p830)]

Until the 1880s medical writers referred to the symptom complex described by Sydenham as either "chorea minor" or "St. Vitus Dance." By the end of the decade increasing numbers of publications referred to "Sydenham's chorea."[22–26] Influenced by the new science of bacteriology, symposia and review articles on the possible connection between rheumatic fever and subsequent movement disorders appeared in diverse medical journals throughout the 1890s.[27] In 1899, Westphal, Wassermann, and Malkoff published evidence of bacterial involvement in a patient suffering from chorea, and in 1913 Poynton and Paine labeled the experimentally verified causal agent *Diplococcus rheumaticus*.[4] But not until 1956 was the connection between the symptom complex and GABHS fully elucidated by Taranta and Stollerman.[28] Two decades later, Husby and his colleagues described the basic mechanisms of antigen antibody response (molecular mimicry) in this movement disorder.[29]

Sydenham's legacy is his specificity. He was the first person to lay out a medically based and empirically detailed account of what had been a vaguely understood, widely varied, and religiously oriented description of movement disorder. His description provided the language later researchers could draw on to refine the catchall choreic category. While we know more now about the etiology of this particular constellation of movement disorder, the current clinical picture of Sydenham's chorea differs little from his 1686 account (quoted earlier):

> The abnormal movements are predominantly distal, and are most apparent when the child attempts to make voluntary movements. In the more severely affected cases all attempted voluntary movements are semipurposeful flinging movements [and] . . . the movements occur simultaneously or successively in multiple locations resulting in a complex pattern of movements . . . Children may attempt to disguise the movements in quasi-purposeful actions (such as flinging back hair) or sit on their hands to prevent the movements from appearing.[1(pp115–116)]

It is important to remember, contrary to some accounts,[4,12] that Sydenham's description of the five convulsive children was not primarily intended to differentiate the broadly defined choreic category. Lacking any other term, he simply applied the label "St. Vitus dance" to the cases he observed. Not until the late nineteenth century would Sydenham's description become equated with a particular complex of choreic symptoms and alternatively labeled "chorea minor." That result more properly stems from the endeavors of Trousseau, Charcot, and others, to construct separate disease categories (based on symptom presentation) for a confusing set of involuntary movement disorders. Sydenham's chorea was one of these new and distinct typologies.

References

1. Garvey M A, Swedo S E. Sydenham's chorea: clinical and therapeutic update. *Adv Exp Med Biol.* 1997;418:115–120.
2. Bannister R. *Brain's Clinical Neurology.* 6th rev ed. Oxford: Oxford University Press; 1986.
3. Swedo S E. Sydenham's chorea: a model for childhood autoimmune neuropsychiatric disorders. *JAMA.* 1994;272:1788–1791.
4. Finger S. *Origins of Neuroscience: A History of Explorations into Brain Function.* New York: Oxford University Press; 1994.
5. Block H. Thomas Sydenham, M D (1624–1689): the father of clinical observation. *J Fam Pract.* 1994; 38:80–81.
6. Haas L F. Neurological stamp. *J Neurol Neurosurg Psychiatry.* 1996;61:465.
7. Meynell G G. *Materials for a Biography of Dr. Thomas Sydenham (1624–1689): A New Survey of Public and Private Archives.* Folkestone: Winterdown Books; 1988.
8. Pearce JMS. Thomas Sydenham "The British Hippocrates." *J Neurol Neurosurg Psychiatry.* 1995;58:292.
9. Bates D G. Book reviews. *Isis.* 1990;81:110–111.
10. Latham R G, trans. *The Works of Thomas Sydenham, M.D., I–II.* London: Sydenham Society; 1848–1850.
11. Dewhurst K. *Dr. Thomas Sydenham (1624–1689): His Life and Original Writings.* Berkeley: University of California Press; 1966.
12. Lohr J B, Wisniewski A A. *Movement Disorders: A Neuropsychiatric Approach.* New York: Guilford Press; 1987.
13. Aron A M, Freeman J M, Carter S. The natural history of Sydenham's chorea: review of the literature and the long-term evaluation with emphasis on cardiac sequelae. *Am J Med.* 1965;38:83–95.

14. Kushner H I. *A Cursing Brain? The Histories of Gilles de la Tourette Syndrome.* Cambridge: Harvard University Press; 1999.
15. English P C. Emergence of rheumatic fever in the nineteenth century. In: Rosenberg C, Golden J, eds. *Framing Disease: Studies in Cultural History.* New Brunswick, NJ: Rutgers University Press; 1991.
16. Stollerman G H. Changing streptococci and prospects for the global eradication of rheumatic fever. *Perspect Biol Med.* 1997;40:165–189.
17. Bright, R. Cases of spasmodic disease accompanying affections of the pericardium. *Trans Med-Chir Soc London.* 1838;22:1–19.
18. Trousseau A; Cormack J R, Bazire P V, trans-eds. *Lectures on Clinical Medicine.* 3rd ed. Philadelphia: Lindsay & Blakiston; 1873.
19. Sée G. De la Chorée. Rapports de Rhumatisme et des Maladies du Coeur avec les Affections Nerveuses et Convulsives (1845). *Mém Acad Méd.* 1850;15:373–525.
20. Itard J. Mémoire Msur Quelques Fonctions Involontaires des Appareils de la Locomotion, de la Préhension et de la Voix. *Arch Gén Méd.* 1825;8:385–407.
21. Sandras CMS. *Traité Pratique des Maladie Nerveuses, I–II.* Paris: Germer-Baillière; 1851.
22. Marie P. Note sur l'existence de l'ovarie dans le Chorée de Sydenham. *Prog Méd.* 1886;2:39.
23. Giuffre L. *Sulla corea del Sydenham; note cliniche ed espozisione d'una nuova teoria.* Palermo: M Amenta; 1886.
24. Laurencin J. Chorée de Sydenham; forme grave; guérison rapide par l'antipyrine. *Lyon Méd.* 1888;57:410–415.
25. Leroux C. La Chorée de Sydenham, son étiologie, sa nature, d' après les faits observés au des pensaire Furtado-Heine. *Rev Mens Méd Chir.* 1890;8:250–266.
26. Charcot J. *Leçons du Mardi à la Salpêtrière Policliniques, 1887–1888.* [Notes de Cours de M M. Blin, Charcot, et Colin] Paris: Bureaux du Progrès Médical; 1887. Handwritten and printed.
27. Kushner H I, Kiessling L S. The controversy over the classification of Gilles de la Tourette's syndrome, 1800–1995. *Perspect Biol Med.* 1996;39:409–435.
28. Taranta A, Stollerman G H. Relationship of Sydenham's chorea to infection with Group A streptococci. *Am J Med.* 1956;20:170–175.
29. Husby G, Van de Rijn I, Zabriskie J B, et al. Antibodies reacting with cytoplasm of subthalamic and caudate nuclei neurons in chorea and rheumatic fever. *J Exp Med.* 1976;1094–1110.

54

VON RECKLINGHAUSEN'S DISEASE

Victor M. Riccardi and Peter J. Koehler

Friedrich Daniel von Recklinghausen was born in Gutersloh, Westphalia, on 2 December 1833.[1–4] He was the son of the sexton and teacher Christoph von Recklinghausen (1805–1849) and his wife Friederike Christiane Zumbusch (1809–1833). Friedrich's mother died a few weeks after his birth. His father married Caroline Jörgens. The town of Gutersloh carried the nickname "Nazareth" because the preacher there, Hermann Volkenig, insisted his flock adhere to a stark maxim: *Ora et labora* (pray and work). A pious Ravensberg movement with a high work ethic found particular resonance in this town and may have influenced Fritz von Recklinghausen.

After his primary education Friedrich went to Gymnasium in the neighboring town of Bielefeld. In 1852 he started his medical studies in Bonn, but he soon moved to Würzburg, which would appear to have been a very important decision. Rudolf Virchow (1821–1902) was professor of pathological anatomy at the University of Würzburg, and there prepared his theory of cellular pathology, replacing the antiquated humoral pathology to explain causes and processes of disease in terms of disordered cells. Every cell is the product of another cell *(omnis cellula e cellula)* was his well-known adage.

Von Recklinghausen followed Virchow to Berlin in 1855. Virchow moved into one of the most modern institutes of pathology, situated on the grounds of the well-known Charité hospital. Von Recklinghausen finished his thesis *De pyaemiae theoriis* at the age of 22 in 1855. He contributed to the explanation of the phenomenon of inflammation. In 1862, he summarized his work on the subject in *Die Lymphgefässe und ihre Beziehungen zum Bindegewebe* [The lymph vessels and their relations to connective tissue]. He demonstrated that inflammation follows the migration of blood cells, similar to leukocytes and lymphocytes. He also described the phenomenon of phagocytosis. In 1864 he was called to the chair of pathological anatomy in Königswinter, and six months later, to Würzburg to take the chair previously held by Virchow. During this period he published on hematological subjects.

After the Franco-German War (1870–1871), Von Recklinghausen was called to the newly founded University of Strassburg in Elsass-Lotharingen. He took part in the preparation of a new institute for anatomic pathology, which was opened in 1877. He was instrumental in the call to Strassburg of Ernst von Leyden (1832–1910), Friedrich Leopold Goltz (1834–1902), and Wilhelm von Waldeyer (1837–1921). Following the example of Virchow, Von Recklinghausen made an important collection of pathological preparations. Students from all over the world visited his department, including the American William H. Welch (1850–1934), who introduced modern hygiene in the United States, and Karl Albert Ludwig Aschoff (1866–1942), who described the reticuloendothelial system. Von Recklinghausen was dean at the medical faculty several times and from 1883 until 1885 he was rector of the university. He did not accept a call to succeed Karl Freiherr von Rokitansky (1804–1878) in Vienna in 1874 or Julius Cohnheim (1839–1884) at the University of Leipzig, preferring to stay in Strassburg. In 1871, he was nominated honorary doctor by the *Societas Medica Norvegica* in Christiana, the present Oslo. In 1905 he became honorary president of the German Society for Pathology. He retired in 1906, being succeeded by Hans Chiari (see Chapter 42).

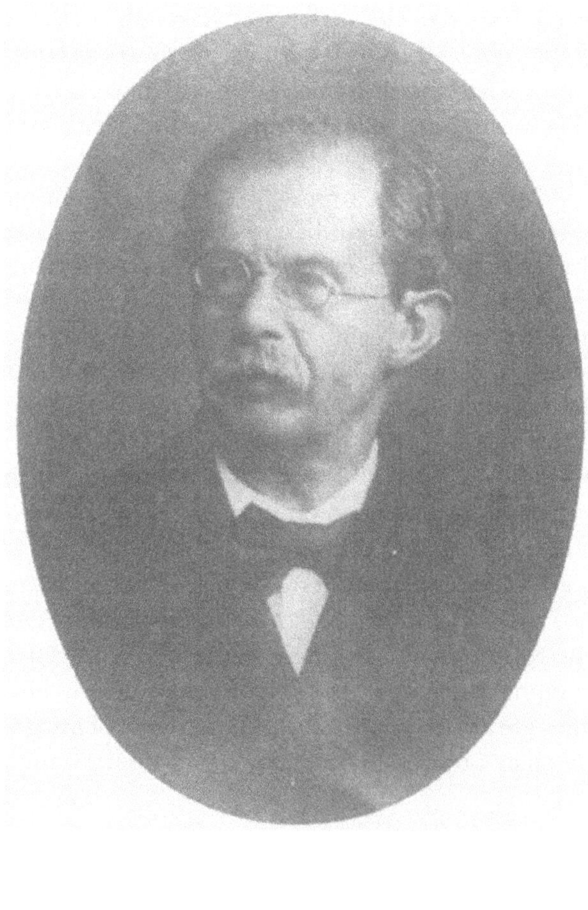

Figure 54–1. Daniel Friedrich von Recklinghausen (1833–1910). Courtesy of Medizinhistorisches Institut, Zurich, Switzerland.

His colleagues and pupils depicted him as self-assured, deliberate, unshakable, and straightforward. His work took priority over family and personal affairs. His wife Marie Jacobsen, whom he married in 1865, took care of their social commitments. She also helped improve his scientific publications. They had three sons and a daughter. The eldest son, Heinrich, became a physician and helped his father finish his last book, *Untersuchungen über Rachitis und Osteomalacie.* In the introduction to this book, Heinrich wrote:

> Denn auch als Emeritus arbeitete er vom frühen Morgen bis spät in die nacht. Es unterstützte ihn dabei eine eiserne Gesundheit: seine Arbeitskraft kam seiner Arbeitsfreudigkeit gleich, und die Last der zunehmende Jahre hatte sie nicht vermindert . . . als eines Morgens ein Herzschlag rasch und sanft seinem Leben ein Ende machte, da war sein Buch in allen wesentliche Teilen vollendet, so dass das wenige, was noch zu tun übrig blieb, von anderen getan werden könnte.[1]

[Even as emeritus, he worked from early in the morning until late at night. He was supported by an iron health: his working power was equal to his working pleasure, and the burden of increasing age had not dimished these . . . when, one morning, a heart attack ended his life, swiftly and gently, his book was finished in all essential parts, in such a way that the finishing touch could be performed by others.]

Friedrich Daniel von Recklinghausen died at the age of 76 on 18 August 1910. He was buried at the Saint-Louis cemetery in Strassburg-Robertsau. A few years after his death, a statue was unveiled in the city of Strassburg. He is still considered one of the most outstanding nineteenth-century pathologists of Germany.

Von Recklinghausen's name is now associated with two totally distinct disorders: neurofibromatosis and osteitis fibrosa cystica. The latter disease is characterized by changes in bones accompanying primary hyperparathyroidism. Here, our focus is on neurofibromatosis. In 1882, Von Recklinghausen published *Ueber die multiplen Fibrome der Haut und ihre Beziehung zu den multiplen Neuronomen.*[5] The monograph was dedicated to his teacher Rudolf Virchow and published as a Festschrift for the occasion of the twenty-fifth anniversary of the Institute of Pathology. Von Recklinghausen described two cases and provided a literature review of many other cases with skin fibromas and multiple neurinomas (schwannomas). In the introduction he stated that he had autopsied the first case three years previously. It was "eine besondere Gunst, dass sich mir die Gelegenheit darbot, die schon auf anatomischem Wege gewonnene Erkenntnis in einem zweiten Falle auch am Lebenden zu erproben." [It was particularly auspicious that I had the opportunity to check the knowledge that had been obtained from anatomy in a second case, which was still alive.] Moreover, it was important that he had been interested in the neighboring field of oncology, at least in the comparison of skin tumors arising in connective tissue.

The first patient, a 55-year-old woman, who was admitted because of lung hemorrhages, died a few hours after admission to the hospital and was autopsied. Skin tumors had been present since the age of three. At autopsy the following findings were noted:

> Zahllose Knoten, fast an der ganzen äusseren Haut . . ., grösstentheils gestielt, andere breitbasig aufsitzend, meist einfach kuglig, in allen möglichen Grössen, besonders aber die grösseren polypös gestaltet, bis zu 5 Ctm. lang und 4 Ctm. dick,

> sämmtlich mit vollständig intacter, fast glatter Haut bedeckt; nur auf dem Kreuzbein ist ein flachgedrückter, pilzförmiger Knoten, welcher an seiner Oberfläche leicht ulcerirt ist, ausserdem noch an der linken Seite des Rumpfes ein kleiner ulcerirter Knoten.[5(p3)]

An English translation was published in 1981:

> Innumerable nodules, almost over the entire outer skin layer . . ., for the most part on stalks, while others sat on broad bases and were mostly simple spheres in all possible sizes. The larger ones, however, were especially polypous, up to 5 cm long and 4 cm thick, all covered with completely intact, almost smooth skin; although on the sacrum there was a flatly pressed, mushroom-shaped nodule, lightly ulcerated on its surface, while another small ulcerated nodule appeared on the left side of the trunk.[6]

The case study continued:

> Im Allgemeinem hat die Haut des ganzen Körpers ein schmutzig bräunliches Colorit; genauer betrachtet, existiren an den meisten Theilen, namentlich am Rumpf und Hals zahllose linsengrosse, braune Pigmentflecke.[5(p4)]
>
> Links im Nervus cruralis, in der Mitte des Oberschenkels, schon im Anfang des N. saphenus ein Tumor, spindelförmig, 32 Mm. Lang, 7 Mm. dick, der Nerv an seiner hinteren Seite verlaufend. In der Höhe des Knie am Saphenus ein anderer kleiner Tumor. Kleine Tumoren in den muskelästen des Cruralis. Der Cutaneus lateralis (Femoro-cutaneus) hat 2 Tumore, der eine unterhalb der Theilungsstelle am oberen Ast, der andere handbreit oberhalb . . .
>
> Rückenmark und Gehirn boten gar nichts Besonderes, auch nicht bei der mikroskopischen Untersuchung.[5(p7)]

> In general, the skin of the entire body had a dirty brown color; closer examination revealed the existence in many places, particularly on the trunk and throat, of innumerable brown pigmentation spots.
>
> On the left side, on the femoral nerve, in the middle of the thigh below the origin of the saphenous nerve, there was a spindle-shaped tumor 32 mm long, 7 mm thick, running along the posterior side of the nerve. At the knee was another small tumor on the saphenous nerve. There were small tumors on the muscle rami of the femoral nerve. The lateral cutaneous (femorocutaneous) nerve exhibited two tumors, one below the branching point on the upper ramus, the other a hand-width above it . . .
>
> The spinal cord and brain were unremarkable, even under microscopic examination.[6]

> Die Epicrise des Falles musste hiernach lauten: Multiple weiche Fibrome der äusseren Haut, auch des subcutanen Gewebes, multiple fibromatöse Neurome der Hautnerven, der Stämme und Zweige der Nerven der Extremitäten, vorwiegend der unteren, so wie der Plexus sacrales, der Vagi und Bauchsympathici, der Stirnhautäste der Trigemini, einzelner Muskeläste der N obturatorii . . . Tod durch Pneumorrhagie aus einem Pulmonalarterien-Aneurysma.[5(p8)]

> The summary of this case should be as follows: multiple soft fibromas of the outer skin, also of the subcutaneous tissue; multiple fibromatous neurinomas of the nerves of the skin, the trunks and branches of the nerves of the extremities, predominantly of the lower extremities, as well as of the sacral plexus, the vagus

> nerve distribution, the sympathetic nervous system of the abdomen, the branches of the trigeminal nerve in the skin of the forehead, and isolated muscle rami of the obturator nerve . . . Death resulted from pulmonary hemorrhage from a pulmonary artery aneurysm.[6]

The patient also showed signs of tuberculosis of the lungs and intestines. The autopsy report and case history was followed by a description of the microscopic features of the neurofibromas. There were no signs of nerve fiber neoplasia or "fatty deneration." Even in larger neurinomas, the nerve fibers could be distinguished. Though still myelinated, some fibers showed an increase of connective tissue.

Von Recklinghausen also discussed his ideas about the possible evolution of neurofibromas. He presented a second case history of a 47-year-old man with unaffected parents, stepbrothers, and stepsisters (Fig. 54–2).[5(p34)] The patient could remember the number of skin tumors had increased since he was 15. Von Recklinghausen was particularly interested in examining the peripheral nerves, in which he found enlargements that could be distinguished from skin fibromas with certainty, because of the location and the way the tumors could be moved underneath the skin. Von Recklinghausen could not find any sensory disturbances.

He had his colleague Friedrich Jolly (1844–1904) examine the patient: "Die Schmerzempfindlichkeit, sowie Erregbarkeit der Muskeln bei electrischer Reizung des Medianus ganz normal, wenigstens dem Durchschnittsmenschen entsprechend."[5(p38)] [The sensibility for pain as well as the irritability of the muscle by electric stimulus of the median nerve entirely normal, at least corresponding to average persons.] Four small nodules were taken from the patient's back and examined microscopically, with the same result as in the first case. He concluded that the smaller tumors are neurofibromas. "Fibrome, welche in kleinen Cutisnerven nach dem Typus der Fibrome in den grösseren Stämmen mit Verlagerung, aber anfänglicher Erhaltung der Primitivfasern gebildet sind.[5(p41)] [Fibromas that are formed in small cutaneous nerves following the type of fibromas in the greater trunks in layers, but at first started in primitive nerve fibers.] (Fig. 54–3)

In the second part of the book, Von Recklinghausen goes into the differential diagnosis and provides some thoughts about the cause of neurofibromas. Finally, he reviews previous case histories with multiple fibromas (in 35 papers, several of which had been published by Virchow and his pupils) and neurinomas from the medical literature. Clearly, not all papers discussed refer to cases with Von Recklinghausen's disease.

Friedrich von Recklinghausen was not the first clinician or pathologist to describe what has since become known as neurofibromatosis type I (NF1). However, his description was both exceptionally detailed and chronologically positioned to warrant assignation of his name to the disorder, thus the eponym of "von Recklinghausen's disease"—both a mouthful and a cause for concern for those who realized early on that there is more than one form of neurofibromatosis (NF).

The year 1592 may be the first in which a person with NF was described.[7] Almost two centuries later, in 1768, Akenside published the first English-language description of a case of NF1.[8] Twenty-five years later Tilesius provided excellent color

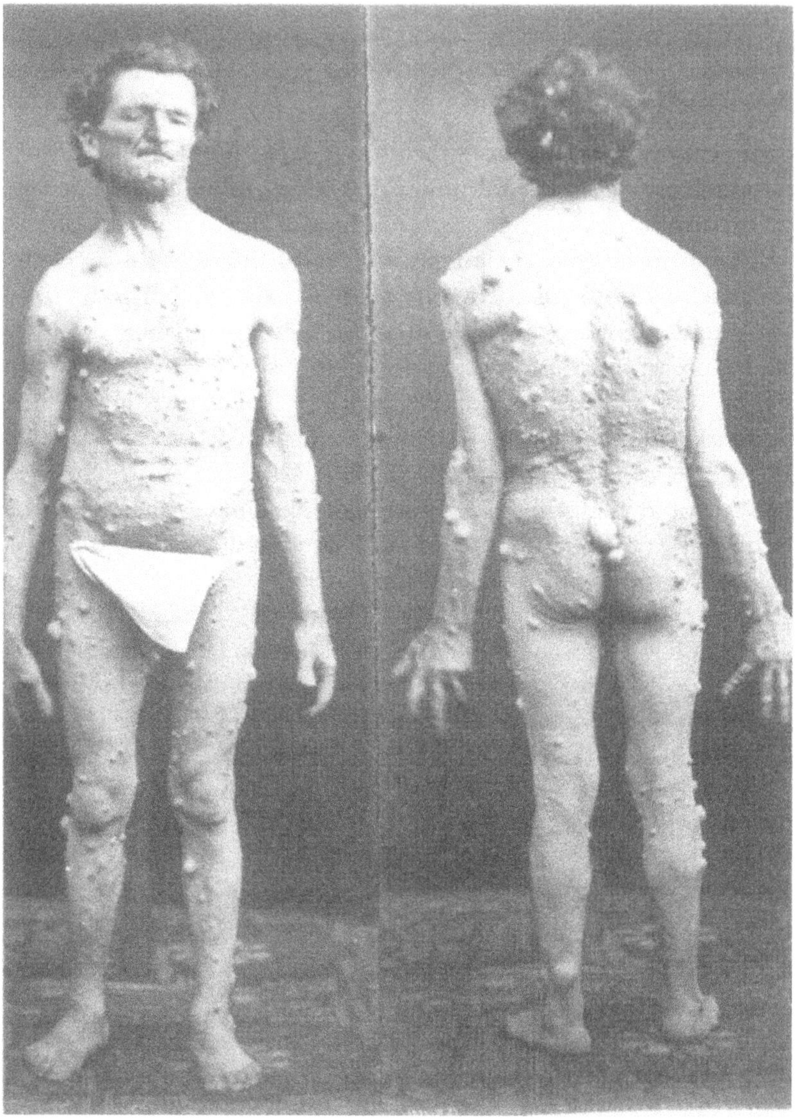

Figure 54–2. Case II from Ref. 5, Plate II.

illustrations of the skin tumors characterizing the disorder.[9] Von Recklinghausen referred to him.

In 1982, the first author of this paper (VMR) first proposed that there were multiple forms of NF, the most clear-cut of which were NF1 and NF2, respectively, von Recklinghausen's disease and bilateral acoustic neurinomas (vestibular schwannomas).[10] In July 1987, the American National Institutes of Health Consensus Conference program adopted and promulgated this nomenclature.[11] The formal recognition was on Bastille Day, Saturday, 14 July 1987, which the first of the present authors (VMR) remembers well by virtue of celebrating the occasion in a French restaurant

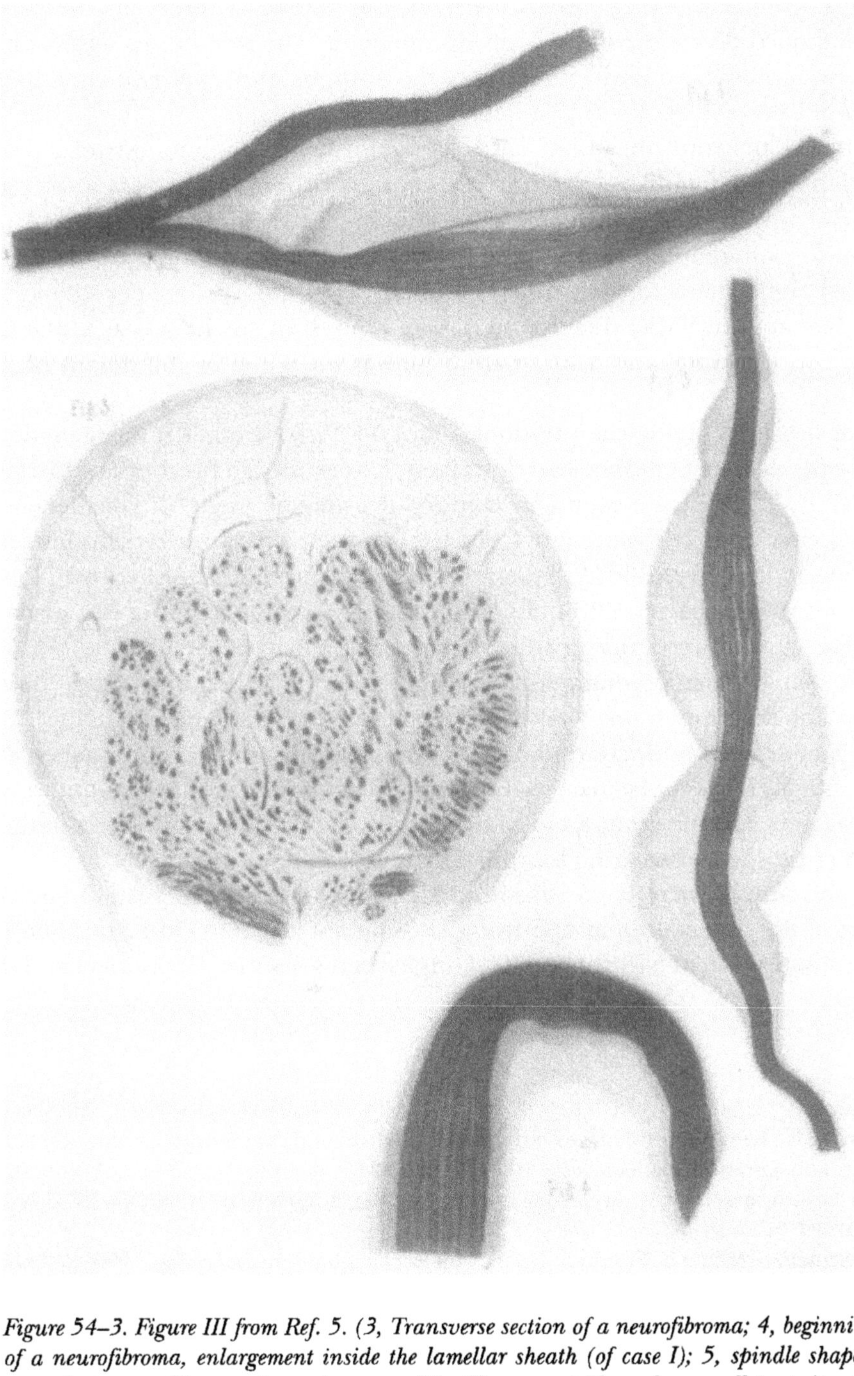

Figure 54–3. Figure III from Ref. 5. (3, Transverse section of a neurofibroma; 4, beginning of a neurofibroma, enlargement inside the lamellar sheath (of case I); 5, spindle shaped, wound-up neurofibroma, the main mass of the fibroma outside, only a small part situated inside the nerve fiber bundle (case I); 6, spindle-shaped neurofibroma, a nerve fiber bundle dissecting the tumor mass, interference of the tumor with the neighboring branch of the nerve (case I).

that evening, ironically mixing French, German, and American history into the international potpourri deserving of the neurofibromatoses. The result was a significantly increased recognition and understanding of the disorder, and a perhaps lamentable discarding of a coveted eponym; Von Recklinghausen's disease.

The term "neurofibromatosis" and its eponym are tongue twisters. Thus many patients and families were not resistant to dropping the not-so-coveted eponym. But what's in a name? Does the attachment of the name of Friedrich Daniel von Recklinghausen to NF1 contribute to our understanding of the disorder or our commitment to such understanding? We think so. In February 1972, when the first author(VMR) decided to devote himself to NF, he was as much fascinated by von Recklinghausen the man as he was intrigued by the details of the disorder itself.

One of the early biological questions about NF1 was whether it was genetic in origin. As early as 1818 Schiffner had described the disorder in brothers, as Virchow did in 1847.[5(p132–133)] In the twentieth century, the genetic origin of von Recklinghausen's disease and its distinction from the disorder characterized by bilateral acoustic neurinomas (vestibular schwannomas) were firmly established by various biochemical and molecular techniques. And with new developments we risk neglecting the importance of recognizing and characterizing the disease clinically.[12,13]

Von Recklinghausen preeminently contributed to the notion that cogent observation and apt description are vital to understanding disease and pathology. The spirit of his endeavors both contradicts and compliments modern approaches. On the one hand, NF1, the molecularly defined disorder, seems to be paramount to various investigators. On the other hand, the clinically and pathologically characterized disorder is critical to those caring for individuals with the disorder.

Plain and simply, there is no substitute for cogent clinical observation and the enshrining of the observation in eponyms. Thus we apologize to Herr Friedrich for proposing substitution of NF1 for von Recklinghausen's disease. The respect and the love remain.

References

1. Murken A H. Der Begründer der Entzündungslehre und Namensgeber der Recklinghausenschen Krankheiten. *Pathologe.* 1996;17:307–331.
2. Delling G, Kummerfeldt K. Friedrich Daniel von Recklinghausen. *Dtsch Med Wochenschr.* 1991;116:1976–1979.
3. Kummerfeldt K, Delling G. Friedrich Daniel von Recklinghausen. *Pathologe.* 1996; 17:78–82.
4. Warkany J. Friedrich Daniel von Recklinghausen and his times. *Adv Neurol.* 1981; 29 :251–257.
5. Von Recklinghausen F. *Ueber die multipten Fibrome der Haut und ihre Beziehung zu den multiplen Neuronomen.* Berlin: Hirschwald; 1882.
6. Crump T. Translation of case reports in "Ueber die multiplen Fibrome der haut und ihre Beziehung zu den multiplen Neuromen" by F. v. Recklinghausen. *Adv Neurol.* 1981;29: 259–275.
7. Aldrovandi J. *Monstrorum Historia cum Paralipomenis Historiae Omnium Animalium, Bononiae.* Typis Nicolai Tibaldini; 1642.

8. Akenside M. Observations on cancers (first reported case of NF-1). *Med Trans Coll Physicians London.* 1785;1:64–92.
9. Tilesius W G. *Historia Pathologica Singularis Cutis Turpitudinis.* Leipzig: Crusius; 1793:1–11.
10. Riccardi V M. Neurofibromatosis: clinical heterogeneity. *Curr Probl Cancer.* 1982;7:1–34.
11. National Institutes of Health. National Institutes of Health Consensus Development Conference statement: neurofibromatosis. *Neurofibromatosis.* 1988;1:172–178.
12. Riccardi V M. Von Recklinghausen neurofibromatosis. *N Engl J Med.* 1981;305:1617–1627.
13. Riccardi V M. *Neurofibromatosis: Phenotype, Natural History and Pathogenesis.* 2nd ed. Baltimore: Johns Hopkins University Press; 1992.

55

WILSON'S DISEASE

John M. S. Pearce

Samuel Alexander Kinnier Wilson (1878–1937) was born in Cedarville, New Jersey, on 6 December 1874. When he was a child his family moved to Scotland, where he was educated at George Watson's College and qualified in medicine in 1902 at Edinburgh University. He became house physician to Byrom Bramwell, whose strong leanings toward neurology probably encouraged Wilson later to extend his training with Pierre Marie and Joseph Babinski in Paris.

He returned to England in 1904, working as house physician at the National Hospital, Queen Square. His evident ability led to further training under the supervision of John Hughlings Jackson, William Gowers, Henry-Charlton Bastian, and Victor Horsley. In 1912 he published his M.D. thesis, *Progressive Lenticular Degeneration*, for which he was awarded the Edinburgh University gold medal. He was elected assistant physician in 1913 and full physician in 1925. Wilson was also assistant physician and dean at the Westminster Hospital until 1919, when he was appointed neurologist to King's College Hospital; he was given full charge of the neurological department in 1928.

He became a prolific and gifted writer, adopting a terse but lucid style. He assiduously collected the neurological literature and, unusually for his era, was able to study papers in German and French, as well as classical literature. Hepatolenticular degeneration was an early contribution. He was to write many other important and influential papers. "The Old Motor System and the New" showed his critical, scholarly powers. He gave the Croonian Lectures in 1925 on "Disorders of Motility and Muscle Tone," and he gave his Harveian Lecture in 1926 on "The Epilepsies." These admirable papers were included in his volume of collected papers, dedicated "to the memory of Dr J Hughlings Jackson," revised and modified in *Modern Problems in Neurology*.[1]

In 1920 he founded the *Journal of Neurology and Psychopathology*, becoming its first editor. His two-volume *Neurology* (published posthumously in 1940), edited by Ninian Bruce, his son-in-law, is one of the greatest neurology texts ever written. It

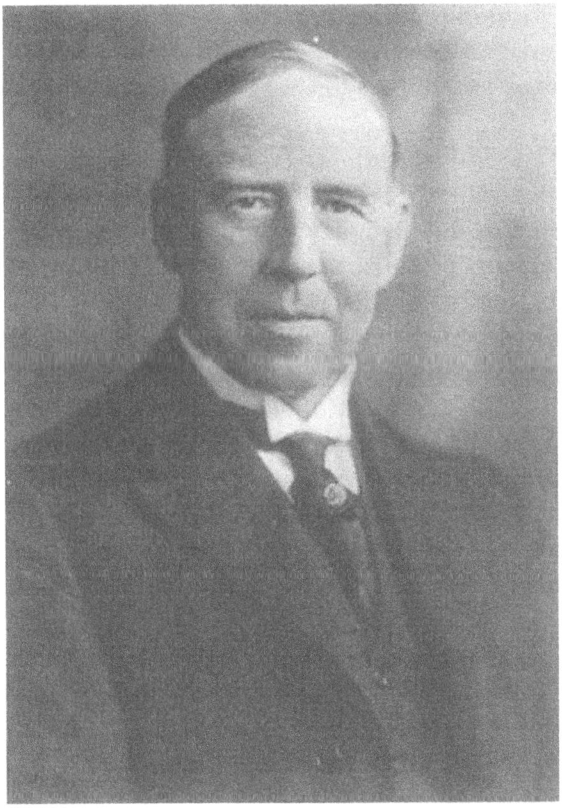

Figure 55–1. Samuel Alexander Kinnier Wilson (1878–1937). Courtesy of the Institute of Neurology, National Hospital, Queen Square, London.

is the last of the single-author texts encompassing almost the whole of neurology and is to be ranked with Gowers's *Diseases of the Nervous System* (1886–1888) and with Hermann Oppenheim's *Lehrbuch der Nervenkrankheiten* (1894).

Wilson's clinical papers ranged over apraxia, aphasia, epidemic encephalitis, and tics and allied conditions. He was fascinated by the pathological laughing and crying and the related paralysis of emotional facial movements, in which Gowers had discerned a dissociation between emotional and voluntary innervation. Brainstem disorders were a particular interest, at a time when their clinical hallmarks were incompletely recognized.

He was both a brilliant clinical observer and a theatrically impressive teacher. Those who came into contact with him described a large imposing man with a memorable voice whose grandiose gestures and mannerisms made his teachings unforgettable. A contemporary remembered:

> This large man with "ham-like" hands would slowly roll up the collar of his white coat, with infinite grace, bringing the lapels together beneath his chin, cross his arms on his expansive chest—this series of movements was a mannerism of his—and with his resonant voice and penetrating eye would transfix his audience by telling them the story of the disorder, putting each character into proper perspective.[2]

His lectures were lucid, closely reasoned in argument, and had an urgent, dramatic aspect that attracted students from all over the world.[3]

Derek Denny-Brown once asked Wilson his opinion on the essential aspects of "hepatolenticular degeneration," whereupon Wilson eyed him with circumspection and, starting to walk away, asked, perhaps with tongue in cheek, "Do you mean Kinnier Wilson's disease?"

Although his satirical style masked a sensitive and restless spirit, he was not the most discreet or tactful physician. While visiting Foster Kennedy, he spent three frustrating hours examining a patient with a lateral medullary syndrome, in which the signs failed to match the anatomy; to Kennedy's embarrassment, he suddenly asked the patient, "Will you see to it that I get your brain when you die?"

In 1913 he married Annie Louisa, whose father was Alexander Bruce, M.D., of Edinburgh. While at the peak of his powers, Wilson died of cancer, just before *Neurology* was finished. My late chief, Hugh Garland, was one of many distinguished neurologists trained by Wilson; each passed on the Jackson–Gowers–Wilson traditions of clinical methods: the keen-edged, critical, reasoned dissection of neurological problems seen at the bedside and in the clinic. Apart from golf and gardening at his Thorpeness home, neurology filled his life—sometimes, one suspects, at the cost of his family. The many neurologists whom he trained, his methods, and his unique book are his lasting legacy.

In his textbook *Neurology*, Wilson looks back on the roots of the disease that bears his name: "My monograph of 1912 described a disease unknown to the medical profession at that time."[4] While summarizing the essential features he emphasizes the familial but not congenital nature of the illness, which lasted a few months in acute cases, many years in chronic cases:

> The object of this paper is to give a full description of a rare nervous disease, of which, as far as I am aware, no instance has been recorded during the last twenty years—a disease to which, for reasons which will hereinafter become evident, the name of "Progressive Lenticular Degeneration" may be conveniently applied . . . This affection, where it occurs in an uncomplicated form is an extrapyramidal motor disease, the importance of which is apparent not only because of its rarity, but also by reason of the light it sheds on such diseases as paralysis agitans . . .
>
> Progressive lenticular degeneration, as the disease may be called, is not one with which the medical profession is familiar. As far as I can discover, no case has been recorded since 1890, with the very doubtful exception of one reported by Anton, of Halle, under the title of "Dementia Choreoasthenica, with Juvenile Nodular Cirrhosis of the Liver," some three years ago. In all probability this case was one of congenital syphilis. The total number of cases of the disease that have been published amounts to six only. Of these, two (brother and sister) were reported by Gowers in 1888 under the name of "Tetanoid Chorea, associated with Cirrhosis of the Liver"; one by Ormerod in 1890; three (two brothers and a sister) by Homen, of Helsingfors, also in 1890 . . .
>
> In this paper will be described four cases of the affection which have been personally observed and diagnosed (in all but one the diagnosis was made during life), in three of which it has been possible to make a post-mortem examination.
>
> The first patient (S.T.) came under observation in 1905, and died on July 28, 1908. At the autopsy bilateral degeneration of the lenticular nucleus was found, coupled with cirrhosis of the liver.

> The second patient (D. P.) came under observation in 1906, and died on March 3, 1907. Here also, cirrhosis of the liver and a slighter degree of lenticular change were discovered.
>
> The third patient (E. P.), a brother of the above, came under notice in 1907. This patient was exhaustively examined in the summer of 1910. He died on September 20, 1910, and in his case identical findings were obtained at the autopsy.
>
> The fourth patient (M. To.) came under observation in the autumn of 1911, and at the time of writing she is still living.
>
> In addition to these four personal cases the record of two other cases of the disease has been obtained, one of which occurred in the family described by Gowers, but has not hitherto been published, as the notes were lost years ago. By a piece of good fortune I was able to trace the mother of the family, an old lady aged 70 and to obtain from her the clinical details of this new case. The other is one referred to by Ormerod in his paper of 1890, the notes, not hitherto published, are preserved in the National Hospital Queen Square.[5]

This paper formed part of a thesis for the medical degree of the University of Edinburgh in July 1911, for which a gold medal was awarded. Wilson related that this, his most celebrated paper, the basis of his M.D. thesis, "contained references to six old and previously obscure cases (none later than 1890)."[4]

A full description is to be found in his paper[5] and his textbook,[4] which includes an account of the corneal ring first reported by Bernard Kayser in a case diagnosed as multiple sclerosis, then by Bruno Fleischer, who realized its diagnostic significance. Wilson describes the clinical picture:[4]

> Initial jaundice is fairly often specified in case-reports, together with ascites perhaps, yet customary symptoms and signs of cirrhosis very seldom occur indeed.

He mentions terminal hematemesis in one case, and he notes,

> More usual is swelling of the spleen, enough to render it palpable . . . The clinical features of an advancing case are highly characteristic. With mouth often held open, and a stereotyped smile, or, if not laughing or smiling, a vacant or fatuous look, the patient sits and leans to one or the other side, or back, all four limbs agitated by tremor, mostly quick and rather fine; fingers and hands are contracted in flexion, trunk is held stiffly, and willed movements are slowly performed, to the accompaniment of wilder tremulousness. Though saliva may drip from the parted lips and facies almost silly, the eyes are alert and intelligent. Youth may impart a curiously complacent aspect to the features. Fluidity and fixity of symptoms are both evident to the observer; tremors wax and wane, leave one part for another, or alter their type in the same segment according as it is being used or not, but behind the changing phenomena is a general postural stiffness and contraction-attitude, while the physiognomy, too, is apt to become set.

The salient features he summarized as a combination of cerebral and visceral lesions, that is, bilateral softening or degeneration of lenticular nucleus and to a lesser degree of globus pallidus, with hepatic cirrhosis.

Wilson's ideas about its etiology show his frustrations with the limitations of available knowledge.[6] He refers to the classic Eck's fistula as establishing a link between liver and brain; and he observes "that the liver first becomes affected, that the lenticular lesions follow, and that this hepatitis has something to do with the continuance of toxic effects." He considered toxic metallic poisons, but "the evidence is scant."

Wilson acknowledged Gowers's earlier description.[7] In 1888, Gowers had reported

> a ten year old boy with a brother and three other relations having suffered maladies resembling chorea. The boy suffered from tonic spasm which was continuous . . . affecting the face producing a constant peculiar smile. The tongue was pressed back against the palate in such a manner as to impede swallowing and prevent speech. The arms were extended, pronated and rotated inwards . . . fingers extended and slowly moved in the irregular way characteristic of athetosis. The legs were extended . . . feet overextended in talipes equinovarus.

He died within seven months. Autopsy showed neither naked eye nor microscopic abnormality in the central nervous system.

Eighteen years later Gowers provided the full histories of the 10-year-old Sydney M. and his 15-year-old sister, Charlotte, noting: "The liver was 'firm, hard and lobular and was evidently sclerosed. His sister developed a similar illness . . . lip hanging down and was easily excited . . . as well as having movements similar to those of her brother."[8]

Wilson's *Neurology* notes that Joseph Ormerod had also described bilateral putaminal softenings in a "Case of Cirrhosis of the Liver in a Boy with Obscure and Fatal Nervous Symptoms";[9] Homén reported a "Peculiar Disease Occurring in Three Members of a Family in the Form of a Progressive Dementia Probably Lues Hereditaria Tarda".[10] However, Wilson strenuously discounted those instances of "pseudosclerosis" described by Westphal and Strümpell, which he regarded as "non specific, with no evidence of liver disease, and heterogeneous"—a view confirmed later by Greenfield.

Thus, although the separate constituent parts of the syndrome had been described, apart from Gowers's descriptions[6] there had been no unifying account of the disorder of liver and brain. Wilson rather harshly and critically denounced the other cases, many of which were probably not examples of hepatolenticular degeneration. All the evidence shows he was correct, and since his own account of the syndrome could hardly be bettered, the eponym is rightly his.

In 1939 Samuel Kinnier Wilson died of cancer, before the discoveries of the defect of ceruloplasmin by Scheinberg in 1952 with consequent copper overloading of the liver, cornea, and brain. His inquiring mind would have been fascinated by the later discovery of the autosomal recessive gene linked to markers on chromosome 13. He would indeed have been gratified by the efficacy of penicillamine shown by Walshe in 1956[11] and later by the effects of trientine and zinc.

References

1. Wilson SAK. *Modern Problems in Neurology*. London: Edward Arnold; 1928.
2. Haymaker W, Schiller F, eds. *The Founders of Neurology*. 2nd ed. Springfield, Ill: Charles C Thomas, 1970:535–539.
3. *Munks Role, Lives of the Fellows of the Royal College of Physicians of London*. Compiled by G H Brown. Lonpdon: Royal College of Physicians; 1955;4:540.

4. Wilson SAK. *Neurology*. London: Edward Arnold; 1940;2:806–831.
5. Wilson SAK. Progressive lenticular degeneration: a familial nervous disease associated with cirrhosis of the liver. *Brain*. 1912;34:295–509.
6. Pearce JMS. Wilson's disease. *J Neurol Neurosurg Psychiatry*. 1997;63:174.
7. Gowers W R. Tetanoid chorea. In: *A Manual of Diseases of the Nervous System*. London: Churchill; 1888;2:656.
8. Gowers W R. On tetanoid chorea and its association with cirrhosis of the liver. *Rev Neurol Psychiatry*. 1906;4:249–258.
9. Ormerod J. Case of cirrhosis of the liver in a boy with obscure and fatal nervous symptoms. *St Bartholomew's Hospital Reports*. 1890;26. Cited by Wilson SAK in: *Modern Problems in Neurology*. London: Edward Arnold; 1928:806.
10. Homén E A. A peculiar disease occurring in three members of a family in the form of a progressive dementia probably Lues hereditaria tarda. *Arch Psychiat Nervenkrankh*. 1892;24. Cited by Wilson SAK in: *Modern Problems in Neurology*. London: Edward Arnold; 1928:806.
11. Walshe J M, Yealland M. Wilson's disease: the problem of delayed diagnosis. *J Neurol Neurosurg Psychiatry*. 1992; 55:692–696.

INDEX

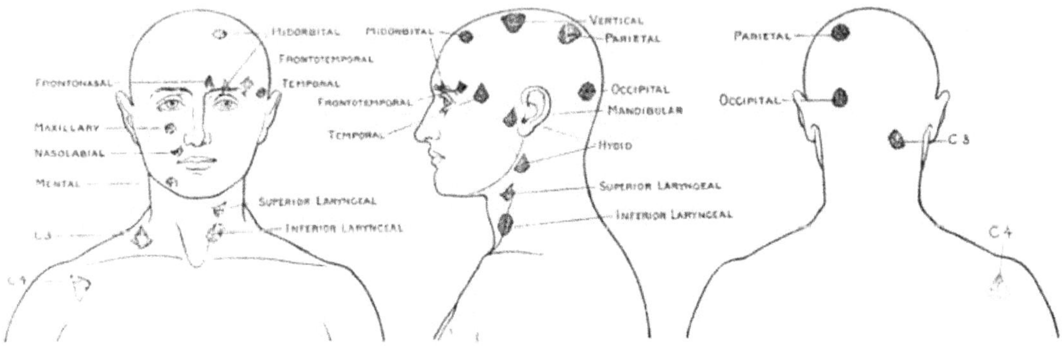
Midorbital
Frontotemporal
Frontonasal
Temporal
Maxillary
Nasolabial
Mental
Superior Laryngeal
Inferior Laryngeal
C3
C4
Midorbital
Vertical
Parietal
Occipital
Frontotemporal
Mandibular
Temporal
Hyoid
Superior Laryngeal
Inferior Laryngeal
Parietal
Occipital
C3
C4

1.

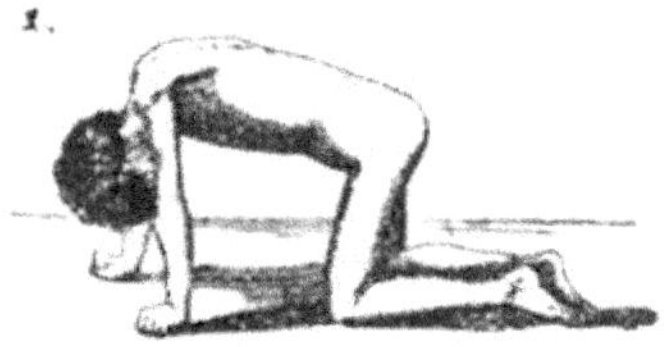

2.

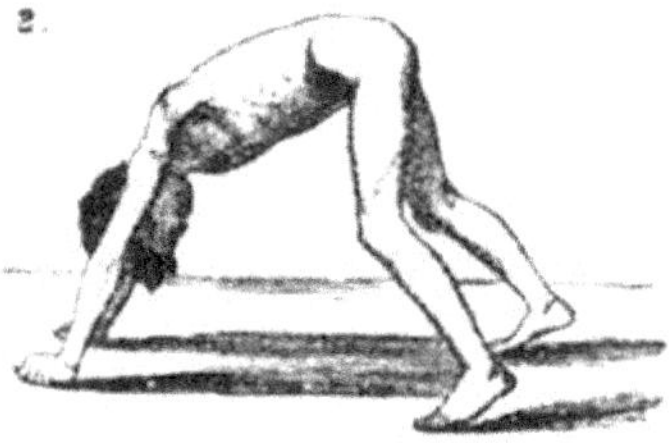

3.

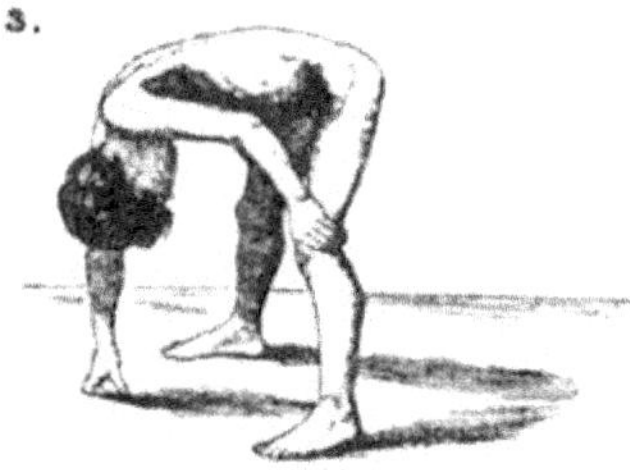

www.ingramcontent.com/pod-product-compliance
Ingram Content Group UK Ltd.
Pitfield, Milton Keynes, MK11 3LW, UK
UKHW052229270726
14060UKWH00004B/671

9 780195 133660